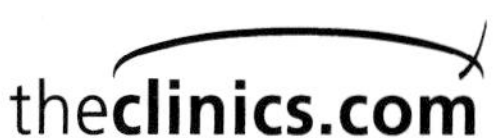

UROLOGIC CLINICS OF NORTH AMERICA

Testicular Cancer

GUEST EDITOR
Joel Sheinfeld, MD

CONSULTING EDITOR
Martin I. Resnick, MD

May 2007 • Volume 34 • Number 2

SAUNDERS

An Imprint of Elsevier, Inc.
PHILADELPHIA LONDON TORONTO MONTREAL SYDNEY TOKYO

W.B. SAUNDERS COMPANY
A Division of Elsevier Inc.

1600 John F. Kennedy Boulevard • Suite 1800 • Philadelphia, Pennsylvania 19103-2899

http://www.theclinics.com

UROLOGIC CLINICS OF NORTH AMERICA
May 2007
Editor: Kerry Holland

Volume 34, Number 2
ISSN 0094-0143
ISBN-13: 978-1-4160-4585-4
ISBN-10: 1-4160-4585-6

Urologic Clinics of North America (ISSN 0094-0143) is published quarterly by Elsevier Inc., 360 Park Avenue South, New York, NY 10010-1710. Months of issue are February, May, August, and November. Business and Editorial Offices: 1600 John F. Kennedy Blvd., Suite 1800, Philadelphia, PA 19103-2899. Customer Service Office: 6277 Sea Harbor Drive, Orlando, FL 32887-4800. Periodicals postage paid at New York, NY and additional mailing offices. Subscription prices are $231.00 per year (US individuals), $358.00 per year (US institutions), $264.00 per year (Canadian individuals), $429.00 per year (Canadian institutions), $308.00 per year (foreign individuals), and $429.00 per year (foreign institutions). Foreign air speed delivery is included in all *Clinics* subscription prices. All prices are subject to change without notice. **POSTMASTER:** Send address changes to *Urologic Clinics of North America*, Elsevier Periodicals Customer Service, 6277 Sea Harbor Drive, Orlando, FL 32887-4800. **Customer Service: 1-800-654-2452 (US). From outside the US, call 1-407-345-4000.**

Urologic Clinics of North America is covered in *Index Medicus, Excerpta Medica, Current Contents/Clinical Medicine, Science Citation Index,* and *ISI/BIOMED.*

Printed in the United States of America.

CONSULTING EDITOR

MARTIN I. RESNICK, MD, Lester Persky Professor and Chairman, Department of Urology, Case Medical Center, Cleveland, Ohio

GUEST EDITOR

JOEL SHEINFELD, MD, Vice Chairman, Department of Urology, Sidney Kimmel Center for Prostate and Urologic Cancers, Memorial Sloan-Kettering Cancer Center; and Professor of Urology, Department of Urology, Weill College of Medicine, New York, New York

CONTRIBUTORS

HIKMAT AL-AHMADIE, MD, Department of Urology and Pathology, Memorial Sloan-Kettering Cancer Center, New York, New York

JACK BANIEL, MD, Head of Urology Section, Department of Urology, Rabin Medical Center–Beilinson Campus, Petah Tikva; and Professor of Urology, Sackler Medical School, Tel Aviv University, Tel Aviv, Israel

STEPHEN D.W. BECK, MD, Department of Urology, Indiana University School of Medicine, Indiana Cancer Pavilion, Indianapolis, Indiana

RICHARD BIHRLE, MD, Department of Urology, Indiana University School of Medicine, Indiana Cancer Pavilion, Indianapolis, Indiana

BRETT S. CARVER, MD, Department of Urology and Pathology, Memorial Sloan-Kettering Cancer Center, New York, New York

SAM S. CHANG, MD, Associate Professor, Department of Urologic Surgery, Vanderbilt University, Nashville, Tennessee

TONI K. CHOUEIRI, MD, Fellow, Section of Urologic Oncology, Glickman Urological Institute, Cleveland Clinic Foundation, Cleveland, Ohio

IVAN DAMJANOV, MD, PhD, Professor of Pathology and Laboratory Medicine, Department of Pathology, University of Kansas School of Medicine, Kansas City, Kansas

JOHN P. DONOHUE, MD, Department of Urology, Indiana University School of Medicine, Indiana Cancer Pavilion, Indianapolis, Indiana

YARON EHRLICH, MD, Department of Urology, Rabin Medical Center–Beilinson Campus, Petah Tikva, Israel

LAWRENCE H. EINHORN, MD, Department of Urology, Indiana University School of Medicine; and Department of Medicine, Section of Hematology and Oncology, Indiana University School of Medicine, Indiana Cancer Pavilion, Indianapolis, Indiana

ANTONIO FINELLI, MD, MSC, FRCSC, Assistant Professor of Surgery, Division of Urology, Department of Surgical Oncology, University Health Network, Princess Margaret Hospital, Toronto, Ontario, Canada

HARRY FISCH, MD, Clinical Professor of Urology, Male Reproductive Center, Department of Urology, Columbia University, College of Physicians and Surgeons, New York Presbyterian Hospital, New York, New York

NEIL FLESHNER, MD, MPH, FRCSC, Associate Professor of Surgery, and Chief of Urology, Division of Urology, Department of Surgery, Princess Margaret Hospital, University Health Network, University of Toronto, Toronto, Canada

RICHARD S. FOSTER, MD, Department of Urology, Indiana University School of Medicine, Indiana Cancer Pavilion, Indianapolis, Indiana

TIMOTHY GILLIGAN, MD, Attending Staff, Department of Solid Tumor Oncology, Taussig Cancer Center, Cleveland Clinic Foundation, Cleveland, Ohio

RYAN J. GROLL, MD, Resident, Division of Urology, Department of Surgery, University of Toronto, Toronto, Ontario, Canada

ROBERT J. HAMILTON, MD, MPH, Resident, Division of Urology, Department of Surgery, University of Toronto, University Health Network, Princess Margaret Hospital, Toronto, Ontario, Canada

JEFFERY M. HOLZBEIERLEIN, MD, Assistant Professor of Urology, Department of Urology, University of Kansas School of Medicine, Kansas City, Kansas

MICHAEL A.S. JEWETT, MD, Professor, Division of Urology, Department of Surgical Oncology, Princess Margaret Hospital and the University Health Network, Toronto, Ontario, Canada

MICHAEL E. KARELLAS, MD, Urology Fellow, Department of Surgery, Division of Urology, Memorial Sloan Kettering Cancer Center, New York

MARK H. KATZ, MD, Resident in Urology, Department of Urology, Columbia University, College of Physicians and Surgeons, New York Presbyterian Hospital, Columbia University Medical Center, New York, New York

MELISSA R. KAUFMAN, MD, PhD, Department of Urologic Surgery, Vanderbilt University, Nashville, Tennessee

ERIC A. KLEIN, MD, Professor, Section of Urologic Oncology, Glickman Urological Institute, Cleveland Clinic Foundation, Cleveland, Ohio

G. VARUNI KONDAGUNTA, MD, Assistant Attending Physician, Genitourinary Oncology Service, Division of Solid Tumor Oncology, Department of Medicine, Memorial Sloan-Kettering Cancer Center; and Department of Medicine, Joan and Sanford I. Weill Medical College of Cornell University, New York, New York

SARAH M. LAMBERT, MD, Urology Resident, Male Reproductive Center, Department of Urology, Columbia University, College of Physicians and Surgeons, New York Presbyterian Hospital, New York, New York

PAUL H. LANGE, MD, FACS, Professor and Chair, Department of Urology, University of Washington, Seattle, Washington

DANIEL W. LIN, MD, Assistant Professor, Department of Urology, University of Washington, Seattle, Washington

JAMES M. McKIERNAN, MD, Assistant Professor of Urology, Department of Urology, Columbia University, College of Physicians and Surgeons, New York Presbyterian Hospital, Columbia University Medical Center, New York, New York

ROBERT J. MOTZER, MD, Attending Physician, Genitourinary Oncology Service, Division of Solid Tumor Oncology, Department of Medicine, Memorial Sloan-Kettering Cancer Center; and Department of Medicine, Joan and Sanford I. Weill Medical College of Cornell University, New York, New York

JUDD W. MOUL, MD, FACS, Professor and Chief, Division of Urologic Surgery, and Director, Duke Prostate Center, Duke University Medical Center, Durham, North Carolina

MISCHEL NEILL, MD, Fellow in Urologic Oncology, Division of Urology, Department of Surgery, Princess Margaret Hospital, University Health Network, University of Toronto, Toronto, Canada

JOEL SHEINFELD, MD, Vice Chairman, Department of Urology, Sidney Kimmel Center for Prostate and Urologic Cancers, Memorial Sloan-Kettering Cancer Center; and Professor of Urology, Department of Urology, Weill College of Medicine, New York, New York

HONG GEE SIM, MBBS, MRCSEd, MMED, FAMS, Fellow, Department of Urology, University of Washington, Seattle, Washington

PRAMOD SOGANI, MD, FACS, Attending, Department of Urology, Sidney Kimmel Center for Prostate and Urologic Cancers, Memorial Sloan-Kettering Cancer Center; and Professor of Urology, Department of Urology, Weill College of Medicine, New York, New York

ANDREW J. STEPHENSON, MD, Assistant Professor, Section of Urologic Oncology, Glickman Urological Institute, Cleveland Clinic Foundation, Cleveland, Ohio

GUY C. TONER, MBBS, MD, FRACP, Associate Professor of Medicine, University of Melbourne, Melbourne; and Head, Department of Medical Oncology, Peter MacCallum Cancer Centre, East Melbourne, Victoria, Australia

DAVID J. VAUGHN, MD, Associate Professor of Medicine, Division of Hematology/Oncology, Abramson Cancer Center of the University of Pennsylvania, Philadelphia, Pennsylvania

PADRAIG WARDE, MD, Professor of Radiation Oncology, and Deputy Head of Radiation Oncology, Division of Urology, Department of Surgery, Princess Margaret Hospital, University Health Network, University of Toronto, Toronto, Canada

CONTENTS

GOAL STATEMENT

The goal of *Urologic Clinics of North America* is to keep practicing urologists and urology residents up to date with current clinical practice in urology by providing timely articles reviewing the state of the art in patient care.

ACCREDITATION

The *Urologic Clinics of North America* is planned and implemented in accordance with the Essential Areas and Policies of the Accreditation Council for Continuing Medical Education (ACCME) through the joint sponsorship of the University of Virginia School of Medicine and Elsevier. The University of Virginia School of Medicine is accredited by the ACCME to provide continuing medical education for physicians.

The University of Virginia School of Medicine designates this educational activity for a maximum of *15 AMA PRA Category 1 Credits*™. Physicians should only claim credit commensurate with the extent of their participation in the activity.

The American Medical Association has determined that physicians not licensed in the US who participate in this CME activity are eligible for *15 AMA PRA Category 1 Credits*™.

Credit can be earned by reading the text material, taking the CME examination online at http://www.theclinics.com/home/cme, and completing the evaluation. After taking the test, you will be required to review any and all incorrect answers. Following completion of the test and evaluation, your credit will be awarded and you may print your certificate.

FACULTY DISCLOSURE/CONFLICT OF INTEREST

The University of Virginia School of Medicine, as an ACCME accredited provider, endorses and strives to comply with the Accreditation Council for Continuing Medical Education (ACCME) Standards of Commercial Support, Commonwealth of Virginia statutes, University of Virginia policies and procedures, and associated federal and private regulations and guidelines on the need for disclosure and monitoring of proprietary and financial interests that may affect the scientific integrity and balance of content delivered in continuing medical education activities under our auspices.

The University of Virginia School of Medicine requires that all CME activities accredited through this institution be developed independently and be scientifically rigorous, balanced and objective in the presentation/discussion of its content, theories and practices.

All authors/editors participating in an accredited CME activity are expected to disclose to the readers relevant financial relationships with commercial entities occurring within the past 12 months (such as grants or research support, employee, consultant, stock holder, member of speakers bureau, etc.). The University of Virginia School of Medicine will employ appropriate mechanisms to resolve potential conflicts of interest to maintain the standards of fair and balanced education to the reader. Questions about specific strategies can be directed to the Office of Continuing Medical Education, University of Virginia School of Medicine, Charlottesville, Virginia.

The authors/editors listed below have identified no professional or financial affiliations for themselves or their spouse/partner:
Hikmat Al-Ahmadie, MD; Jack Baniel, MD; Steven D. W. Beck, MD; Richard Bihrle, MD; Brett S. Carver, MD; Sam S. Chang, MD; Toni K. Choueiri, MD; Ivan Damjanov, MD, PhD; John P. Donahue, MD; Yaron Ehrlich, MD; Lawrence H. Einhom, MD; Antonio Finelli, MD, MSc; Harry Fisch, MD; Neil Fleshner, MD, MPH, FRCSC; Richard S. Foster, MD; Timothy Gilligan, MD; Ryan J. Groll, MD; Robert J. Hamilton, MD, MPH; Kerry K. Holland (Acquisitions Editor); Jeffery M. Holzbeierlein, MD; Michael A. S. Jewett, MD; Michael E. Karellas, MD; Mark H. Katz, MD; Melissa R. Kaufman, MD, PhD; Eric A. Klein, MD; G. Varuni Kondagunta, MD; Sarah M. Lambert, MD; Paul H. Lange, MD; Daniel W. Lin, MD; James M. McKiernan, MD; Robert J. Motzer, MD; Judd W. Moul, MD, FACS; Mishcel Neill, MD; Hong Gee Sim, MRCSEd, MMED, FAMS; Pramod C. Sogani, MD; Andrew J. Stephenson, MD; David J. Vaughn, MD; and, Padraig Warde, MD.

The authors/editors listed below identified the following professional or financial affiliations for themselves or their spouse/partner:
Joel Sheinfeld, MD (Guest Editor) is employed by Memorial Sloan-Kettering.
Guy C. Toner, MBBS, MD, FRACP is on the advisory committee and has received travel/conference sponsorship from Pfizer.

Disclosure of Discussion of non-FDA approved uses for pharmaceutical products and/or medical devices:
The University of Virginia School of Medicine, as an ACCME provider, requires that all faculty presenters identify and disclose any "off label" uses for pharmaceutical and medical device products. The University of Virginia School of Medicine recommends that each physician fully review all the available data on new products or procedures prior to instituting them with patients.

TO ENROLL

To enroll in the Urologic Clinics of North America Continuing Medical Education program, call customer service at 1-800-654-2452 or visit us online at www.theclinics.com/home/cme. The CME program is available to subscribers for an additional fee of $195.00.

FORTHCOMING ISSUES

August 2007

Urolithiasis
Margaret Pearle, MD, PhD, *Guest Editor*

November 2007

Sexual Dysfunction
Allen Seftel, MD, *Guest Editor*

RECENT ISSUES

February 2007

Urologic Issues and Pregnancy
Deborah R. Erickson, MD, *Guest Editor*

November 2006

Overactive Bladder
Michael B. Chancellor, MD, *Guest Editor*

August 2006

Urologic Imaging
Pat Fox Fulgham, MD, *Guest Editor*

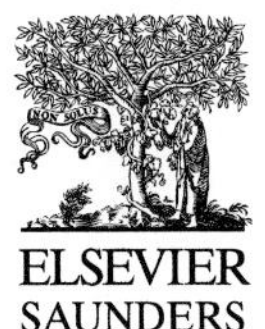

ELSEVIER
SAUNDERS

Urol Clin N Am 34 (2007) xv

UROLOGIC
CLINICS
of North America

Foreword

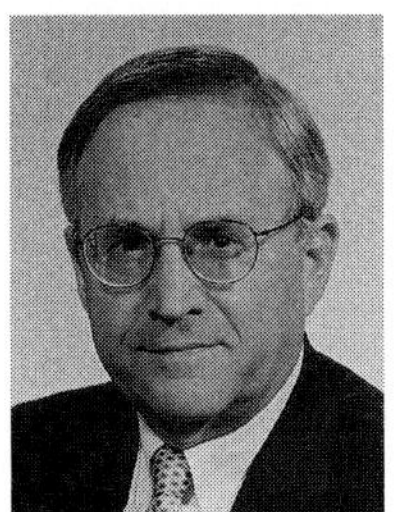

Martin I. Resnick, MD
Consulting Editor

Testicular tumors are the most common solid malignancies of young men; fortunately the majority of patients can expect their therapy to be curative in most instances. Based on tumor stage and histological type, these tumors, in distinction of other genitourinary malignancies, are amenable to multiple forms of therapy including surgery, radiation therapy, and chemotherapy. Additionally, with the development of new staging techniques including imaging and tumor markers, surveillance is also an option in the properly selected patient.

In this issue of *Urologic Clinics of North America*, Dr. Sheinfeld has brought together recognized experts in the evaluation and treatment of these patients. Not only are the newly evolving techniques of retroperitoneal lymph node dissection discussed but also the management of patients with recurrent disease, which has proven to be successful in many. Additionally, the associated complications and morbidity of treatment is appropriately reviewed.

All physicians managing these patients, including urologists, radiation therapists, and medical oncologists will find the information in this monograph to be of value in caring for these patients. The information presented is up to date and is of significant clinical relevance.

Martin I. Resnick, MD
Department of Urology
University Hospitals Case Medical Center
Cleveland, OH

E-mail address: martin.resnick@case.edu

doi:10.1016/j.ucl.2007.04.001

urologic.theclinics.com

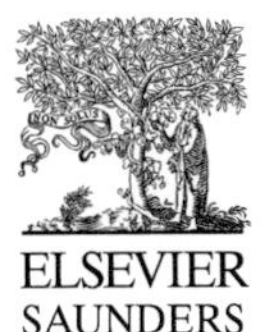
ELSEVIER
SAUNDERS

Urol Clin N Am 34 (2007) xvii

UROLOGIC CLINICS of North America

Preface

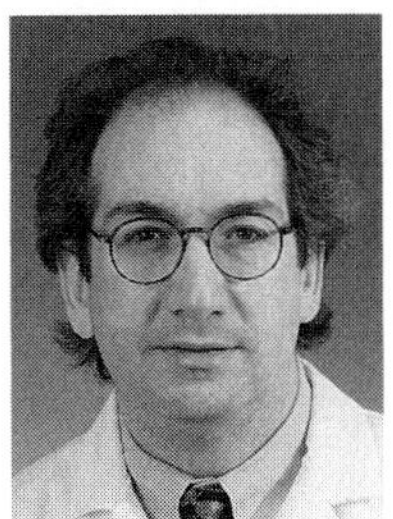

Joel Sheinfeld, MD
Guest Editor

Each year there are approximately 8000 new cases of testicular cancer diagnosed in the United States, resulting in almost 400 deaths. The incidence of testicular cancer, the most common solid tumor in men between the ages of 20 and 35 years, is increasing in the United States and Europe. The management of patients who have testicular cancer has evolved significantly over the past 25 years, representing a model in the successful multidisciplinary approach to a solid malignancy with the appropriate integration of surgery and cisplatin-based chemotherapy resulting in improvements in survival from 60% to 65% in the 1960s to greater than 95% at present. Given the high probability of achieving cure, considerable effort has been focused on individualizing therapy for specific patients in an attempt to minimize morbidity and preserve quality of life without adversely impacting survival. This has been possible because of refinements in histologic, serologic, and radiographic parameters that have resulted in improved risk assessment for patients of all stages. Surgical techniques and the development of less toxic and more effective chemotherapy regimens have also played a critical role. The apparent overtreatment of many patients and the availability of multiple approaches that achieve cure have resulted in several significant controversies in the management of testicular cancer. The long-term survival of patients has identified significant issues that appear to have been underappreciated in the past, such as late relapse, reoperative surgery, and the long-term sequelae of treatment, particularly chemotherapy. Some of these problems have prompted us to re-examine and challenge previously accepted treatment paradigms. This issue of the *Urologic Clinics of North America* describes the current state-of-the-art therapy for testicular cancer and specifically addresses some of the important controversies faced by clinicians today. This has been possible because of the insight and expertise of an exceptional group of distinguished urologists, medical and radiation oncologists, and pathologists.

Joel Sheinfeld, MD
Department of Urology
Sidney Kimmel Center for Prostate and Urologic Cancers
Memorial Sloan-Kettering Cancer Center
353 East 68th Street
New York, NY 10021, USA

E-mail address: sheinfej@mskcc.org

doi:10.1016/j.ucl.2007.02.017

urologic.theclinics.com

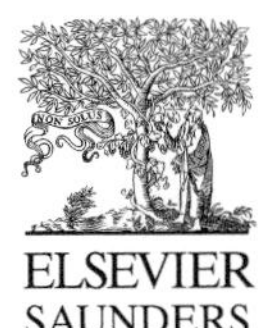

ELSEVIER
SAUNDERS

Urol Clin N Am 34 (2007) 109–117

UROLOGIC
CLINICS
of North America

Timely Diagnosis of Testicular Cancer

Judd W. Moul, MD, FACS

Division of Urologic Surgery, Duke Prostate Center, Duke University Medical Center, Durham, NC, USA

Screening for testicular cancer, like any true disease-screening effort, involves evaluation of an asymptomatic population for the disease in question. The goal of any cancer screening effort is to diagnose the disease at an early, more easily treatable stage with the ultimate goal of improving the disease-specific survival and minimizing treatment morbidity. Screening efforts can also be directed toward population groups most at risk for the disease to improve cost effectiveness, which is becoming increasingly important as we face the aging of the "Baby Boom" generation.

Although testicular cancer is an uncommon neoplasm, it is the most common solid tumor in men between the ages of 20 and 34, and the incidence is increasing [1]. Because of the known and continuing problem of delayed diagnosis, which is discussed later, screening might be considered for this disease. Conversely, with most patients now being cured, the screening goal of increasing disease-specific survival may be impossible to improve substantially. The goal of early detection to minimize morbidity of treatment may be an obtainable goal.

Particularly relevant to testicular cancer is the concept of true screening of an entire asymptomatic population versus case finding in at-risk or symptomatic men. Akin to case finding is the concept of testicular self-examination (TSE) and increasing awareness of this disease among young men.

Importance of early detection

The common sense importance of early detection and diagnosis of testicular cancer has been known for many years. Before the advent of curative therapy, this was one of the few ways (if not the only way) to prevent deaths in the usually young and otherwise healthy men who are affected. In the current era of effective chemotherapy, most (but not all) patients can be salvaged despite delays in diagnosis and, consequently, more advanced disease [2]. This salvage, however, generally requires much more extensive chemotherapy or surgery, and the potential morbidity of these more heroic efforts must not be underestimated. Expedient diagnosis of these neoplasms affords the opportunity to treat these patients at their earliest stage of disease and therefore to minimize long-term morbidity.

Despite this worthy goal of early diagnosis, pitfalls in the early and accurate diagnosis of testicular tumors are common. Delay in diagnosis of testicular cancer is well documented [2–30]. Table 1 illustrates that the mean delay (26 weeks) has varied little over the last 75 years from various series throughout the world. It is interesting that this approximate 5-month delay from initial symptoms to a surgical diagnosis has remained constant in these reports. Despite this consistency, some investigators have shown a trend toward a decreased delay in more recent years [2,12]. Dieckmann and colleagues [12] found that the number of patients in whom diagnosis was made improved within 2 weeks from 13.6% to 25.4% between 1969 to 1976 and 1982 to 1986. Similarly, Moul and colleagues [2] found that the mean symptomatic interval decreased from 22.7 to 16.4 weeks between the 1970 to 1974 and the 1985 to 1987 intervals. Conversely, Nikzas and colleagues [22] found no decrease in delay between 1980 and 1987 in 232 patients studied in Great Britain. Even if delay time has improved somewhat, in some series it remains a significant

E-mail address: judd.moul@duke.edu

doi:10.1016/j.ucl.2007.02.003

Table 1
Delay in diagnosis of testicular cancer: review of the literature

Study	Time period of review	No. of patients	Mean duration of symptoms (wk)
Weissbach et al [3]	1926–1973	182	40
Host and Stokke [4]	1932–1953	289	33.6
Patton et al [5]	1940–1956	510	20
Thompson et al [6]	1940–1960	178	87
Bosl et al [7]	1941–1978	335	12
Kurohara et al [8]	1945–1965	196	25.4
Borski [9]	1953–1973	150	26.1
Seib et al [10]	1960–1973	50	20
Ware et al [11]	1965–1977	100	17.3
Dieckmann et al [12]	1969–1986	156	24.3
Kulig [13]	1970–1979	27	24
Moul et al [2]	1970–1987	148	21.1
Leyh [14]	1971–1982	101	21.8
Kuhne et al [15]	1971–1982	50	30.5
Scher et al [16]	1972–1979	123	8
Fischer [17]	1973–1981	182	20
Heising [18]	1976–1981	1344	19.6
Jones and Appleyard [19]	1976–1982	121	19.8
Thornhill et al [20]	1980–1985	217	40
Chilvers et al [21]	1980–1986	257	16
Nikzas et al [22]	1980–1987	232	22
Total	—	4948	26

problem. Patients and health care providers may contribute to delay in diagnosis. Patient-mediated delays owing to ignorance, embarrassment, fear of cancer, or fear of emasculation are well known [23,28]. Dieckmann and colleagues [12] found that delay was related to educational level. College-educated men in whom both seminoma and nonseminoma were diagnosed were found to have shorter mean and median delays. The less informed or less educated patient may actually believe that a larger testicle makes a more virile man [23]. Patients who have testicular cancer may be more inclined than other cancer patients to delay or even refuse seeking medical attention or treatment [31]. Testicular cancer affects young and usually otherwise healthy men who may be unable to acknowledge the threat of fatal disease. Instead of seeking evaluation, they may hold fast to their normal routine as a denial mechanism termed the *flight into health* [32]. Furthermore, that testicular cancer involves the loss of an external sexual organ during a time in the patient's life when sexuality is very important is an added stressor [31]. Jones and Appleyard [19] point out that it is often the partner and not the patient himself who insists that medical attention be sought.

Physician-mediated delay most commonly results from the misdiagnosis of a testis tumor as an infection. Unfortunately for the clinician, the classic painless testicular mass or swelling is the presenting symptom in only approximately half of patients in whom testicular cancer ultimately is diagnosed (Table 2). Scrotal pain with or without a mass occurs in up to 50% of testicular cancer presentations and has been attributed to hemorrhage into the tumor [5,25,33].

This painful presentation is not uncommonly responsible for a false diagnosis of epididymitis. In one study of 335 testicular cancer patients, one third were treated initially with antibiotics or local treatments for presumed epididymitis, and most of these were delayed from appropriate orchiectomy for more than 2 weeks [7]. In another study of 133 men who had testicular cancer, 23 (17%) were treated initially for epididymitis [26]. Most were delayed for 2 or 3 months, and 5 patients were delayed from 6 to 22 months.

Because nonseminomas generally are considered a more rapidly growing neoplasm than seminomas, they may be more commonly associated with a painful presentation. Sandeman [24] found that 109 (47%) nonseminoma patients initially presented with pain, whereas only 102 (38%) seminoma patients had a similar presentation. Seminomas are usually a more indolent-growing neoplasm, and a painless mass or swelling is the most common presentation. It is the nonseminoma patient who might benefit the most from early diagnosis but who also may be more difficult to distinguish from a patient who has an inflammatory lesion.

In my prior practice at the Walter Reed Army Medical Center and now at Duke University, we frequently see young men who are prime candidates for testicular cancer or epididymitis. Our policy is to assume malignancy until proved otherwise. Urinalysis usually demonstrates pyuria when epididymitis is present and, in most cases, epididymal tenderness and swelling are distinguishable from the testis proper. When more severe orchitis or swelling is present and suspicion for tumor persists, a 1% lidocaine cord block can allow for a more meaningful examination. If we

Table 2
Presenting signs and symptoms of testicular tumors in various series

Signs and symptoms	Percentage presenting							
	Patton et al [5] (n = 491)	Robson et al [33] (n = 360)	Sandeman [24] (n = 502)	Bosl et al [7] (n = 335)	Dieckmann et al [12] (n = 180)	Thornhill et al [20] (n = 217)	Wishnow et al [27] (n = 154)	Meffan et al [30] (n = 79)
Painless mass or swelling	NS	56.9	54	NS	51.2	32	57	43
Painful scrotum with or without mass or swelling	NS	26.4	42	45	32.8	31	40	50
Incidental finding	5	4.3	4	NS	NS	23	NS	NS
Associated with trauma	7	13[a]	NS	11.2[b]	NS	10	NS	3
Symptoms and signs of metastases	10	5.2	NS	10.7	6.3	19	NS	5
Gynecomastia or tenderness	NS	NS	NS	5	1.1	2	3	1.3

Abbreviation: NS, not stated.
[a] Hernia, traumatic orchitis, or torsion.
[b] Trauma, hydrocele, or benign tumor.

still have any index of suspicion for a tumor, we proceed directly to scrotal sonography.

Serum tumor markers, such as β–human chorionic gonadotropin and α-fetoprotein, usually are also useful to obtain in this setting and are absolutely essential to obtain before orchiectomy. The differential diagnosis of testicular masses has been aided by cytologic examination of seminal fluid obtained by ejaculation or prostatic massage [34,35]; however, this is not in widespread clinical use. Even if the clinician is sure of a diagnosis of epididymitis or orchitis, it is still prudent to insist that the patient be seen in follow-up in 7 to 10 days after the inflammation has subsided to re-examine the testis for an occult neoplasm. This follow-up of presumed infection is crucial especially if the diagnosis of epididymitis is not certain.

In addition to presumed infection, trauma frequently may cloud an accurate and early diagnosis of testicular cancer. Stephen [25] cites trauma as "a wolf in sheep's clothing" with respect to complicating the diagnosis of testicular cancer. Up to 10% of testicular cancer patients initially receive a diagnosis of posttraumatic pain or swelling (see Table 2). It is presumed that the enlarged tumorous testis is more susceptible to trauma or that less significant trauma might more easily precipitate symptoms. Patton and colleagues [5] claim that the trauma is coincidental in attracting the patient's attention to an already existing lesion. Stephen [25] has described an interesting sign whereby the lack of sickening pain at the moment of injury, because of prior destruction or partial destruction of the testis from neoplasm, is an important point to elicit from the patient. The pitfall is a less-than-adequate evaluation for tumor in a patient presenting with trauma. One should be especially wary when the swelling or pain is out of proportion to what would be considered minor trauma, or vice versa. Again, in the setting of trauma, a high index of suspicion for tumor is necessary and scrotal sonography, exploration, or compulsive follow-up frequently is indicated.

Up to 19% of patients present with signs or symptoms of metastases (see Table 2). Back pain, abdominal mass, lymphadenopathy, and weight loss are the most prevalent constitutional symptoms. An additional 1% to 5% of patients present with gynecomastia or breast tenderness. The major pitfall in these presentations is to fail to examine the genitalia and so miss an obvious testicular tumor, and thereby delay, misdiagnose, or mistreat a metastatic germ cell cancer. Oliver [28] has stated that the most severe delays in diagnosis occur in patients undergoing investigation of symptoms that are subsequently shown to have been caused by metastases. Inappropriate laparotomy in the case of an obvious testicular tumor remaining in situ is not rare [23]. Patients who have back pain have been subjected to osteopathic therapy while a testicular cancer went unsuspected [26]. Prout and Griffin [26] have even reported two patients being subjected to mastectomy for gynecomastia before any evaluation for testicular cancer. Surprising as this may be, we have also seen a patient who had bilateral subcutaneous mastectomy and soon thereafter received a diagnosis of obvious testicular cancer [36].

For seminoma patients, delay in diagnosis is not necessarily associated with more advanced disease or decreased survival. Many investigators have noted that seminomas can have a protracted indolent growth, and symptom duration does not correlate with disease stage [2,12,24]. Because of slow growth characteristics, stage I seminoma can be associated with very long symptomatic intervals. Moul and colleagues [2] found the mean symptomatic interval for stage I seminomas to be 39 weeks, whereas that for stage II disease ranged from 11 to 18.5 weeks. Dieckmann and colleagues [12] found that stage I patients had a 228-day mean delay in diagnosis, compared with 129 days for the stage II seminomas. Regarding survival and delay for seminoma patients, the longer period of delay has not been shown statistically to affect survival, although deaths from seminoma have been associated with very long delays [2].

For the nonseminoma patient, there is a clearer association between delay in diagnosis and advanced disease. Bosl and colleagues [7] found a median delay of 75, 101, and 134 days for stages I, II, and III testicular cancer, respectively (24% seminomas included). Thornhill and colleagues [20] noted that stage I patients had a mean duration of symptoms of 2.2 months, whereas stage II cases were delayed 4.7 months (stage III and IV were delayed 3.4 and 4.5 months, respectively). Chilvers and colleagues [21], reporting on 257 nonseminomatous germ cell tumor (NSGCT) patients seen between 1980 and 1986, found that of those who sought medical advice within 100 days of onset of symptoms, 54% had stage I tumors compared with 41% who delayed longer (P = .05 by χ^2 analysis). The Wishnow and colleagues [27] study of 154 NSGCT patients compared patients in whom tumor was diagnosed within 1 month (n = 65, group 1) to patients delayed longer than 1 month (n = 89, group 2). Sixty-two percent of group 1 presented with stage I disease compared with only 28% of group 2 (P<.001). Similarly, only 8% of group I patients had stage III disease, compared with 39% of group 2 patients (P<.001, χ^2). Moul and colleagues [2] found the mean symptomatic interval for stages I, IIA, and IIB nonseminomas to range between 8.5 and 9.7 weeks, whereas for stages IIC and III the delay was 26.4 weeks.

Increased delay has also traditionally been associated with decreased survival for nonseminoma patients. Sandeman [24] reported a progressively decreased 3-year disease-free interval as delay increased. Post and Belis [23] reported a 69% 3-year survival for patients in whom NSGCT was diagnosed within 3 months, versus a 47% survival if the delay was greater than 3 months. Prout and Griffin [26] noted a 0% crude death rate for men in whom diagnosis was made within 1 month, compared with a 27.6% death rate when delay was longer than 1 month. Oliver [28] found that the average delay was 2 months in patients who remained free of disease, 4 months in those who relapsed but were salvaged, and 7 months in those who died of drug-resistant disease. Thornhill and colleagues [20], studying 217 cases of testicular cancer in Ireland, found delay to be statistically associated with metastases, diminished prospects of cure, and mortality. The median duration of symptoms was 4 months in those who died of disease, compared with 2.5 months in those patients who were alive. Wishnow and colleagues [27] noted that only 1 of 65 patients in whom diagnosis was made within 1 month died of disease, whereas 11 of 89 (12.4%) delayed beyond 1 month died of testicular cancer (P = .0072, χ^2). In a study of 232 patients treated between 1980 and 1987, Nikzas and colleagues [22] found an 8% mortality in patients in whom tumor was diagnosed within 6 months, compared with 16% in those with a longer delay (P<.01).

Moul and colleagues [2] found that a delay greater than 16 weeks had a strong statistical adverse effect on survival for nonseminoma patients treated between 1970 and 1987. When these investigators separated patients treated during the more contemporary "cisplatin era" (1979–1987), the impact of delay on survival was attenuated and no longer was statistically significant. These authors concluded that effective chemotherapy salvages many patients who in the past would have been at a disadvantage as a consequence of delayed diagnosis. Other investigators also have found that delay in diagnosis does not necessarily influence survival for NSGCT patients in the contemporary era. In their study of 257 NSGCT patients between 1980 and 1986, Chilvers and colleagues [21] actually found an inverse relationship between delay and survival. Patients in whom diagnosis was made within 0 to 49 days had a lessened relapse-free survival compared with patients in whom diagnosis was made later (P<.05, log rank test for trend). The authors concluded that faster-growing, more aggressive tumors are more likely to produce symptoms leading to medical consultation. Similarly, Meffan and colleagues [30], in a small study of 79 patients (40 seminomas, 39 NSGCT) treated between 1976 and 1985 in New Zealand, found no relation between delay and prognosis. They concluded that all cases in their series were being diagnosed too late and that is why no association was seen.

Although contemporary chemotherapy may salvage most patients despite delay in diagnosis and more advanced disease, deaths still result from delay. Furthermore, effective chemotherapy may be a double-edged sword in that clinicians may become more lax in expediently caring for these patients and so delay may increase [27]. The potentially higher morbidity associated with the more intensive therapy that is required to salvage patients as a consequence of delay must not be underestimated. Efforts to decrease delay in diagnosis may be the most cost-effective method to improve further the survival of testicular cancer patients and to lessen treatment morbidity.

True screening

True screening would involve evaluating an entire asymptomatic population for testicular cancer. With the overall high curability and low incidence of this disease, it is debatable whether we should invest in screening programs for testicular cancer. The principal screening test for testicular cancer is palpation of the testis by an examiner [37]. The sensitivity, specificity, and positive predictive value of the testicular examination in asymptomatic individuals are unknown. False-negative and false-positive examinations because of epididymal and testicular changes from infections, trauma, and cysts are common even among urologists and would be significantly higher among other practitioners. Varicoceles and hydroceles, relatively common conditions, also would pose accuracy problems for screening physical examinations. Alternatively, scrotal sonography might be more accurate in general widespread screening, but the cost-effectiveness of this modality for this uncommon neoplasm is questionable [38].

Despite these concerns regarding testicular examination, the American Cancer Society and the National Cancer Institute [39,40] recommend that it be included as part of the periodic health examination of men. The Canadian Task Force and the US Preventive Services Task Force, however, recommend that screening examinations should be performed only on patients who have risk factors, such as those with a history of cryptorchidism or testicular atrophy [37,41]. Aside from age, the only currently known main risk factors for testicular cancer include cryptorchidism, Caucasian race [42], prior testicular tumor, and family history. Screening of these risk groups may be beneficial, although the value has not been proved.

Because of the rarity of this disease and the inaccuracy of the screening test (scrotal examination by physician), routine screening examinations of the genitalia of all asymptomatic men would have a low yield and would not be cost effective. From the available information, general screening of the population is not indicated, but a testicular examination should be part of the male physical examination, and periodic screening for men with risk factors may be beneficial.

Case finding and testicular self-examination

Case finding is similar to screening but involves detecting disease in a symptomatic patient or one who presents to the physician with concerns that he might have the disease in question. As can be surmised from the prior discussion regarding delay in diagnosis, case finding for testicular cancer is critically important for the man who presents with scrotal symptoms, such as a mass, pain, or swelling, or after trauma. As previously noted, testicular cancer should not be overlooked when initial signs or symptoms are related to distant metastases. Case finding may be enhanced by patient education about testicular cancer and by TSE.

TSE is the process of instructing patients to examine themselves periodically for testicular masses, swelling, and other changes, and is patterned on the well-accepted concept of breast self-examinations [43–56]. The American Cancer Society and the National Cancer Institute [57,58] recommend that all postpuberal males perform a monthly TSE. Not all authorities agree that TSE is beneficial, however. The US Preventive Services Task Force [37] contends that there is insufficient evidence for or against counseling patients to perform periodic TSE. This group contends that reliable information on the accuracy of TSE is lacking and that it is unknown whether counseling men to perform TSE actually motivates them to adopt the practice or to perform it correctly [37]. Others, citing the lack of evidence that TSE is effective, advised physicians against routinely devoting time to discussing TSE [59,60]. Some have argued that the yield does not offset the increased anxiety that emphasis on TSE causes among men in an age group that already has many bodily concerns [47]. Conversely, Friman and Finney [61] point out that TSE would not cause excess anxiety but would reduce anxiety with regular practice. Furthermore, teaching young men to conduct TSE may result in these men taking increased responsibility for their own health care [61].

Despite the knowledge and perceived benefit of TSE by most health care professionals, little of this knowledge has been transferred to the public. Sheley and colleagues [62] studied 415 men from different regions of the United States and found that only 2% reported correctly performed, monthly TSE. These investigators concluded that there was a technology transfer problem regarding awareness of testicular cancer and TSE, teaching proper TSE, and conveying a benefit to the individual for performing TSE. Dachs and colleagues [63] similarly found that only 4.7% of New England college students performed monthly TSE in the mid-1980s. Even after being provided written material and a lecture on TSE by a physician, only 36% of the students changed their behavior and began performing monthly TSE [63].

Brubaker and Wickersham [64] postulate that the reason for this failure of TSE education is based on the theory of reasoned action, which proposes that performance of a behavior, such as TSE, is a direct result of a person's reasoned intention to perform that behavior. Behavioral intention, in turn, is a function of the individual's attitude toward the behavior and his or her perception of whether significant others would approve. Attitude toward the behavior reflects salient beliefs about the outcomes of performing the behavior, weighted by the value of each outcome. Brubaker and Wickersham [64] studied 232 college men exposed to educational lectures, reading materials, and posters about TSE. A student's attitude about the potential benefit of TSE and the perceived value of TSE by other peers affected his intention to perform TSE. Likewise, intention helped to determine who actually performed TSE. Clearly, we must convey a benefit to performing TSE to change a young man's intention to carry through with the behavior. Simple education without conveying a benefit of the behavior will not succeed in increasing the practice of TSE.

Having concluded that TSE may be beneficial at least for men who have risk factors for testicular cancer, if not for all young men, its teaching should emphasize the following points. First, men must gain familiarity with the surface, texture, and consistency of their testicles in the normal state. Second, the ideal time for TSE is during or after a warm bath or shower. Third, the man examining himself should rotate both testicles between thumb and forefinger until he determines that the entire surface of each is free of lumps. Fourth, the man should learn the location of the epididymis and that this structure is not a tumor. Fifth, any detected lump should be reported to a physician immediately [65]. Most importantly, as noted earlier, physicians must convey the benefit of TSE to affect the intention to perform it regularly. Education must include possible consequences of not performing TSE, such as delay in diagnosis with resulting advanced stage of disease; the need for intensive treatment, such as chemotherapy; and death. One approach may be to have a testicular cancer survivor discuss his experiences to convey the benefit of TSE [51]. Regarding the actual technical procedure itself, the message is that TSE is easily learned and should be practiced regularly [61]. Studies have shown that TSE teaching improves knowledge and performance of the self-examination [53,64,66].

Public awareness

Despite the controversy regarding physician-conducted screening and TSE, there seems to be a consensus that increased awareness about testicular cancer among young men is necessary [66]. Those who advocate TSE programs must be mindful that these cannot succeed unless education and awareness can impart a value to the behavior. Numerous recent studies have demonstrated that young men generally are ignorant regarding testicular cancer and TSE (Table 3). On average, less than two thirds of young men had ever heard of testicular cancer and only approximately one third knew that it primarily affects young men. Less than one third were aware of TSE, and less than 10% perform TSE [38,43,62,63,67–75]. Most of these studies were of college and graduate students, implying that the general population knows little or nothing about this disease [38,67–69]. The largest survey of more than 7,000 European students found that 87% never practiced TSE and only 3%

Table 3
Knowledge of testicular cancer among young people

Study	No. of subjects	Ever heard of testicular cancer (%)	Aware that young men are at risk (%)	Aware of TSE (%)	Practice of TSE (%)	Aware that testicular cancer usually is curable (%)
Conklin et al [43]	90	25	NS	0	0	NS
Cummings et al [67]	266	NS	42	16	5	NS
Goldenring and Purtell [38]	147	NS	13	9.5	6	NS
Thornhill et al [68]	365	68	13	8	1.3	14
Blesch [69]	129	61	NS	31	9.5	NS
Reno [70]	126	NS	NS	13	9.5	NS
Dachs et al [63]	633	NS	57	39	4.7	NS
Klein et al [71]	66	47	15	23	1.5	NS
Raghavan [72]	80	<15	10	NS	NS	NS
Pendered [73]	Men, 79	63	29	35	27	59
	Women, 96	72	50	48	—	82
Sheley et al [62]	415	NS	30	NS	16	NS
Singer et al [74]	717	NS	30	30	8	6
Wardle et al [75]	7,304	NS	NS	NS	9	NS

Abbreviation: NS, not stated.

reported regular monthly TSE [75]. Even among health care providers, knowledge is lacking. Stanford [54] found that almost one half of female nurses were not familiar with TSE, and only 5% had taught a patient TSE, although almost two thirds believed it to be part of their job.

Regarding knowledge of signs and symptoms of testicular cancer, Cummings and colleagues [67] also found that more than half of the young men in their study could not identify any correct signs or symptoms of testicular cancer (lump, swelling, enlarged and heavy testis, and pain). Similarly, Thornhill and colleagues [68] found 72% of young men had no knowledge of possible symptoms and actually noted many incorrect symptoms, such as problems with potency or micturition. In one study, young women knew more about testicular cancer than did men of similar age [73].

There are several patient-education brochures available that discuss not only TSE but also the general facts regarding this cancer. These materials are available from the American Cancer Society [57], the National Cancer Institute [58], the American Urological Association [76], and commercial sources [77].

Summary

Mass screening for testicular cancer using physician-conducted scrotal examinations or scrotal sonography is not indicated. Case finding by including a testicular examination as part of a male physical examination is recommended by the American Cancer Society and the National Cancer Institute. Self-screening by TSE may be effective, especially for patients at risk for testicular cancer, although educational efforts must also include and convey the potential value to the individual of such behavior. Awareness of testicular cancer and its signs and symptoms is abysmally poor in young men and undoubtedly contributes to the continued problem of delay in diagnosis. At a minimum, physicians must promote awareness so that men report to their physicians at the first sign or symptom of testicular pathology. Likewise, we must continue to promote education among health care providers.

References

[1] Boring CC, Squires TS, Tong T. Cancer statistics. CA Cancer J Clin 1993;43(1):7–26.
[2] Moul JW, Paulson DF, Dodge RK, et al. Delay in diagnosis and survival in testicular cancer: impact of effective therapy and changes during 18 years J Urol 1990;143:520.
[3] Weissbach L, Bruhl P, Vahlensieck W. Epidermiologie und pravention des hodentumors. Munch Med Wochenschr 1974;116(18):957–8, German.
[4] Host H, Stokke T. The treatment of malignant testicular tumors at the Norwegian Radium Hospital. Cancer 1959;12:323.
[5] Patton JF, Hewitt CB, Mallis N. Diagnosis and treatment of tumors of the testis. JAMA 1959;171:2194.

[6] Thompson IM, Wear J, Almond C, et al. An analytical survey of 178 testicular tumors. J Urol 1961;85: 173.
[7] Bosl GJ, Goldman A, Lange PH, et al. Impact of delay in diagnosis on clinical stage of testicular cancer. Lancet 1981;2:970.
[8] Kurohara SS, George FW, Dykhusen RF, et al. Testicular tumors. Analysis of 196 cases treated at the US Naval Hospital in San Diego. Cancer 1967;20: 1089.
[9] Borski AA. Diagnosis, staging, and natural history of testicular tumors. Cancer 1973;32:1202.
[10] Seib UC, Andres H, Sommerkamp H. Fehldiagnosen beim malignen hodentumor. Aktuelle Urol 1976;7: 302, German.
[11] Ware SM, Al-Askari S, Morales P. Testicular germ cell tumors. Prognostic factors. Urology 1980;15:348.
[12] Dieckmann KP, Becker T, Bauer HW. Testicular tumors: presentation and role of diagnostic delay. Urol Int 1987;42:241.
[13] Kulig JW. Self detection of testicular neoplasms [abstract]. J Adolesc Health Care 1981;2:171.
[14] Leyh H. Anamnese und tastbefun sind die basis der frith-diagnostic von hodentumoren. Med Klin 1984; 79:612, German.
[15] Kuhne U, Andra J, Zacher W. Der maligne hodentumor: ein diagnostisches problem? Z Arztl Fortbild (Jena) 1979;73(6):276–9, German.
[16] Scher H, Bosl G, Geller N, et al. Impact of symptomatic interval on prognosis of patients with stage III testicular cancer. Urology 1983;21:559.
[17] Fischer F. Behandlungsergebnisse bei hodentumorpatienten der Jahrgange 1973–1981 inaugural. Munchen (Germany): Diss Urologische Klinik, Ludwig-Maximilians Universitat; 1983, German.
[18] Heising J. Anamnese. In: Weissbach H, editor. Register und verbundstudie fur odentumoen—Bonn. Munchen (Germany): Zuckschwerdt; 1982. p. 100–9, German.
[19] Jones WG, Appleyard I. Delay in diagnosing testicular tumors. Br Med J 1985;290:1150.
[20] Thornhill JA, Fennelly JJ, Kelly DG, et al. Patients' delay in the presentation of testis cancer in Ireland. Br J Urol 1987;59:447.
[21] Chilvers CED, Saunders M, Bliss JM, et al. Influence of delay in diagnosis on prognosis in testicular teratoma. Br J Cancer 1989;59:126.
[22] Nikzas D, Champion AE, Fox M. Germ cell tumors of testis: prognostic factors and results. Eur Urol 1990;18:242.
[23] Post GJ, Belis JA. Delayed presentation of testicular tumors. South Med J 1980;73:33.
[24] Sandeman TF. Symptoms and early management of germinal tumors of the testis. Med J Aust 1979;2:281.
[25] Stephen RA. The clinical presentation of testicular tumors. Br J Urol 1962;34:448.
[26] Prout GR, Griffin PP. Testicular tumors: delay in diagnosis and influence on survival. Am Fam Physician 1984;29:205.
[27] Wishnow KI, Johnson DE, Preston W, et al. Prompt orchiectomy reduces morbidity and mortality from testicular carcinoma. Br J Urol 1990;65:629.
[28] Oliver RTD. Factors contributing to delay in diagnosis of testicular tumours. Br Med J 1985; 290:356.
[29] Fossa SD, Kupp O, Elgjo RF. The effect of patients' delay and doctors' delay in patients with malignant germ cell tumours. Int J Androl 1981;4:134–45.
[30] Meffan PJ, Delahunt B, Nacey JN. The value of early diagnosis in the treatment of patients with testicular cancer. N Z Med J 1991;104:393.
[31] Moul JW, Paulson DF, Walther PJ. Refusal of cancer treatment in testicular cancer patients. J Natl Cancer Inst 1989;81:1587.
[32] Beisser AR. Denial and affirmation in illness and health. Am J Psychiatry 1979;36:1026.
[33] Robson CJ, Bruce AW, Charbonneau J. Testicular tumors: a collective review from the Canadian Academy of Urological Surgeons. J Urol 1965;94:440.
[34] Czaplicki M, Rojewska J, Pykalo R, et al. Detection of testicular neoplasms by cytological examination of seminal fluid. J Urol 1987;138:787.
[35] Yu DS, Wang J, Chang SY, et al. Differential diagnosis of testicular mass by cytological examination of seminal fluid collected by ejaculation or prostatic massage. Eur Urol 1990;18:193.
[36] Moul JW, Moellman JR. Unnecessary mastectomy for gynecomastia in testicular cancer patient. Mil Med 1992;157:433.
[37] US Preventive Services Task Force. Guide to clinical preventive services: an assessment of the effectiveness of 169 interventions. Baltimore (MD): Williams & Wilkins; 1989.
[38] Goldenring JM, Purtell E. Knowledge of testicular cancer risk and need for self-examination in college students: a call for equal time for men in teaching of early cancer detection techniques. Pediatrics 1984;74:1093–6.
[39] Javadpour N. Germ cell tumor of the testis. CA Cancer J Clin 1980;30:242–55.
[40] National Cancer Institute. Working guidelines for early cancer detection: rationale and supporting evidence to decrease mortality. Bethesda (MD): National Cancer Institute; 1987.
[41] Canadian Task Force on the Periodic Health Examination. The periodic health examination, 1984 update. Can Med Assoc J 1984;130:2.
[42] Moul JW, Schannel FJ, Thompson IM, et al. Testicular cancer in blacks: a multicenter experience. Cancer 1994;72:338.
[43] Conklin M, Klint K, Morway A, et al. Should health teaching include self-examination of the testes? Am J Nurs 1978;78:2073.
[44] Garnick MB, Mayer RJ, Richie JP. Testicular self-examination [letter]. N Engl J Med 1980;302: 297.
[45] Williams HA. Screening for testicular cancer. Pediatr Nurs 1981;7:38.

[46] Marty PJ, McDermott RJ. Teaching about testicular cancer and testicular self-examination. J Sch Health 1983;53:351–6.
[47] Cavanaugh DM. Genital self-examination in adolescent males. Am Fam Physician 1983;28:199.
[48] Anderson EE. Early diagnosis of testicular carcinoma: self-examination of the testicle. N C Med J 1985;46:407.
[49] Carlin PT. Testicular self-examination: a public awareness program. Public Health Rep 1986;101:98.
[50] Scott D. Testicular cancer: the case for self-examination. Postgrad Med 1986;80:175.
[51] Marty PJ, McDermott RJ. Three strategies for encouraging testicular self examination among college-aged males. J Am Coll Health 1986;34:253.
[52] Ramsey FB. Testicular self-examination. Indiana Med 1986;79:36.
[53] Friman PC, Finnery JW, Glasscock SG, et al. Testicular self-examination: validation of a training strategy for early cancer detection. J Appl Behav Anal 1986;19:87.
[54] Stanford T. Testicular self-examination: teaching, learning, and practice by nurses. J Adv Nurs 1987; 12:13.
[55] Walker R, Guyton R. Modeling and guarded practice as a component within a comprehensive testicular self-examination cancer education program J Am Coll Health 1989;37:211.
[56] Neef N, Scutchfield FD, Elder J, et al. Testicular self-examination by young men: an analysis of characteristics associated with practice. J Am Coll Health 1991;39:187.
[57] American Cancer Society. For men only—testicular cancer and how to do testicular self-examination. New York: American Cancer Society; 1984.
[58] National Cancer Institute. Testicular self-examination. Washington, DC: Government Printing Office; 1986 Pub. no. DHHS(NIH) 87–2636.
[59] Westlake SJ, Frank JW. Testicular self-examination: an argument against routine teaching. Fam Pract 1987;4:143.
[60] Goldbloom RB. Self-examination by adolescents. Pediatrics 1985;76:126.
[61] Friman PC, Finney JW. Health education for testicular cancer. Health Educ Q 1990;17:443.
[62] Sheley JF, Kinchen EW, Morgan DH, et al. Limited impact of testicular self-examination promotion J Community Health 1991;16:117.
[63] Dachs RJ, Garb JL, White C, et al. Male college students' compliance with testicular self-examination J Adolesc Health Care 1989;10:295.
[64] Brubaker AG, Wickersham D. Encouraging the practice of testicular self-examination: a field application of the theory of reasoned action. Health Psychol 1990;9:154.
[65] Hongladarom T, Hongladarom G. The problem of testicular cancer: how health professionals in the Armed Services can help. Mil Med 1982;147:211.
[66] Vaz RM, Best DL, Davis SW, et al. Evaluation of a testicular cancer curriculum for adolescents J Pediatr 1989;114:150.
[67] Cummings KM, Lampone D, Mettlin C, et al. What young men know about testicular cancer. Prev Med 1983;12:326.
[68] Thornhill JA, Conroy RM, Kelly DG, et al. Public awareness of testicular cancer and the value of self-examination. Br Med J 1986;293:480.
[69] Blesch KS. Health beliefs about testicular cancer and self-examination among professional men. Oncol Nurs Forum 1986;13:29.
[70] Reno DR. Men's knowledge and health beliefs about testicular cancer and testicular self examination. Cancer Nurs 1988;11:112.
[71] Klein JF, Berry CC, Felice ME. The development of a testicular self-examination instructional booklet for adolescents. J Adolesc Health Care 1990; 11:235.
[72] Raghavan D. Towards the earlier diagnosis of testicular cancer. Aust Fam Physician 1990;19:865.
[73] Pendered L. Cancer of the testicle: an educational problem. Br J Gen Pract 1991;41:81.
[74] Singer AJ, Tichler T, Orvieto R, et al. Testicular carcinoma: a study of knowledge awareness, and practice of testicular self-examination in male soldiers and military physicians. Mil Med 1993;158: 640.
[75] Wardle J, Steptoe A, Burckhardt R, et al. Testicular self-examination: attitudes and practices among young men in Europe. Prev Med 1994; 23:206.
[76] Moul JW. Diagnosis delays impact on testicular cancer. American Urological Association Today 1990; 3(5 May):1.
[77] Testicular self-examination. Daly City (CA): Krames Communications. Publication no. 940243-TSE, 2007.

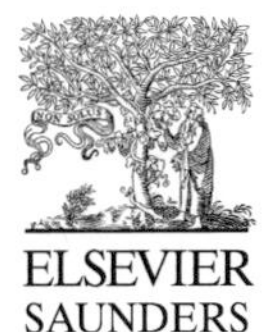
ELSEVIER
SAUNDERS

Urol Clin N Am 34 (2007) 119–125

UROLOGIC
CLINICS
of North America

ITGCN of the Testis, Contralateral Testicular Biopsy and Bilateral Testicular Cancer

Michael E. Karellas, MD[a], Ivan Damjanov, MD, PhD[b], Jeffery M. Holzbeierlein, MD[c,*]

[a]*Department of Surgery, Division of Urology, Memorial Sloan Kettering Cancer Center, 353 E. 68th Street, New York, NY 10021, USA*

[b]*Department of Pathology, University of Kansas School of Medicine, 2017 Wahl Hall West, Mailstop 3045, 3901 Rainbow Boulevard, Kansas City, KS 66160, USA*

[c]*Department of Urology, University of Kansas School of Medicine, 5017 Sudler Hall, Mailstop 3016, 3901 Rainbow Boulevard, Kansas City, KS 66160, USA*

Testicular cancer is the most common solid malignancy in the 20- to 34-year-old male age range. According to the most recent Surveillance Epidemiology and End Results (SEER) data, approximately 8000 men per year will be diagnosed with testicular cancer [1]. The mean age at diagnosis was 34 years of age, while the median age of death was 39.5 years old. The age-adjusted incidence of testicular cancer in the United States for the years from 1998 to 2002 was 5.3 per 100,000 men per year [1]. European data suggest the overall lifetime risk of developing testicular cancer is low at 0.5% to 1% [2]. The overwhelming majority (95%) of testicular tumors are of germ-cell origin (testicular germ-cell tumors [TGCTs]) and are divided into two main types: seminomas and nonseminomas. Nonseminomas are further subdivided into five subtypes and usually consist of a mixture of these subtypes. Additionally, some tumors present as mixed lesions containing both seminomatous and nonseminomatous elements [3]. Despite the variety of TGCT types, it has been well established that almost all TGCTs develop from the precursor lesion of carcinoma in situ (CIS) (Fig. 1), otherwise known as intratubular germ-cell neoplasia (ITGCN), or testicular intraepithelial neoplasia (TIN) [4]. In this review we will focus on the origins of CIS and molecular genetics concerning expression and progression, as well as the current aspects of diagnosis and management of ITGCN, and bilateral TGCTs.

Skakkebæk [5] was the first to describe the presence of a noninvasive precursor lesion that would progress to invasive TGCTs. He found atypical spermatogonia from testicular biopsies in two infertile patients who went on to develop testicular cancers. Over the past three decades since his early report, it is now well established that with the exception of pediatric testicular tumors (yolk sac, mature teratoma) as well as the rare finding of spermatocytic seminoma, almost all TGCTs arise from ITGCN [5]. The presence of ITGCN is present in the testis years before the ultimate tumor becomes clinically evident leading to speculation that early detection of TGCTs is possible with testicular biopsy and immunohistological examination [6]. Multiple studies have shown the prevalence of ITGCN to be consistent with the lifetime risk of developing a TGCT [6,7].

Identification of abnormal cells

Microscopically, ITGCN cells are larger than normal spermatogonia and usually have a prominent irregular nucleus, distinct nucleoli, coarse clumps of chromatin, and abundant cytoplasm (Fig. 2) [8]. As the name suggests, these cells are

* Corresponding author.
E-mail address: jholzbeierlein@kumc.edu (J.M. Holzbeierlein).

doi:10.1016/j.ucl.2007.02.015

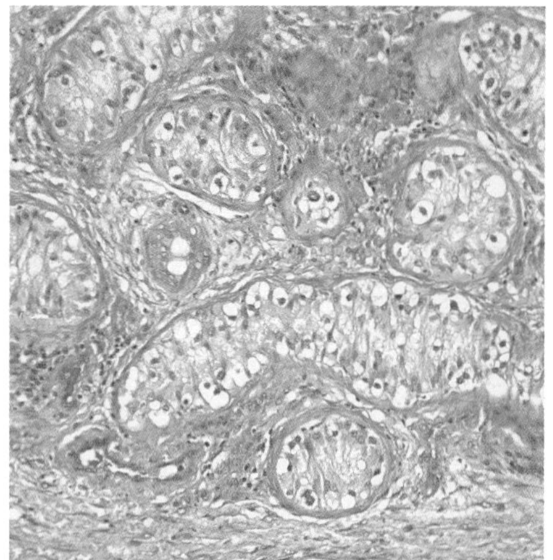

Fig. 1. Low power displaying prominent irregular nucleus, distinct nucleoli, coarse clumps of chromatin, and abundant cytoplasm.

found within the seminiferous tubules, located in a single row at the thickened basement membrane [9]. The tubular architecture is further distorted by having a decreased diameter with an absence of germ cells, making the Sertoli cell the only other cell type present. Tubules with ITGCN are often found in the testicular parenchyma surrounding the invasive cancer, appearing atrophic and with occasional microcalcifications [10]. Other findings associated with ITGCN are lymphocytic invasion, hyaline bodies, or Leydig cell hyperplasia [10]. Immunohistochemical staining for placental-like alkaline phosphatase (PLAP) is the most common method to detect ITGCN cells [11]. Regadera and colleagues [12] have recently published their findings suggesting that detection of *PCPH* oncoprotein could be used as a good early marker to detect testicular neoplasms. They found that *PCPH* expression is substantially increased in human TGCTs, including ITGCN and could serve as a tool to aid in diagnosis.

Pathway to cancer

The malignant transformation to the ITGCN cell is believed to take place in utero during the early development of the germline stem cell. It is believed that this cell would have ultimately differentiated into a gonocyte and has very similar morphologic characteristics [13]. Further immunohistochemical studies have confirmed the presence of proteins in both primordial germ cells and ITGCN cells that are not present in normal adult testes (*KIT*, *OCT3/4*, and *AP-2γ*) (Fig. 3) [14]. Almstrup and colleagues [15] recently published their results describing the expression pattern of *TFAP2C* in neoplastic adult and fetal testes. This protein encodes for the transcription factor *AP-2γ*, which is almost exclusively produced by cells that are not fully differentiated, such as gonocytes and was found to be elevated in ITGCN cells but not in normal germ cells of the adult testis.

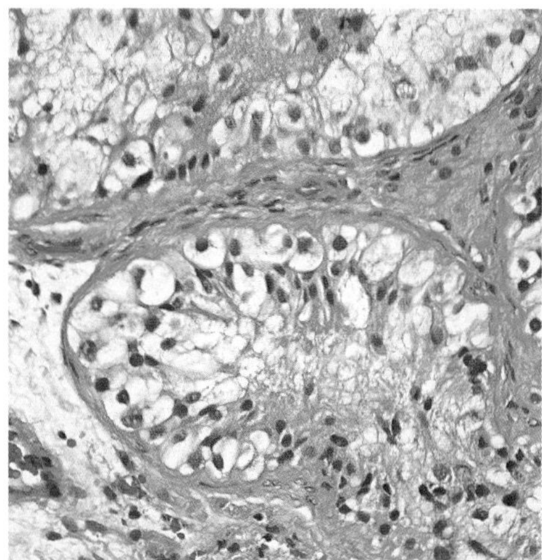

Fig. 2. Higher power displaying prominent nucleoli, abundant cytoplasm, and abnormal spermatogonia.

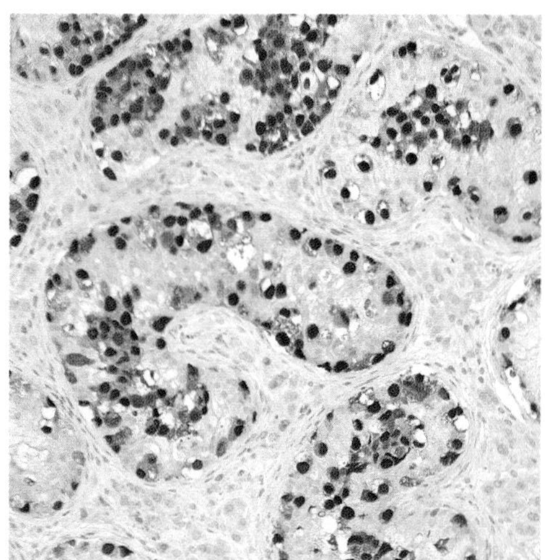

Fig. 3. ITGCN nuclei stained with antibodies to OCT-3, which is specific for ITGCN and embryonal carcinoma.

Various chromosomal abnormalities have been described in ITGCN cells, with polyploidization (DNA index 1.5) and gain of chromosomal material at 12p (as an isochromosome) and 17q being the most common defects [16–18]. Other chromosomes (7, 8, 14, and X) can gain or lose genetic material, but the gain at 12p seems to occur first and correlates with the invasive capability of ITGCN cells [19]. Many other genes that are important to invasive testicular tumors are present on the 12p chromosome (*NANOG*, *STELLA*, and *CCND2*) when studying these tumors via fluorescent in situ hybridization (FISH) or comparative genomic hybridization [20]. Controversy exists concerning the exact role that 12p plays in ITGCN; however, gain of 12p material has been associated with survival of ITGCN cells outside of the seminiferous tubules [6]. The common denominator is that the expression of ITGCN cells is a combination of increased transcriptional activity at some loci and or the loss of silencing of other loci [8]. The exact mechanism of neoplastic transformation of germ cells remains poorly understood. Answering this question has been difficult because of the difficulty of growing ITGCN cells in cell culture, and the lack of an animal model [4]. Research has focused on the observations of increased risk of TGCTs in patients with testicular dysgenesis and the hypothesis that inadequate stimulation of the testes by reproductive hormones during development could disturb normal differentiation and lead to malignant transformation [8]. Another hypothesis suggests that in developed countries exposure to environmental agents leads to an estrogenic effect in utero and could disrupt normal development [21]. Current theory is that once transformed into malignant cells, the tumor cells directly migrate through the basement membrane like other invasive in situ tumors (breast, skin), although recent studies by Donner and colleagues [22] have described a different manner of invasion. Instead of direct extension through the basement membrane, they support the theory of tumor cell proliferation within the tubule and degeneration of the Sertoli cells, followed by conversion of the tubule wall to connective tissue.

Risk factors for ITGCN development

There are several conditions that are believed to predispose an individual to the development of TGCTs. For example, in a patient with a testicular tumor, the contralateral testicle has a 25-fold increased relative risk (RR) of developing another tumor. The finding of contralateral testicular microlithiasis on ultrasound in a patient who has had a TGCT has been reported to increase the risk of having ITGCN by approximately 30 times [23]. The clinical importance of testicular microlithiasis remains a controversial subject. Several studies have shown the prevalence of testicular microlithiasis to be approximately 2% in the asymptomatic population [24,25]. These studies disagree on the association of microlithiasis with TGCTs. Serter and colleagues [24] reported 2.4% of healthy male volunteers (age 17–42) had testicular microlithiasis on screening ultrasound, but none had palpable lesions on physical exam and all had undetectable levels of testicular tumor markers. Other known risk factors are cryptorchidism (RR 4.8), familial testicular cancer (RR 3 to 10) and gonadal dysgenesis (>6%) [26]. Studies of males with first-degree relatives having TGCTs have demonstrated a genetic defect on the X-chromosome at Xq27. Infertility, twin-ship, and testicular atrophy are other factors that have been considered as "probable established associations" with the development of TGCTs. In the infertile population, the highest risk is for those men with extremely low sperm counts ($<3 \times 10^6$/mL) and atrophic testicles (volume <12 mL) [27]. Scrotal trauma was thought to have been linked to testicular cancer but no biologic explanation has been established and data have not supported this association [28]. Likewise, inguinal hernia has been a popular condition thought to predispose to TGCTs. There are conflicting studies on the subject because congenital hernias often occur with cryptorchidism, which is a known risk factor. However, there is no associated risk of TGCTs in patients without an undescended testicle and an inguinal hernia [23].

Diagnosis

Clinical diagnosis of ITGCN is based on surgical biopsy of the testes with immunohistochemical staining for placental alkaline phosphatase (PLAP). It was originally thought that ITGCN was evenly dispersed throughout the testicle and a random biopsy would be adequate for diagnosis. This was challenged by later work that supported a focal or lobule arrangement of ITGCN [29]. Based on this knowledge, biopsy recommendations are to obtain a 3 × 3-mm section of tissue from the craniolateral portion of the testicle, which should minimize the risk to the intratesticular vessels. This size of tissue should be adequate to diagnose ITGCN if at least 10% of the testicular volume is involved [30]. Dieckmann and colleagues [31] determined the false-negative biopsy rate using this method to be less than 0.5%. They followed 1859 cases with a negative biopsy for ITGCN for 7 years, with 42 patients eventually developing TGCTs. Based on their data, testicular biopsy has a 91% sensitivity, and as high as a 99.5% specificity for the detection of ITGCN. Postulated reasons for false-negative biopsies are mechanical trauma to the specimen from surgical instruments, small biopsy size, sampling error, and improper fixation. For example, formalin causes excessive shrinkage of the tubules making the microscopic examination difficult. The preferred fixative is Stieve fluid (formol-sublimate) or Bouin's solution if the former is not available.

Issues concerning contralateral testicular biopsy

Contralateral testicular biopsy in patients with unilateral testis cancer at the time of orchiectomy for the primary tumor is a highly controversial subject. Biopsy patterns differ among countries as well as between high- and low-volume care centers. Contralateral testis biopsy at the time of orchiectomy for unilateral tumor is routinely performed in most large centers in Denmark, Germany, and Austria [32]. Among German urologists at high-volume centers (>20 cases/year), 95% of patients underwent contralateral testicular biopsy at the time of orchiectomy [29]. In contrast, urologists in the United Kingdom, United States, and the Netherlands do not routinely biopsy the contralateral testicle, while urologists in Norway only sample those patients considered high risk. Proponents of contralateral biopsy at the time of orchiectomy argue it is the best possible screening method for ITGCN, has minimal risk, and can offer valuable information if positive while providing reassurance if the biopsy is negative [33]. Additionally, they feel that if a patient has a negative biopsy, then follow-up can be limited to 5 years instead of 25 years or longer [30].

This viewpoint is highly debatable and many others do not advocate routine contralateral biopsy at the time of primary orchiectomy. Overall, contralateral ITGCN occurs in 2% to 5% of patients who have a history of TGCT and at least 50% will progress to a second testicular tumor [34]. Moreover, these patients are at a 25 to 50 fold increased risk for developing a contralateral TGCT. However, routine biopsy remains controversial because of the low numbers of men who actually have ITGCN on biopsy, the potential for undesirable physical and emotional effects of a second orchiectomy, and an excellent prognosis if or when a second tumor develops [35]. In a recent review of the literature on screening of the contralateral testicle, three large studies reported the prevalence of ITGCN to be 4.9%, 5.7%, and 6.1%. On multivariate analysis the highest risk patients were those with testicular atrophy (<12 mL), history of an undescended testicle, and age younger than 30 [28].

Another high-risk group would be those men with abnormal calcifications on ultrasound. Holm and colleagues [23] has reported an association between contralateral testicular microlithiasis on testicular ultrasound and an increased risk of ITGCN (odds ratio 28.6, RR 21.6). These studies would suggest that the majority of men would not have a positive biopsy and would be placed at risk for complications from the procedure. Postsurgical complications include hematoma, edema, and infection in approximately 3% of cases and 15% to 20% will experience pain for a period of time [4,36]. More importantly, exocrine and endocrine function of the remaining testis can be diminished. Trauma from the biopsy may have an adverse effect on spermatogenesis thereby further damaging the patient's fertility [37]. Serum testosterone has been shown to be decreased in men with atrophic testes who have undergone testicular biopsy [38].

Based on these and other studies, most urologists in the United States have not recommended routine biopsy of the contralateral testicle. However, some urologists in the United States, United Kingdom and other countries favor selected biopsy for informed patients who are at high risk for ITGCN (cryptorchidism, testicular atrophy, age, gonadal dysgenesis, testicular microlithiasis). These criteria should limit the number of men who would be subjected to the additional risks of biopsy while selecting those most at risk for ITGCN [28].

Treatment

Treatment for ITGCN can significantly affect a patient's quality of life and further alter reproductive and endocrine functions. Therapeutic options for ITGCN of the contralateral testicle include orchiectomy, radiation, chemotherapy, and observation. However, before treatment for any TGCT or ITGCN is begun, sperm cryopreservation should be discussed with the patient. Treatment depends on a combination of factors such as age, testicular size, fertility, unilateral or bilateral cancer, and patient/physician philosophy. Orchiectomy, the most invasive treatment, is curative, but will leave the patient infertile and dependent on exogenous testosterone. Additionally, the emotional stress of castration can be difficult for any male to handle. Partial orchiectomy has been reported as an option for patients with a solitary testicle who develop a well-demarcated TGCT [39,40]. The goal of partial orchiectomy is to preserve endocrine function and fertility. However, in most cases, ITGCN is diffusely spread throughout the nontumorous portion of the testicle and can eventually develop into another TGCT. Partial orchiectomy for TGCT is currently not considered standard of care and should be performed only in highly selected situations.

ITGCN is radiosensitive and is an excellent treatment option for a positive biopsy. In the past, 20 Gy was the dose given, but up to 25% of men had compromised testosterone synthesis and needed supplementation [41]. Lower dose (14 Gy) treatments have been shown to eradicate ITGCN with preservation of Leydig cell function. Follow-up biopsy usually reveals a Sertoli cell only pattern, but Leydig cell function seems to be preserved, although some recent data suggest that with long-term follow-up, many men will ultimately require androgen replacement [42]. A positive biopsy should not automatically lead to radiating the remaining testicle, especially in patients who might already be at risk for decreased testosterone levels (atrophic testes). The German Testicular Cancer Study Group has advocated drawing pretreatment luteinizing hormone (LH) and testosterone levels in patients with atrophic testes as well as recommending observation as methods to prevent compromised endocrine function following radiation therapy [40].

Cisplatin-based chemotherapy has been shown to be effective against ITGCN but the response can be somewhat variable. While many people have no evidence of ITGCN on follow-up biopsy, the cumulative risk of developing ITGCN in 10 years is as high as 42% [43]. Cisplatin chemotherapy is not a recommended treatment for patients with contralateral ITGCN unless it will be used for treatment of the primary tumor.

Observation is the option that is recommended for men who are not considered high risk and who will be compliant with scheduled follow-up. While this entails regular physician visits and routine testicular ultrasounds, it does not place the patient at further risk from another procedure and does not change endocrine or exocrine function of the remaining testicle. Changes found on self examination or on follow-up ultrasound (mass, microcalcifications) should be biopsied.

Bilateral testicular tumors

Bilateral testicular tumors have been reported with an incidence of 0.5% to 0.7% [44]. In that series, 21 patients of 2088 studied presented with bilateral testicular tumors, 16 patients had metachronous lesions, and 5 had synchronous tumors. Approximately 50% of the metachronous lesions occurred within 5 years. Another large study that included almost 4000 patients found the incidence of bilateral testicular tumors to be slightly higher (1.5%) but had similar findings with regard to metachronous tumors (83%) being the most common bilateral presentation [45]. Of these tumors, the median interval between lesions was 50.5 months; however, 23% of the patients presented more than 10 years after the first tumor. The ten patients in this study who presented with synchronous lesions were all tumor free at a mean follow-up of 29.5 months. Most importantly, patients with bilateral testicular tumors (synchronous or metachronous) had similar outcomes as those with unilateral tumors. A third study that confirms these findings was recently published from Munich. Four percent of their patients developed bilateral tumors, with the majority being metachronous, and without any patient deaths from the second tumor [46]. These findings support the practice of not routinely performing contralateral testicular biopsies in patients with ITGCN, as well as emphasizing the need for long-term follow-up.

Summary

Since the initial discovery by Skakkebæk of ITGCN over 30 years ago, much progress has been made on the role it plays in TGCTs. In the future, new molecular tests might offer a less invasive method to detect ITGCN. At present the role of routine contralateral testicular biopsy in the diagnosis of ITGCN is controversial. While at an increased risk, most men will not develop a second testicular tumor and therefore routine biopsy is not recommended. We recommend a stratified biopsy strategy to for those at high risk, while following the majority of men for many years after their initial tumor. Orchiectomy is considered definitive treatment if ITGCN of the contralateral testicle occurs, while the less invasive option of radiation would also provide acceptable tumor control. Bilateral testicular tumors are a rare occurrence with the majority being metachronous and responding well to traditional treatment.

References

[1] Ries LAG, Eisner MP, Kosary CL, et al (eds). SEER Cancer Statistics Review, 1975–2002. National Cancer Institute; Bethesda (MD). Available at: http://seer.cancer.gov/csr/1975_2002/.

[2] Huyghe E, Matsuda T, Thonneau P. Increasing incidence of testicular cancer worldwide: a review. J Urol 2003;170(1):5–11.

[3] Hoei-Hansen CE, Rajpert-De Meyts E, Daugaard G, et al. Carcinoma in situ testis, the progenitor of testicular germ cell tumours: a clinical review. Ann Oncol 2005;16(6):863–8.

[4] Skakkebæk NE. Possible carcinoma-in-situ of the testis. Lancet 1972;2(7776):2516–7.

[5] Rorth M, Rajpert-De Meyts E, Andersson L, et al. Carcinoma in situ in the testis. Scand J Urol Nephrol Suppl 2000;205:166–86.

[6] Linke J, Loy V, Dieckmann KP. Prevalence of testicular intraepithelial neoplasia in healthy males. J Urol 2005;173(5):1577–9.

[7] Giwercan A, von der Masse H, Skakkebæk NE. Epidemiological and clinical aspects of carcinoma in situ of the testis. Eur Urol 1993;23:104–14.

[8] Almstrup K, Ottesen AM, Sonne SB, et al. Genomic and gene expression signature of the pre-invasive testicular carcinoma in situ. Cell Tissue Res 2005; 322(1):159–65.

[9] Sigg C, Hedinger C. Atypical germ cells of the testis. Comparative ultrastructural and immunohistochemical investigations. Virchows Arch A Pathol Anat Histopathol 1984;402(4):439–50.

[10] Hoei-Hansen CE, Holm M, Rajpert-De Meyts E, et al. Histological evidence of testicular dysgenesis in contralateral biopsies from 218 patients with testicular germ cell cancer. J Pathol 2003;200(3):370–4.

[11] Giwercman A, Cantell L, Marks A. Placental-like alkaline phosphatase as a marker of carcinoma-in-situ of the testis. Comparison with monoclonal antibodies M2A and 43-9F. APMIS 1991;99(7):586–94.

[12] Regadera J, Blanquez MJ, Gonzalez-Peramato P, et al. PCPH expression is an early event in the development of testicular germ cell tumors. Int J Oncol 2006;28(3):595–604.

[13] Skakkebæk NE, Berthelsen JG, Giwercman A, et al. Carcinoma-in-situ of the testis: possible origin from gonocytes and precursor of all types of germ cell tumours except spermatocytoma. Int J Androl 1987; 10(1):19–28.

[14] Rajpert-De Meyts E, Bartkova J, Samson M, et al. The emerging phenotype of the testicular carcinoma in situ germ cell. APMIS 2003;111(1): 267–78.

[15] Almstrup K, Sonne SB, Hoei-Hansen CE, et al. From embryonic stem cells to testicular germ cell cancer—should we be concerned? Int J Androl 2006;29(1):211–8.

[16] de Graaff WE, Oosterhuis JW, de Jong B, et al. Ploidy of testicular carcinoma in situ. Lab Invest 1992;66(2):166–8.

[17] Atkin NB, Baker MC. Specific chromosome change, i(12p), in testicular tumours? Lancet 1982;2(8311): 1349.

[18] Skotheim RI, Lothe RA. The testicular germ cell tumour genome. APMIS 2003;111(1):136–50.

[19] Ottesen AM, Skakkebæk NE, Lundsteen C, et al. High-resolution comparative genomic hybridization detects extra chromosome arm 12p material in most cases of carcinoma in situ adjacent to overt germ cell tumors, but not before the invasive tumor development. Genes Chromosomes Cancer 2003;38(2): 117–25.

[20] Sandberg AA, Meloni AM, Suijkerbuijk RF. Reviews of chromosome studies in urological tumors. III. Cytogenetics and genes in testicular tumors. J Urol 1996;155(5):1531–56.

[21] Hemminki K, Li X. Cancer risks in second-generation immigrants to Sweden. Int J Cancer 2002;99(2): 229–37.

[22] Donner J, Kliesch S, Brehm R, et al. From carcinoma in situ to testicular germ cell tumor. APMIS 2004;112(2):79–88.

[23] Holm M, Hoei-Hanson C, Rajpert-De Meyts E, et al. Increased risk of carcinoma in situ in patients with testicular germ cell cancer with ultrasonic microlithiasis in the contralateral testicle. J Urol 2003;170(4 Pt 1):1163–7.

[24] Serter S, Gumus B, Unlu M, et al. Prevalence of testicular microlithiasis in an asymptomatic population. Scand J Urol Nephrol 2006;40(3):212–4.

[25] Miller FN, Rosairo S, Clarke J, et al. Testicular calcification and microlithiasis: association with primary intra-testicular malignancy in 3,477 patients. Eur Radiol 2007;17(2):363–9. May 2006, [E-pub].

[26] Dieckmann KP, Pichlmeier U. Clinical epidemiology of testicular germ cell tumors. World J Urol 2004;22:2–14.

[27] Moller H, Skakkebæk NE. Risk of testicular cancer in sub-fertile men: case-control study. BMJ 1999; 318:559–62.

[28] Heising J, Engelking R. Malignant tumor of the testicle and trauma: correlative evaluation. Urologe A 1978;17(2):73–5.

[29] Prym C, Lauke H. Carcinoma-in-situ of the human testis: tumor cells are distributed focally in the seminiferous tubules. Andrologia 1994;26:231–4.
[30] Heidenreich A, Moul JW. Contralateral testicular biopsy procedure in patients with unilateral testis cancer: is it indicated? Semin Urol Oncol 2002; 20(4):234–8.
[31] Dieckmann KP, Classen J, Loy V. Diagnosis and management of testicular intraepithelial neoplasia (carcinoma in situ)—surgical aspects. APMIS 2003;111:64–9.
[32] Daugaard G, Giwercman S, Skakkebæk NE. Should the other testis be biopsied? Semin Urol Oncol 1996; 14:8–12.
[33] von der Maase H. Is a contralateral testicular biopsy in patients with unilateral germ cell testicular cancer indicated as a routine procedure? Acta Oncol 2005; 44:523–5.
[34] Dieckmann KP, Loy V. Prevalence of contralateral testicular intraepithelial neoplasia in patients with testicular germ cell neoplasms. J Clin Oncol 1996; 14:3126–32.
[35] Herr HW, Sheinfeld J. Is biopsy of the contralateral testis necessary in patients with germ cell tumors? J Urol 1997;158:1331–4.
[36] Bruun E, Fromhold-Mollr C, Giwercman A, et al. Testicular biopsy as an outpatient procedure in screening for testicular carcinoma in situ: complications and the patient's acceptance. Int J Androl 1987;10:199–202.
[37] Berthelsen JG, Skakkebæk NE. Gonadal function in men with testis cancer. Fertil Steril 1983;39(1): 68–75.
[38] Manning M, Junnemann KP, Alken P. Decrease in testosterone blood concentrations after testicular sperm extraction for intracytoplasmic sperm injection in azoospermic men. Lancet 1998;352:37.
[39] Hughes PD. Partial orchiectomy for malignancy with consideration of carcinoma in situ. ANZ J Surg 2006;76:92–4.
[40] Heidenreich A, Weissbach L, Holtl W, et al. Organ sparing surgery for malignant germ cell tumor of the testis. J Urol 2001;166:2161–5.
[41] Giwercman A, van der Maase H, Berthelsen JG, et al. Localized irradiation of the testes with carcinoma in situ: effects on Leydig cell functionand eradication of malignant germ cells in 20 patients. J Clin Endocrinol Metab 1991;73:596–601.
[42] Petersen PM, Daugaard G, Rorth M, et al. Endocrine function in patients treated for carcinoma in situ in the testis with irradiation. APMIS 2003;111:93–8.
[43] Christensen TB, Daugaard G, Geertsen PF, et al. Effect of chemotherapy on carcinoma in situ of the testis. Ann Oncol 1998;9(6):657–60.
[44] Coogan CL, Foster RS, Simmons GR, et al. Bilateral testicular tumors: management and outcome in 21 patients. Cancer 1998;83(3):547–52.
[45] Holzbeierlein JM, Sogani PC, Sheinfeld J. Histology and clinical outcomes in patients with bilateral testicular germ cell tumors: the Memorial Sloan Kettering Cancer Center experience 1950 to 2001. J Urol 2003;169(6):2122–5.
[46] Hentrich M, Weber N, Bergsdorf T, et al. Management and outcome of bilateral testicular germ cell tumors: twenty-five year experience in Munich. Acta Oncol 2005;44(6):529–36.

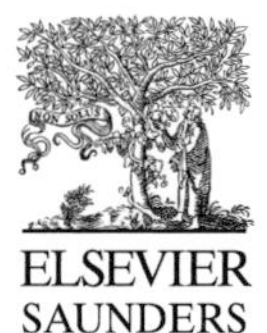

ELSEVIER
SAUNDERS

Urol Clin N Am 34 (2007) 127–136

UROLOGIC CLINICS of North America

Management of Low-Stage Testicular Seminoma

Mischel Neill, MD, Padraig Warde, MD,
Neil Fleshner, MD, MPH, FRCSC*

Division of Urology, Department of Surgery, Princess Margaret Hospital, University Health Network, University of Toronto, 610 University Avenue, Toronto, Canada M5G 2M9

Seminoma of the testicle accounts for approximately 1% of all male cancers [1] and represents an ideal model for a curable human malignancy. It was predicted that approximately 3000 to 4000 American men would be diagnosed with seminoma in 2006 [2]. Incidence rates for seminoma have increased over the past 20 years [3]. Although Americans of African descent are at lower risk for seminoma, a 124.4% increased incidence of seminoma among Black American males has recently been reported [3]. Seminomas represent approximately 50% of germ cell tumors [4] and typically present as an asymptomatic mass among men in their fourth decade of life. Seminoma is sensitive to radiotherapy and chemotherapy, thus cure is an expected outcome among men who have low-stage disease. Because cure rates are so high, current controversies revolve around minimizing treatment-related long-term morbidity and the amount and type of up-front therapy. For the purpose of this article, we focus on men who have clinical stage I (any primary T stage without clinically identifiable lymphatic or visceral metastasis) and stage II (any primary T stage with evidence of metastatic spread to regional lymph nodes, with five or fewer nodes involved and each 2 cm or less in greatest dimension) disease.

* Corresponding author.
E-mail address: neil.fleshner@uhn.on.ca (N. Fleshner).

Ontogeny, histologic subtypes, and pattern of spread

Ontogeny

Seminoma is a malignant tumor of seminiferous tubular epithelium. It is believed to represent a common precursor of other germ cell tumors [5], including all forms of nonseminomatous germ cell tumors (NSGCT). This common origin may have important implications for men because approximately 15% of men who have seminoma may relapse with NSGCT following definitive therapy. One recent CDNA expression profiling study among histologically pure seminoma identified two subgroups of seminoma. One was pure, whereas the other had molecular and immunophenotypic features of embryonal cancer admixed with seminoma [6]. All seminomas are believed to have progressed from an in situ stage, known as intratubular germ cell neoplasia.

Histologic subtypes

Three histologic subtypes of seminoma are described: anaplastic, classic, and spermatocytic. Anaplastic seminoma demonstrates microscopic features of a more aggressive malignancy with enhanced mitosis, nuclear pleomorphism, and higher nuclear to cytoplasmic ratio. Although anaplastic seminomas present at higher stage, the stage for stage prognosis is equivalent to that of classic seminoma [5].

Spermatocytic seminoma is a unique human neoplasm. It accounts for 1% to 2% of cases and elderly men (over age 50) typically present with this disease [7]. The metastatic potential of spermatocytic seminoma is minimal, although rare

doi:10.1016/j.ucl.2007.02.009

cases of sarcomatous dedifferentiation [8] and frank metastases from the seminoma itself have been reported [9]. Men who have spermatocytic seminoma generally do not require additional therapy post-orchidectomy. It is now well accepted that the nonspermatocytic forms of seminoma and spermatocytic seminoma originate from different pathways. Spermatocytic seminoma is currently believed to arise from a more mature [10] germ cell, such as a spermatogonium or spermatocyte, and have different patterns of DNA flow cytometry, genetic karyotyping, and comparative genomic hybridization [11] compared with classic and anaplastic seminomas.

Patterns of spread

Compared with NSGCT, seminoma has a favorable natural history and indolent growth pattern. It is estimated that 70% [12] of seminomas present with clinical stage I disease. Seminomas typically spread by way of the testicular lymphatics to the retroperitoneal lymph nodes. On the left side these are principally para-aortic and on the right side, interaortocaval. The second level of spread after the retroperitoneum is the mediastinal lymph nodes. Visceral spread to lung, liver, and other organs is uncommon.

Clinical management

Clinical presentation

Seminoma most commonly presents as a painless testicular mass in the fourth decade of life [13]. Distant to the primary tumor, metastases may manifest particularly as a palpable mass of the abdomen or neck, gynecomastia with or without tenderness, and respiratory symptoms, such as shortness of breath or, less commonly, hemoptysis. It is a well-recognized phenomenon of testicular cancer that the interval between the onset of symptoms and diagnosis is often prolonged. A combination of factors, including patient embarrassment and delays in investigation owing to such factors as treatment of presumptive epididymitis, postpone the correct diagnosis by 3 months on average [14,15].

Initial evaluation involves ultrasonography of the testes, a modality well suited to this purpose because of ease of access, lack of radiation, and high sensitivity and specificity for intratesticular lesions [16]. Before surgical management of the primary lesion, the serum tumor markers α-fetoprotein (AFP), human chorionic gonadotropin (HCG), and lactate dehydrogenase (LDH) are evaluated and chest (plain radiograph or CT) and abdominal (CT) imaging is performed. Testicular biopsy is avoided on general principle, because the disruption of lymphatic integrity that may occur with scrotal violation has been associated with an absolute increase in local recurrence rates of up to 2.5% [17].

Orchidectomy

Standard surgical management of the primary tumor involves radical orchidectomy by way of an inguinal approach with high ligation of the spermatic cord at the deep inguinal ring using a nondissolvable suture as a potential future marker for retroperitoneal exploration. Partial orchidectomy remains an option in the setting of a solitary testis or bilateral testicular masses if small, to preserve testicular function [18]. The long-term fate of this approach in endocrine function and cancer control remains unknown.

Radical orchidectomy serves not only to provide local control but also to establish the pathologic nature, grade, and stage of the primary tumor. With increasing subspecialization and interhospital referral of patients for postorchidectomy management, the importance of central histopathologic review has recently been highlighted [19]. On pathologic review Delaney and colleagues [19] found a 4% discrepancy in tumor type, of which roughly one half were recategorized from seminomatous to nonseminomatous germ cell tumor. Additionally there was a 10% difference in the identification of lymphovascular invasion and further differences in the description of nonseminomatous tumor elements. Discrete from the increased metastatic potential of NSGCT, some centers have identified the presence of vascular invasion and rete testis invasion as risk factors for metastatic recurrence in seminoma [20]. The importance of establishing the exact nature of the tumor primary is clear in determining the most appropriate option for clinical management of the disease. This determination is most important in early-stage disease in which treatment options vary considerably based on the assignment of a particular case as a seminoma or NSGCT.

Imaging

Imaging of the primary echelon retroperitoneal lymph nodes is routinely performed with CT scanning of the abdomen and pelvis. In seminoma patients, abdominal CT scans are normal in 70% [16]. Of those patients who have germ cell tumors and CT-detectable lymph nodes between 5 and 10 mm in maximal diameter, tumor is detected in 50%; between 10 and 20 mm this figure increases to 70% [21]. In an effort to refine the accuracy of clinical staging, other imaging modalities have been assessed. MRI offers the benefit over CT of avoiding radiation; however, metastatic evaluation is currently based on lymph node size criteria in the same way and therefore prediction of disease is similar. There is potential for improved detection of metastatic lymph node disease with MRI using paramagnetic iron oxide contrast agents; however, this awaits further investigation in the field of testicular cancer [22,23].

Positron emission tomography (PET) relies on the differential metabolism of ^{18}fluoro-2-deoxy-D-glucose (FDG) by tumor cells to distinguish them from normal tissue. FDG is taken up more avidly by seminoma than NSGCT and it was initially expected that this would enhance clinical management [24]. The acuity of this technique is limited by false positives from inflammatory and granulomatous tissues and false negatives for small lesions (<5–10 mm) and mature teratoma [25]. In a recent review of PET scanning in germ cell cancers, only two of nine trials reported improvement with a higher sensitivity and negative predictive value for PET over CT during staging at presentation [25]. Currently there is no clear role for PET scanning in the initial staging of seminoma.

Tumor markers

The role of tumor markers in seminoma is perhaps less pronounced than in NSGCT. AFP is not secreted by seminoma. Men who have elevated AFP regardless of tumor histology should thus be treated as an NSGCT. HCG, produced by syncytiotrophoblasts, is elevated in only 10% to 15% of cases. LDH is a nonspecific marker elevated in up to 80% of seminomas and 60% of nonseminomas when advanced, but also in many benign conditions. Specifically, AFP is useful to identify the presence of NSGCT elements when elevated and HCG may be used to follow response to treatment and for surveillance of recurrence in that fraction of patients who have disease that produces it. In contradistinction to NSGCT, tumor markers were not found to be useful for risk stratification in patients who had seminoma as described by the International Germ Cell Cancer Collaborative Group [26]. This finding has been confirmed subsequently by several authors in the setting of low-stage seminoma. Although elevated levels of HCG have been associated with larger tumor volumes, this does not seem to translate into differences in treatment outcome [27,28]. Because of a lack of specificity and a tendency to become elevated only with more advanced disease, the relevance of LDH as a surveillance tumor marker has recently been contested [29].

Staging

With information garnered from the pathologic analysis of the orchidectomy specimen, tumor markers, examination, and imaging, a clinical stage may be assigned. Management of seminomatous germ cell tumors is tailored to this and the pertinent factors in decision making vary by stage. Table 1 contains the most relevant staging system for testicular germ cell tumor.

Stage I seminoma: surveillance versus treatment

The prognosis for stage I seminoma is excellent, with long-term cure rates approaching 100% [30–33]. Stage I is that most commonly assigned to new presentations of seminoma, making up 70% of all incident cases [34]. Seminoma is highly radiosensitive and chemosensitive. Traditionally stage I disease has been most commonly managed with orchidectomy and adjuvant radiotherapy.

Of clinical stage I disease, a percentage of patients have occult micrometastases undetectable by imaging. This observation is borne out by surveillance series in which 15% to 20 % of patients experience disease relapse [34–39]. A combination of the advent of highly effective salvage chemotherapy for recurrent disease and ethical

Table 1
2002 TNM stage grouping of testicular cancer

Stage	Definition
I	Any T stage, N0, M0
IIA	Any T stage, N1 (≤5 lymph nodes ≤2 cm maximal diameter), M0
IIB	Any T stage, N2 (lymph nodes >2 cm but ≤5 cm maximal diameter), M0
IIC	Any T stage, N3 (lymph nodes >5 cm maximal diameter), M0
III	Any T stage, any N stage, M1

considerations with regard to the consequences of overtreating 80% to 85% of patients in this group has called the original treatment paradigm into question.

Efficacy of surveillance

No randomized controlled trials exist to compare the outcome of surveillance and salvage treatment if required to adjuvant treatment with radiotherapy or chemotherapy following orchidectomy. Given the excellent prognosis and likely small differences in long-term outcome, such a trial is unlikely to be conducted. There have been several prospective, nonrandomized studies of surveillance published over the last 2 decades with similar results [20,34–38]. The study from Princess Margaret Hospital in Toronto followed 241 patients for a median of 7.3 years and disease-free 5-year survival rates of 86% were reported [34]. The Danish Testicular Carcinoma Study Group (DATECA) had a 19% failure rate at a median of 48 months follow-up [20]. In each study, most recurrences (89% and 82%, respectively) occurred in the retroperitoneum (specifically the para-aortic and interaortocaval lymph nodes) at a median of 12 to 18 months. Late relapses more than 5 years from original diagnosis are well known to seminoma surveillance and protocols generally follow patients for at least 10 years from the point of diagnosis [39]. The Princess Margaret Hospital seminoma surveillance protocol is appended (Table 2).

Patients who have disease relapse from these studies have generally been treated with salvage radiotherapy. Secondary relapse following radiotherapy occurred in 19% in the PMH series and 11% in the DATECA series. Virtually all cases who had relapse beyond the retroperitoneum or following radiation were salvaged with chemotherapeutic regimens.

Cost

The financial cost of surveillance protocols may be difficult to estimate in a general manner given that expenses vary depending on the protocol used, the local medical economic climate, and regional costs and choices in treating relapse and secondary malignancies. Warde and colleagues [40] evaluated the economic cost of the Princess Margaret Hospital surveillance protocol, including the cost of salvage treatment. Over a 10-year period, surveillance resulted in the expenditure of approximately $2500 Canadian more than adjuvant radiotherapy. A study from the University of Wisconsin estimated the cost of surveillance at $20,487 as opposed to $14,722 for adjuvant radiation [41]. Although the absolute values differ, surveillance seems to be consistently more expensive than adjuvant radiotherapy.

Toxicity issues

The testicular germinal epithelium is exquisitely sensitive to ionizing radiation so that in an effort to maintain hormonal and reproductive function in the remaining testis, scrotal shielding is routinely used. Despite this, some radiation scatter is still experienced and persistent oligospermia has been reported in 8% [42]. There seems to be no increase in the incidence of children who have genetic anomalies born to men who have undergone radiation treatment of testicular malignancy [43].

Commonly experienced acute side effects of radiation include nausea, vomiting, and diarrhea, whereas late gastrointestinal toxicity, usually in

Table 2
Princess Margaret Hospital stage I seminoma surveillance protocol

Year	Month 2	Month 4	Month 6	Month 8	Month 10	Month 12
1		TM, CT		TM, CXR CT		TM, CT
2		TM, CXR CT		TM, CT		TM, CXR CT
3		TM, CT		TM, CT		TM, CXR CT
4			CT			CT, CXR
5			CT			CT, CXR
6			CT			CT, CXR
7			CT			CT, CXR
8						CT, CXR
9						CT, CXR
10						CT, CXR

Abbreviations: CT, computed tomography of the abdomen and pelvis; CXR, chest radiograph; TM, tumor markers.

the form of peptic ulcer disease, occurs in around 5% [43]. Grade II to IV hematologic toxicity is seen in 5% to 15% [44]. Studies of men from early radiation populations have raised concerns of cardiac toxicity and excess risk for death from cardiac events. Risk for events was increased by a factor of 1.8 to 2.4 [44,45]. Although the magnitude of these estimates may not pertain to modern radiotherapy practice, this remains an issue when considering adjuvant treatment.

Although the long-term psychologic effects of the diagnosis and management of seminoma are generally minimal, isolated patients develop significant psychologic symptoms [46]. Comparisons between adjuvant radiation and surveillance are limited; however, it has been suggested that men on surveillance have fewer sexual issues than men who have received adjuvant treatment [47].

Second malignancies

Seminoma patients are already at greater risk for further malignancies, such as contralateral testicular cancers, than the general populace presumably because of a combination of genetic predisposition and environmental exposures [48]. One of the central concerns in the debate between surveillance and adjuvant radiotherapy is the issue of iatrogenically induced late second malignancy following radiation. In the largest study to date, Travis and colleagues [49] looked at 40,576 men surviving more than 1 year following their diagnosis of testicular cancer. Details were extracted from 14 North American and European databases and the mean follow-up was 11.3 years. Overall 2285 solid tumors were observed compared with an expected 1619 (relative risk [RR] = 1.4) and by 10 years the relative risk increased to 1.6. The estimated cumulative risk for developing a second malignancy assuming diagnosis at 35 years of age and follow-up for 40 years was 36% for the seminoma population, 31% for the NSGCT population, and 23% for the general population. Being diagnosed at 20 years of age added approximately 10% to these figures. Relative risk also varied by type of treatment, whether radiation (RR = 2), chemotherapy (RR = 1.8), or both (RR = 2.9). Cancer rates were higher for organs within radiation fields (eg, bladder, stomach, pancreas, ureter) but also increased for other organs (eg, pleural, esophageal) and leukemias. Although it is difficult to predict with precision the impact of a policy of routine surveillance on these figures, a significant reduction in events would be expected.

Compliance

For surveillance to be a viable option for the management of stage I seminoma following orchidectomy, patients and medical personnel must be resolved to undertake the rigors of intensive follow-up imaging and outpatient visits. Given that the patient population predominantly consists of young men, this may not necessarily be possible. Changes in study, work, and personal circumstances may lead to relocation, whereas cancer diagnosis denial or perhaps a minimization of perceived risk in the medium to longer term may all contribute to a decline in attendance rates. Hao and colleagues [50] reported compliance with office visits declined from 61% in the first year to 35% in the second and that imaging protocols fared even more poorly with only 25% and 12%, respectively, undergoing all scans. Patients lost to follow-up in the surveillance arm of another study totaled 20.9% by the median follow-up time of 54 months [51]. These data lead to concern about the external validity of widespread surveillance protocols as opposed to those based in cancer centers. They also emphasize the need for, and provide an impetus to, the refinement of patient selection. The impact of poor compliance on overall survival is unknown but would be difficult to quantify given high cure rates in advanced disease.

Patient selection

Warde and colleagues [52] performed a pooled analysis of four published series involving 638 patients who had a median of 7 years surveillance. Only the first two univariate prognostic factors, from tumor size greater than 4 cm, rete testis invasion, lymphovascular invasion, and anaplastic versus classic seminoma, retained significance on multivariate analysis. The estimated 5-year relapse rates were 12%, 16%, and 32% if zero, one, or two factors were present, respectively. Restricting surveillance to only those patients who had one or fewer prognostic variables and irradiating the remainder would eliminate 20% from surveillance but avoid unnecessary treatment in 70%. This plan may present the best compromise for those patients considered to be compliant candidates for surveillance.

Para-aortic strip versus dog-leg radiotherapy

For more than 50 years, the standard of therapy for treatment of men who had Stage I/IIa seminoma was adjuvant irradiation (30 Gy in 15 fractions) of the ipsilateral pelvic and para-aortic nodes. Using this approach, disease-specific survival rates approach 100%. Recent revelation of a 20% failure rate among men placed on surveillance protocols (with their certain salvageability) coupled with concerns of long-term cardiac toxicity, fertility, and secondary malignancies [44] has led investigators to attempt to minimize exposure to radiation. One such maneuver has been to omit the ipsilateral inguinal radiotherapy. The rationale for this makes logical sense from an embryonic and anatomic point of view. The other change has been to lower doses to as low as 20 Gy in 10 fractions.

The impact of these dose-reduction strategies has been minimal in relapse-free survival and certainly in overall survival. In addition, less hematologic, gastrointestinal, and gonadal toxicity have been recognized [53]. Men who have scrotal violation or prior inguinal or scrotal surgery should not be offered para-aortic strip radiotherapy alone [54]. The EORTC completed a large randomized trial of 30 Gy versus 20 Gy as adjuvant therapy. The long-term results among the 625 randomized subjects revealed the same rate of relapse in both assigned treatment arms [53]. Additional follow-up data among other large cohorts have confirmed these findings [42,54]. Niazi and colleagues [55] reported the McGill University experience using 25 Gy in a paraaortic strip field among 71 patients. At 75-month follow-up, 68 were free of relapse. One patient failed in the ipsilateral pelvic area. The German testicular cancer study group performed a nonrandomized trial of para-aortic–only radiation among 675 patients (26 Gy). At 8 years follow-up, 26 patients relapsed, of which 24 were salvaged. Only 1.6% of patients failed in the ipsilateral pelvis [56]. These data are consistent with those published in other centers [57–59].

Recently some concern has been expressed regarding the long-term success of 20 Gy dose plus para-aortic strip only treatment with case reports of pelvic recurrences with significant clinical sequelae [60,61]. Long-term follow-up will be required at these doses and fields to ensure equivalence to historical norms.

Stage I: emerging role of chemotherapy

One of the more recent controversial topics in the management of patients who have stage I seminoma is the use of chemotherapy as an alternative to radiotherapy among men routinely or among those who do not elect surveillance. The use of one or two cycles of adjuvant carboplatin has been investigated by Oliver and colleagues [62] and other investigators [63–65] for more than a decade.

A recent phase III trial has been completed comparing single-dose carboplatin to radiotherapy (para-aortic strip or dog-leg) among 1477 patients in 14 countries [62]. The primary outcome measure was relapse-free survival with the power to detect a 3% absolute difference. At 4 years median follow-up, relapse rates were the same in both groups (95.9% radiotherapy versus 94.8 % carboplatin). Patients given carboplatin were less lethargic and attended their employment more reliably. Ten new primary testicular tumors were noted among men randomized to radiotherapy versus two among men randomized to carboplatin ($P = .04$). This study has demonstrated noninferiority of carboplatin in relation to radiotherapy and may have an added benefit of sterilizing smaller contralateral tumors. Although this study has greatly increased our understanding of early-stage seminoma we must exercise some caution in using single-dose carboplatin as the new standard of therapy. First, we must recognize that 80% to 85% of these patients never required chemotherapy at all, thus relapse has been decreased from 15% to less than 5% at most. Second, relapses in the retroperitoneum have been reported postchemotherapy, necessitating continuous imaging of the abdomen posttreatment. This finding contrasts to the rare in-field recurrence following dog-leg radiotherapy. Finally, late relapses cannot be excluded as a possibility, although recent data from phase II studies among 243 patients followed over 5 years (including 82 followed over 10 years) suggest that relapse after 3 years does not occur [60]. Finally, the long-term morbidity of subjecting 80% of patients to unnecessary chemotherapy with unknown long-term toxicity must be kept in mind. Adjuvant carboplatin may benefit patients not eligible for surveillance and is a reasonable alternative to standard radiotherapy regimens. A pragmatic approach may represent that taken by the Spanish Germ Cell Cancer group, which advocates surveillance among low-risk patients (<4 cm tumor and no rete testis involvement) and two cycles of adjuvant carboplatin among higher-risk patients. In their experience with 100 men, 13 have relapsed using this strategy [37] and overall survival is 100%. The criticism of this approach is that far too many men who do not require chemotherapy at all do get treated.

Management of stage IIA seminoma

Approximately 15% to 20% of patients who have seminoma are classified as having clinical stage II disease, or metastatic spread limited to the retroperitoneum [7]. Most have low- to moderate-volume disease and are therefore sub-staged as either IIA or B.

Radiotherapy

There have been no randomized controlled trials to confirm the optimal radiation dose for stage II seminoma. By consensus most centers manage stages IIA and sometimes B with radiation alone, administering 25 to 30 Gy to the retroperitoneum and pelvis with a further 5- to 10-Gy boost to areas of disease [54]. Although a randomized controlled trial demonstrates similar efficacy between 20 Gy and 30 Gy in stage I disease, this may not necessarily be extrapolated to Stage IIA or greater [53]. Some centers have added prophylactic radiation to the left supraclavicular fossa in an attempt to reduce relapse rates in that region [66]. This practice has not been widely adopted because less than 3% of patients within this group are likely to receive any material benefit [67,68]. The earlier practice of prophylactic radiotherapy to the mediastinum has been discarded because of minimal patient benefits and an associated increased risk for treatment-related death if salvage chemotherapy is required later [67].

The most important prognostic variable for stage II outcome overall is the volume of lymph node involvement. For men who have stage IIA disease, relapse after therapy occurs in 0% to 15% [66,69–71]. Specifically, long-term relapse rates between 0% to 8% may be expected in modern practice, with in-field recurrences on the order of 0% to 2% [66,69,70]. Once again cure is achieved in virtually 100% with salvage chemotherapeutic regimens if relapse occurs following radiotherapy treatment in stage IIA seminoma.

As tumor burden in the retroperitoneum increases, the likelihood of cure with radiation alone diminishes. In the Princess Margaret Hospital experience, 5-year relapse-free survival was 91% if nodal disease with maximal diameter less than 5 cm was present compared with only 44% if greater than 5 cm [70]. Furthermore, patients who had nodes smaller than 2 cm experienced disease recurrence 11% of the time, whereas for patients who had nodes 2 to 5 cm in diameter this increased to 9% to 18%.

Chemotherapy

The toxicity profile of chemotherapeutic combinations, efficacy of radiotherapy in achieving cure, and ability of patients who have disease relapse following radiotherapy to be effectively salvaged with chemotherapy have all contributed to the current standard of care being radiotherapy for stage IIA seminoma.

Recently the Royal Marsden Hospital published their results using a combination of a single cycle of carboplatin and radiotherapy for the treatment of stage II seminoma [71]. This addition prevented recurrence in 31 of 33 patients who had stage IIA and B disease. The overall 6% recurrence rate at a median of 2 years follow-up compares favorably with results from this center before the initiation of the protocol change. Previously stage IIA and B recurrence rates were reported as 15% and 30%, respectively. This study stands alone to date and the regimen requires further verification but may herald a change in the paradigm of stage II seminoma in the longer term.

Chemotherapy alone is generally not used for stage IIA disease unless there are factors complicating the delivery of radiotherapy, such as previous radiation or higher-than-usual risk for visceral organ injury as may be seen with disease beyond the primary echelon nodes.

Follow-up

Men who have early-stage seminoma require long-term follow-up and follow-up protocols for stage IIA seminoma generally do not differ from those used for patients who have treated stage I disease. Reasons for need for follow-up include chance of relapse (especially among surveillance patients), risk for contralateral testicular tumor [48],and long-term sequelae of seminoma or its therapy, including second malignancy and cardiovascular disease. Surveillance for relapse should last for 10 years.

References

[1] Jemal A, Siegel R, Ward E, et al. Cancer statistics, 2006. CA Cancer J Clin 2006;56(2):106–30.

[2] Chung P, Warde P. Surveillance in stage I testicular seminoma. Urol Oncol 2006;24(1):75–9.

[3] McGlynn KA, Devesa SS, Graubard BI, et al. Increasing incidence of testicular germ cell tumors among black men in the United States. J Clin Oncol 2005;23(24):5757–61.

[4] McGlynn KA, Devesa SS, Sigurdson AJ, et al. Trends in the incidence of testicular germ cell tumors in the United States. Cancer 2003;97(1):63–70.

[5] Ulbright TM, et al. Testicular and paratesticular tumors. In: Mills SE, Greenson JK, Oberman HA, et al, editors. Sternberg's diagnostic surgical pathology. 4th edition. Philadelphia: Lippincott Williams & Wilkins; 2004. p. 2168.

[6] Hofer MD, Browne TJ, He L, et al. Identification of two molecular groups of seminomas by using expression and tissue microarrays. Clin Cancer Res 2005; 11(16):5722–9.

[7] Cheville JC. Classification and pathology of testicular germ cell and sex cord-stromal tumors. Urol Clin North Am 1999;26(3):595–609.

[8] Eble JN. Spermatocytic seminoma. Hum Pathol 1994;25(10):1035–42.

[9] Steiner H, Gozzi C, Verdorfer I, et al. Metastatic spermatocytic seminoma—an extremely rare disease. Eur Urol 2006;49(1):183–6 [Epub 2005 Nov 8].

[10] Looijenga LH, Hersmus R, Gillis AJ, et al. Genomic and expression profiling of human spermatocytic seminomas: primary spermatocyte as tumorigenic precursor and DMRT1 as candidate chromosome 9 gene. Cancer Res 2006;66(1):290–302.

[11] Verdorfer I, Rogatsch H, Tzankov A, et al. Molecular cytogenetic analysis of human spermatocytic seminomas. J Pathol 2004;204(3):277–81.

[12] Clinical Oncology Information Network (CION) Guidelines. Guidelines on the management of adult testicular cancer. J Clin Oncol 2000;12(5):S173–210.

[13] Weir HK, Marrett LD, Moravan V. Trends in the incidence of testicular germ cell cancer in Ontario by histologic subgroup, 1964–1996. CMAJ 1999;160: 201–5.

[14] Bosl G, Goldman A, Lange P, et al. Impact of the delay in diagnosis on clinical stage of testicular cancer. Lancet 1981;2:970–3.

[15] Moul J, Paulson D, Dodge R, et al. Delay in diagnosis and survival in testicular cancer: impact of effective therapy and changes during 18 years. J Urol 1990;143:520–3.

[16] Carver BS, Sheinfeld J. Germ cell tumors of the testis. Ann Surg Oncol 2005;12:871–80.

[17] Capelouto C, Clark P, Ransil B, et al. A review of scrotal violation in testicular cancer: is adjuvant local therapy necessary? J Urol 1995;153:1397–401.

[18] Oliver RT, Ong J, Blandy JP, et al. Testis conservation in germ cell cancer justified by improved primary chemotherapy response and reduced delay, 1978–1994. Br J Urol 1996;78:119–24.

[19] Delaney RJ, Sayers CD, Walker MA, et al. The continued value of central histopathological review of testicular tumors. Histopathology 2005;47:166–9.

[20] von der Maase H, Specht L, Jacobsen GK, et al. Surveillance following orchidectomy for stage I seminoma of the testis. Eur J Cancer 1993;29A:1931–4.

[21] Hilton S, Herr H, Teitcher J, et al. CT detection of retroperitoneal lymph node metastases in patients with clinical stage I testicular non-seminomatous germ cell cancer: assessment of size and distribution criteria. AJR Am J Roentgenol 1997;169:521–5.

[22] Anzai Y, Piccoli CW, Outwater EK, et al. Evaluation of neck and body metastases to nodes with ferumoxtran 10-enhanced MR imaging: phase III safety and efficacy study. Radiology 2003;228: 777–88.

[23] Harisinghani MG, Barentsz J, Hahn PF, et al. Noninvasive detection of clinically occult lymph-node metastases in prostate cancer. N Engl J Med 2003; 348:2491–9.

[24] Wilson CB, Young HE, Ott RJ, et al. Imaging metastatic germ cell tumors with 18FDG positron emission tomography: prospects of detection and management. Eur J Nucl Med 1995;22:508–13.

[25] De Santis M, Pont J. The role of positron emission tomography in germ cell cancer. World J Urol 2004;22:41–6.

[26] International Germ Cell Cancer Collaborative Group. International Germ Cell Consensus Classification: a prognostic factor-based staging system for metastatic germ cell cancers. J Clin Oncol 1997;15: 594–603.

[27] Weissbach L, Bussar-Maatz R, Lohrs U, et al. Prognostic factors in seminomas with respect to HCG: results of a prospective multicenter study. Eur Urol 1999;36:601–8.

[28] Bruns F, Raub M, Schaefer U, et al. No predictive value of β-hCG in patients with stage I seminoma—results of a long-term follow-up study after adjuvant radiotherapy. Anticancer Res 2005;25:1543–6.

[29] Ackers C, Rustin GJS. Lactate dehydrogenase is not a useful marker for relapse in patients on surveillance for stage I germ cell tumors. Br J Cancer 2006; 94:1231–2.

[30] Dosmann MA, Zagars GK. Post-orchiectomy radiotherapy for stages I and II testicular seminoma. Int J Radiat Oncol Biol Phys 1993;26:381–90.

[31] Fossa SD, Aass N, Kaalhus O. Radiotherapy for testicular seminoma stage I: treatment results and long term post-irradiation morbidity in 365 patients. Int J Radiat Oncol Biol Phys 1989;16:383–8.

[32] Giaccheti S, Raoul Y, Wibault P, et al. Treatment of stage I testis seminoma by radiotherapy: long-term results-a 30 year experience. Int J Radiat Oncol Biol Phys 1993;27:3–9.

[33] Warde P, Gospodarowicz MK, Panzarella T, et al. Stage I testicular seminoma: results of adjuvant radiation and surveillance. J Clin Oncol 1995;13:2255–62.

[34] Steele GS, Richie JP, Stewart AK, et al. The national cancer database report on patterns of care for testicular carcinoma, 1986–1996. Cancer 1999;86: 2171–83.

[35] Horwich A, Alsanjari N, Ahern R, et al. Surveillance following orchidectomy for stage I testicular seminoma. Br J Cancer 1992;65:775–8.

[36] Ramakrishnan S, Champion AE, Doreen MS, et al. Stage I seminoma of the testis: is post-orchidectomy

surveillance a safe alternative to routine post-operative radiotherapy? Clin Oncol (R Coll Radiol) 1992; 4:284–6.

[37] Aparicio J, Muro G, Maroto P, et al. Multicenter study evaluating a dual policy of postorchiectomy surveillance and selective adjuvant single-agent carboplatin for patients with clinical stage I seminoma. Ann Oncol 2003;14:867–72.

[38] Choo R, Thomas G, Woo T, et al. Long term outcome of postorchidectomy surveillance for stage I testicular seminoma. Int J Radiat Oncol Biol Phys 2005;61:736–40.

[39] Michael H, Lucia J, Foster RS, et al. The pathology of late recurrences of testicular germ cell tumors. Am J Surg Pathol 2000;24:257–73.

[40] Warde P, Gospodarowicz M, Panzarella T, et al. Issues in the management of stage I testicular seminoma. Int J Radiat Oncol Biol Phys 1997;39: 156–9.

[41] Sharda NN, Kinsella TJ, Ritter MA. Adjuvant radiation vs. observation: a cost analysis of alternate management schemes in early-stage testicular seminoma. J Clin Oncol 1996;14:2993–9.

[42] Fossa SD, Horwich A, Russell JM, et al. Optimal planning target volume for stage I testicular seminoma: a Medical Research Council randomized trial. J Clin Oncol 1999;17:1146–54.

[43] Senturia YD, Peckham CS, Peckham MJ. Children fathered by men treated for testicular cancer. Lancet 1985;2:766–9.

[44] Zagars GK, Ballo MT, Lee AK, et al. Mortality after cure of testicular seminoma. J Clin Oncol 2004;22: 640–7.

[45] Huddart RA, Norman A, Shahidi M, et al. Cardiovascular disease as a long-term complication of treatment for testicular cancer. J Clin Oncol 2003; 21:1513–23.

[46] Caffo O, Amichetti M, Tomio L, et al. Quality of life after radiotherapy for early-stage testicular seminoma. Radiother Oncol 2001;59:13–20.

[47] Tinkler SD, Howard GC, Kerr GR. Sexual morbidity following radiotherapy for germ cell tumors of the testis. Radiother Oncol 1992;25:207–12.

[48] Fossa SD, Chen J, Schonfeld SJ, et al. Risk of contralateral testicular cancer: a population based study of 29,515 US men. J Natl Cancer Inst 2005;97: 1056–66.

[49] Travis LB, Fossa SD, Schonfeld SJ, et al. Second cancers among 40,576 testicular cancer patients: focus on long-term survivors. J Natl Cancer Inst 2005; 97:1354–65.

[50] Hao D, Seidel J, Brant R, et al. Compliance of clinical stage I non-seminomatous germ cell tumor patients with surveillance. J Urol 1998;160:768–71.

[51] Alomary I, Samant R, Gallant V. Treatment of stage I seminoma: a 15 year review. Urol Oncol 2006;24: 180–3.

[52] Warde P, Specht L, Horwich A, et al. Prognostic factors for relapse in stage I seminoma managed by surveillance: a pooled analysis. J Clin Oncol 2002; 20:4448–52.

[53] Jones WG, Fossa SD, Mead GM, et al. Randomized trial of 30 versus 20 Gy in the adjuvant treatment of stage I Testicular Seminoma: a report on Medical Research Council Trial TE18, European Organisation for the Research and Treatment of Cancer Trial 30942 (ISRCTN18525328). J Clin Oncol 2005;23(6): 1200–8.

[54] Schmoll HJ, Souchon R, Krege S, et al. European consensus on diagnosis and treatment of germ cell cancer, a report of the European Germ Cell Cancer Consensus Group (EGCCCG). Ann Oncol 2004; 15:1377–99.

[55] Niazi TM, Souhami L, Sultanem K, et al. Long-term results of para-aortic irradiation for patients with stage I seminoma of the testis. Int J Radiat Oncol Biol Phys 2005;61(3):741–4.

[56] Classen J, Schmidberger H, Meisner C, et al. German Testicular Cancer Study Group (GTCSG) Para-aortic irradiation for stage I testicular seminoma: results of a prospective study in 675 patients. A trial of the German testicular cancer study group (GTCSG). Br J Cancer 2004;90(12):2305–11.

[57] Niewald M, Waziri A, Walter K, et al. Low dose radiotherapy for stage I seminoma: early results. Radiother Oncol 1995;37:164–6.

[58] Kiricuta IC, Sauer J, Bohndorf W. Omission of pelvic irradiation on stage I testicular seminoma: a study of postorchiectomy para-aortic radiotherapy. Int J Radiat Oncol Biol Phys 1009;35:293–298.

[59] Logue JP, Harris MA, Livsey JE, et al. Short course para-aortic radiation for stage I seminoma of the testis. Int J Radiol Oncol Biol Phys 2003;57:1304–9.

[60] Oliver T. One-dose carboplatin in seminoma [correspondence]. Lancet 2005;366:1526.

[61] Power RE, Kennedy L, Crown J, et al. Pelvic recurrence in stage I seminoma: a new phenomenon that questions modern protocols for radiotherapy and follow-up. Int J Urol 2005;l2:378–82.

[62] Oliver RT, Mason MD, Mead GM, et al. Radiotherapy versus single-dose carboplatin in adjuvant treatment of stage I seminoma: a randomized trial. Lancet 2005;366:293–300.

[63] Dieckmann KP, Bruggeboes B, Pichlmeier U, et al. Adjuvant treatment of clinical stage I seminoma: as a single course of carboplatin sufficient? Urology 2000;55:102–6.

[64] Steiner H, Holtl I, Witenberger W. Long term experience with carboplatin monotherapy for clinical stage I seminoma: a retrospective single center study. Urology 2002;60:324–8.

[65] Reiter WJ, Brodowicz T, Alavi S, et al. Twelve year experience with two courses of adjuvant single-agent carboplatin therapy for clinical stage I seminoma. J Clin Oncol 2001;19:101–4.

[66] Zagars GK, Pollack A. Radiotherapy for stage II testicular seminoma. Int J Radiat Oncol Biol Phys 2001;51:634–9.

[67] Chung PW, Warde PR, Panzerella T, et al. Appropriate radiation volume for stage IIA/B testicular seminoma. Int J Radiat Oncol Biol Phys 2003;56:746–8.

[68] Loehrer P, Birch R, Williams S, et al. Chemotherapy of metastatic seminoma: the Southeastern Cancer Study Group experience. J Clin Oncol 1987;5:1212–20.

[69] Claasen J, Schmidberger H, Meisner C, et al. Radiotherapy for stages IIA/B testicular seminoma: final report of a prospective multicenter clinical trial. J Clin Oncol 2003;21:1101–6.

[70] Chung PW, Gospodarowicz MK, Panzarella T, et al. Stage II testicular seminoma: patterns of recurrence and outcome of treatment. Eur Urol 2004;45:754–9.

[71] Patterson H, Norman AR, Mitra SS, et al. Combination carboplatin and radiotherapy in the management of stage II testicular seminoma: a comparison with radiotherapy treatment alone. Radiother Oncol 2001;59:5–11.

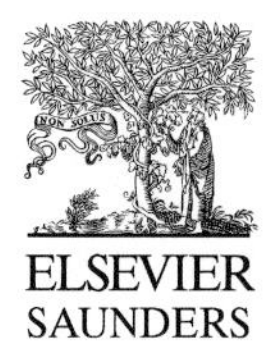

ELSEVIER
SAUNDERS

Urol Clin N Am 34 (2007) 137–148

UROLOGIC CLINICS of North America

Management of Clinical Stage I Nonseminomatous Germ Cell Testicular Cancer

Toni K. Choueiri, MD[a], Andrew J. Stephenson, MD[b], Timothy Gilligan, MD[a], Eric A. Klein, MD[b,*]

[a]*Department of Solid Tumor Oncology, Taussig Cancer Center, Cleveland Clinic Foundation, 9500 Euclid Avenue, R35, Cleveland, OH 44195-0001, USA*

[b]*Section of Urologic Oncology, Glickman Urological Institute, Cleveland Clinic Foundation, 9500 Euclid Avenue, Desk A100, Cleveland, OH 44195-0001, USA*

Approximately one third of patients who have nonseminomatous germ cell testicular cancer (NSGCT) have clinical stage (CS) I disease at diagnosis, defined as normal postorchiectomy serum levels of the tumor markers α-fetoprotein (AFP), human choriogonadotropin (HCG), and lactate dehydrogenase (LDH) without evidence of metastatic disease on imaging studies of the chest, abdomen, and pelvis. The optimal management of these patients continues to generate controversy. Surveillance, retroperitoneal lymph node dissection (RPLND), and chemotherapy with two cycles of bleomycin-etoposide-cisplatin (BEP×2) are established treatment options for CS I and all are associated with long-term survival rates of 97% or greater. Contributing to the controversy is the fact that occult metastases in the retroperitoneum or at distant sites are present in only 25% to 35% of patients overall. Any intervention after orchiectomy, with its associated short- and long-term morbidity, represents over-treatment for the 65% to 75% of patients who have disease limited to the testis.

NSGCT follows a predictable pattern of metastatic spread that has contributed to its successful management. With the exception of choriocarcinoma, the most common route of disease dissemination is by way of lymphatic channels from the primary tumor to the retroperitoneal lymph nodes and subsequently to distant sites (most commonly the lung, posterior mediastinum, and left supraclavicular fossa). Choriocarcinoma has a propensity for hematogenous dissemination. The retroperitoneum is the initial site of metastatic spread in 70% to 80% of patients who have testicular cancer. Detailed mapping studies from RPLND series have increased our understanding of the testicular lymphatic drainage and identified the most likely sites of metastatic disease [1]. For right-sided testicular tumors, the primary drainage site is the interaortocaval lymph nodes, followed by the paracaval and para-aortic nodes. The primary "landing zone" for left-sided tumors is the para-aortic lymph nodes, followed by the interaortocaval nodes [2]. Contralateral spread is common with right-sided tumors but is rarely seen with left-sided tumors and usually is associated with bulky disease. More caudal deposits of metastatic disease usually reflect retrograde spread to distal iliac and inguinal lymph nodes secondary to large volume disease and, more rarely, aberrant testicular lymphatic drainage.

Risk assessment

Considerable attention has been devoted to identifying clinical and pathologic parameters associated with the presence of occult metastasis in the retroperitoneum or at distant sites to better select patients for additional therapy after orchiectomy. The retroperitoneum continues to be the most difficult area to stage clinically and

* Corresponding author.
E-mail address: kleine@ccf.org (E.A. Klein).

doi:10.1016/j.ucl.2007.02.001

a consistent 25% to 35% rate of clinical understaging has been reported over the last 4 decades for CS I NSGCT despite the advent of third- and fourth-generation computed tomography (CT) scanners. In contrast, pulmonary metastases 5 mm in size are easily identified by contemporary imaging modalities. There is no consensus regarding size criteria for retroperitoneal lymph nodes that constitute a "normal" abdominal CT scan. A size cutoff of 10 mm is frequently used to identify enlarged lymph nodes, but false-negative rates up to 63% have been reported when this size criterion is used.

An understanding of the primary drainage sites for left- and right-sided tumors has led to efforts to increase the sensitivity of abdominal CT imaging by decreasing the size criteria for clinically positive lymph nodes in the primary landing zone and size criterion as small as 4 mm have been proposed. Leibovitch and colleagues [3] showed that using a size cutoff of 4 mm in the primary landing zone and 10 mm outside this region was associated with a sensitivity and specificity for pathologic stage II disease of 91% and 50%, respectively. In a similar study, Hilton and colleagues [4] reported a sensitivity and specificity of 93% and 58%, respectively, using a cutoff of 4 mm for lymph nodes in the primary landing zone that were anterior to a horizontal line bisecting the aorta. Based on this evidence, patients who have retroperitoneal lymph nodes greater than 4 mm in the primary landing zone, particularly if they are anterior to the great vessels on transaxial CT images, should be considered for additional therapy after orchiectomy given the high probability of regional metastasis. Of note, investigations of positron emission tomography with fluorine-18 fluorodeoxyglucose (FDG-PET) in the staging of patients who have low-stage NSGCT have been disappointing and there is currently no role for FDG-PET in the routine staging of CS I NSGCT.

The most commonly reported risk factors for occult metastasis are the presence of lymphovascular invasion (LVI) and a predominant component of embryonal carcinoma (EC). The definition of EC predominance in the literature varies from 45% to 90%. The reported rate of relapse or pathologic stage II for patients who have LVI and EC predominance varies from 50% to 90% and 30% to 80%, respectively [5–14]. In the absence of these two risk factors, the reported rate of occult metastasis is less than 20%. Other identified risk factors include advanced pT stage, absence of mature teratoma, absence of yolk sac tumor, presence of EC, percentage of MIB-1 staining, increasing primary tumor size, and older patient age. In a pooled analysis of 23 studies assessing predictors of occult metastasis in CS I NSGCT, Vergouwe and colleagues [14] identified LVI (odds ratio [OR] 5.2), MIB-1 staining greater than 70% (OR 4.7), and EC predominance (OR 2.8) as the strongest predictors, and these factors were present in 36%, 55%, and 51% of CS I patients, respectively.

Numerous risk groups and prognostic indices have been proposed based on the presence or absence of several of these risk factors, most commonly on the basis of LVI and EC predominance. These risk stratification schemes classify patients as low, intermediate, or high risk based on the presence of none, some, or all of these parameters. A summary of these risk stratification tools is listed in Table 1 [15]. These risk stratification tools are most useful for predicting a low risk for occult metastasis to identify patients who are optimal candidates for surveillance. Between 18% and 64% of patients are classified as low-risk in these series and the metastasis rate for these patients is less than 20% in all reported series (range, 0% to 19%).

The usefulness of these tools to guide treatment decisions in patients who have intermediate- and high-risk features is less clear. In most of the models in which 25% or more of patients are identified as high risk, the reported relapse rate ranges from 48% to 64%. Mandating treatment for all high-risk patients would expose 36% to 52% of patients to potential treatment-related toxicity unnecessarily. Some models predict a risk for relapse greater than 70% for patients who have adverse features, although often only a small proportion of patients (<10%) are classified as such. The usefulness of these models for intermediate-risk patients is even less clear. In general, between 30% and 50% of patients are classified as intermediate risk on the basis of one or two risk factors, and the reported occult metastasis rate ranges from 23% to 48%.

Caution must be exercised when using these models to guide treatment decisions for the individual patient, particularly if he is classified as intermediate or high risk. Data from prospective studies of patients staged and evaluated in a standardized and rigorous fashion are needed to develop optimal prediction tools for CS I NSGCT and they must be based on all potentially important variables. External validation of these

Table 1
Summary of published risk stratification models for occult metastasis in clinical stage I nonseminomatous germ cell testicular cancer and the proportion of patients classified as low, intermediate, and high risk

	Low risk			Intermediate risk			High risk		
	Features	Mets (%)	Cohort (%)	Features	Mets (%)	Cohort (%)	Features	Mets (%)	Cohort (%)
Albers et al [5]	No LVI, EC <50%, MIB <70%	19	18		—	53	LVI, EC >50%, MIB >70%	64	29
Alexandre et al [6]	No LVI, teratoma	0	31	LVI or no teratoma	29	39	LVI, no teratoma	61	26
Freedman et al [47]	0–1 of LI, VI, EC, or no YS	9	38	2 risk factors	24	38	3–4 risk factors	58	24
Heidenreich et al [7]	No LVI, EC <45%	8	48	LVI or EC >45%	48	18	LVI, EC >45%	91	38
Hermans et al [8]	No LVI, EC <50%	16	31	LVI or EC >50%	29	37	LVI, EC >50%	62	33
Leibovitch et al [15]	EC volume, MIB-1, LN size	2	45		—	—	EC volume, MIB-1, LN size	88	55
Nicolai et al [9]	No LVI, EC <90%	14	54	LVI or EC >90%	30	32	LVI, EC >90%	48	14
Read et al [46]	0–1 of LI, VI, EC, or no YS	17	39	2 risk factors	23	39	3–4 risk factors	48	23
Sogani et al [11]	No LVI, EC <50%	12	64	LVI or EC >50%	44	30	LVI, EC >50%	71	7
Stephenson et al [12]	No LVI, EC <50%	—	35	LVI or EC >50%	47	45	LVI, EC >50%	63	20

Abbreviations: EC, embryonal carcinoma; LI, lymphatic invasion; LN, lymph node; LVI, lymphovascular invasion; Mets, regional or distant metastasis; VI, vascular invasion; YS, yolk sac.

models in independent cohorts is essential to reliably assess their anticipated performance in future patients.

Surveillance

Early interest in surveillance for CS I NSGCT was based on two key developments: (1) the finding that 65% to 75% of patients who had CS I NSGCT were cured by orchiectomy alone and therefore did not need any additional therapy, and (2) the demonstration that cisplatin-based chemotherapy could cure almost all patients who had favorable-prognosis metastatic disease. Surveillance thus seemed to offer the promise of minimizing treatment toxicity by restricting treatment to those who had a proven need for it. Studies of surveillance have reported overall and disease-specific survival rates indistinguishable from the rates seen with RPLND and primary chemotherapy. As a result, initial surveillance for CS I NSGCT with deferred chemotherapy at relapse is now widely accepted as a standard treatment option for CS I NSGCT.

Published studies of surveillance have reported results on more than 1800 men, with a mean relapse risk of 28% and 1.2% disease-specific mortality. The nine largest trials, including more than 100 patients per trial, are summarized in Table 2 [16–19]. More than 90% of relapses occur within the first 2 years following orchiectomy but late relapses (>5 years) are seen in up to 1% of patients and have represented as many as 5% of relapses in some reports [20]. With the use of cisplatin-based chemotherapy at relapse, more than 98% of patients managed with surveillance are alive without evidence of disease 5 years after diagnosis. Roughly 30% to 40% of relapses are retroperitoneal only with normal serum tumor markers, whereas about 20% to 30% have normal imaging but elevated serum tumor markers. Most remaining relapses manifest as retroperitoneal

Table 2
Published reports of surveillance for clinical stage I nonseminomatous germ cell testicular cancers

Study	Number of patients	Relapses	Median follow-up (months)	Median time to relapse, range (months)	Systemic relapse[a] (%)	Dead of testis cancer
Read et al [46]	373	100 (27%)	60	3 (1.5–20)	39	5 (1.3%)
Daugaard et al [20]	301	86 (29%)	60	5 (1–171)	66	0
Freedman et al [47]	259	70 (32%)	30	Not reported	61	3 (1.2%)
Colls et al [16]	248	70 (28%)	53	Not reported	73	4 (1.6%)
Francis et al [17]	183	52 (28%)	70	6 (1–12 [46])	54	2 (1%)
Gels et al [18]	154	42 (27%)	72	4 (2–24)	71	2 (1%)
Sharir et al [19]	170	48 (28%)	76	7 (2–21)	79	1 (0.5%)
Sogani et al [11]	105	27 (26%)	136	5 (2–24)	37	3 (3%)
Pooled data	1793	495 (28%)	—	—	59	20 (1.1%)

[a] Systemic relapse defined as relapse with elevated serum tumor markers or relapse in tissue other than retroperitoneal lymph nodes.

adenopathy with elevated serum tumor markers. Supradiaphragmatic relapses are markedly less common but are the first sign of relapse in about 8% of relapsing patients. Because most patients have elevated serum tumor markers, extra-retroperitoneal metastases, or clinical stage IIB or greater retroperitoneal disease at relapse, systemic chemotherapy is the standard treatment for relapsing patients. Nonetheless, patients who have normal serum tumor markers and relapses limited to small volume retroperitoneal adenopathy (clinical stage IIa) may be managed with RPLND.

The surveillance schedule used in published series is highly variable and no schedule has been demonstrated to be superior to another regarding survival. All studies noted that the relapse rate is highest within the first 2 years of follow-up, with about half of all relapses occurring within the first 6 months, 76% to 90% occurring in the first year, and 87% to 100% occurring within 2 years. This finding supports a more frequent surveillance schedule early on with gradually increasing intervals between examinations over time. We use the following schedule: physical examination, chest radiograph, and serum tumor markers (BHCG, AFP, and LDH) every 1 to 2 months during the first year, every 2 months in year two, every 3 months in year three, every 4 months in year four, every 6 months in year five, and annually thereafter. We recommend abdominal-pelvic CT scans every 3 months in year one, every 4 months in year two, every 6 months in years three and four, and annually thereafter. Thoracic relapses in the setting of normal STMs and normal abdominal imaging are rare and chest CT scans are not routinely performed. The most appropriate duration of surveillance has not been defined. Any benefit from prolonged surveillance beyond 5 to 7 years must be balanced against the potential risk resulting from radiation exposure during surveillance imaging.

A successful surveillance program depends on compliance from the patient, which cannot be taken for granted. Suboptimal compliance with surveillance has been reported [21], and noncompliant patients may relapse with advanced disease less amenable to cure with salvage therapy at that time. Nonetheless, as noted above, multiple studies have documented the feasibility of achieving sufficient compliance to result in 98% disease-specific survival.

Surveillance represents an alternative to RPLND or primary chemotherapy in patients who have CS I NSGCT. It offers the benefit of restricting postorchiectomy treatment to those who have a proven need for it. Most CS I patients undergoing surveillance are thus spared the treatment-related morbidity of RPLND and chemotherapy. Surveillance may result in greater anxiety because of the greater risk for relapse compared with surgery or primary chemotherapy. Moreover, those patients who do relapse on surveillance typically require three to four cycles of cisplatin-based chemotherapy for disseminated disease, which carries more risk for short- and long-term side effects than either RPLND or the two cycles of postorchiectomy chemotherapy offered to men who have CS I disease. Surveillance is most appropriate for patients who do not have a high risk for relapse. It must be emphasized, however, that patient compliance with follow-up surveillance schedules is a prerequisite for a successful surveillance strategy. In patients for whom there are questions about motivation and compliance with surveillance, treatment with either primary RPLND or BEP×2 chemotherapy should be recommended.

Retroperitoneal lymph node dissection

In the United States and parts of Europe, the conventional approach to patients who have CS I NSGCT has been bilateral infrahilar RPLND. The main factors in favor of RPLND are that the retroperitoneum is the initial site of metastatic spread in 70% to 80% of patients who have occult metastasis, retroperitoneal lymph nodes often harbor chemotherapy-resistant teratomas, and there is a low rate of relapse following RPLND [12]. The argument for RPLND is thus that the therapeutic focus for CS I patients should be control of the retroperitoneum, and RPLND is the most effective way to achieve this goal.

The four largest series that have described the outcome of CS I patients managed by primary RPLND at centers of excellence are listed in Table 3. The rate of pathologic stage II in these series ranges from 19% to 28%. Of the patients who have pathologic stage II, an estimated 66% to 81% were cured after RPLND alone, demonstrating the therapeutic efficacy of RPLND. Improvements in clinical staging and patient selection have had a favorable impact on the extent of retroperitoneal metastasis among patients who have low-stage NSGCT. In the Memorial Sloan-Kettering series, approximately two thirds of patients who had pathologic stage II disease had low-volume (pN1) retroperitoneal disease (five or fewer involved nodes, none greater than 2 cm, no extranodal extension), and an estimated 90% were cured after RPLND alone [12]. Most RPLND series have reported retroperitoneal recurrences in less than 2% of patients, demonstrating its efficacy for control of regional metastasis. Patients undergoing this operation should be referred to a surgeon who has extensive RPLND experience to achieve comparable results.

The route of metastatic spread for NSGCT is primarily by way of lymphatics to the retroperitoneum. Hematogenous dissemination that bypasses the retroperitoneum is uncommon in germ cell testicular cancer (GCT) and is usually heralded by elevated serum tumor markers. The rate of occult systemic disease in CS I NSGCT is low. Of the 70% to 81% of patients who have pathologically negative retroperitoneal lymph nodes (pathologic stage I) at RPLND, relapses are reported in 6% to 12%. Among patients who have pathologic stage II, an estimated 20% to 35% have occult systemic disease [12].

The retroperitoneum is the most frequent site of chemoresistant GCT elements and failure to control the retroperitoneum surgically during the initial treatment phase may compromise patient curability. In autopsy studies of patients who died of NSGCT, visceral metastases were late events in the course of the disease and most patients had concomitant (and usually bulky) uncontrolled retroperitoneal disease. Approximately 20% to 30% of CS I patients who have pathologic stage II disease have retroperitoneal teratoma, which is relatively resistant to chemotherapy [12,22,23]. The absence of teratoma in the primary tumor does not reliably predict for its absence in the retroperitoneum among patients who have pathologic stage II [23]. Although histologically benign, the biologic potential of teratoma is unpredictable and it may grow and become unresectable, undergo malignant transformation, or result in late relapse. All of these events may have lethal consequences. The retroperitoneum is also the most frequent site of chemoresistant malignant GCT elements (most commonly yolk sac or EC). In post-chemotherapy RPLND series, 10% to 20% of patients who have metastatic NSGCT have viable malignancy in the retroperitoneum following induction chemotherapy for metastatic

Table 3
Summary of published series of retroperitoneal lymph node dissection for clinical stage I nonseminomatous germ cell testicular cancer

Study	Patients	PS II (%)	Retroperitoneal teratoma (%)	Relapse PS I (%)	Relapse PS II (%)	Adjuvant chemotherapy (%)	Dead of testis cancer (%)
Donohue et al [26]	378	113 (30)	15	12	34	13	3 (0.8)
Hermans et al [8]	292	67 (23)	NR	10	22	12	1 (0.3)
Nicolai et al [9]	322	61 (19)	NR	NR	27	NR	4 (1.2)
Stephenson et al [12]	297	83 (28)	15	6	19	15	0

Abbreviations: NR, not reported; PS, pathologic stage.

disease [24,25]. For patients who have clinical stage IIA and IIB NSGCT, the incidence of chemoresistant malignancy is estimated to be as high as 8% [12]. RPLND may thus be the best way to ensure long-term cancer control in patients who have metastatic NSGCT.

An important consideration regarding RPLND is that patients who relapse are "chemotherapy-naïve" and can be cured with "good-risk" cisplatin-based chemotherapy regimens and resection of any residual masses in virtually all cases. In the cisplatin era, the cancer-specific survival after primary RPLND for CS I in the Memorial Sloan-Kettering and Indiana University experience is 100% (297 patients) and 99.4% (666 of 670 patients), respectively [8,26]. In addition, the risk for retroperitoneal relapse after RPLND is less than 2%. By clearing the retroperitoneum of all GCT elements, the risk for late relapse after RPLND is substantially reduced. Over a median follow-up of almost 5 years, the late relapse rate among 297 CS I patients treated by RPLND at Memorial Sloan-Kettering was 0.3%.

The debate over RPLND is most contentious with regard to patients who have high-risk CS I NSGCT. Relapse rates between 23% and 37% after RPLND have been reported for patients who have CS I with EC predominance or LVI in the primary tumor and pathologic stage I disease [8,9]. Proponents of BEP×2 for CS I have questioned the appropriateness of performing such a major operation in patients who would be left with such a high postoperative risk for relapse [27]. In a review of 267 patients who had CS I and IIA NSGCT with EC predominance or LVI treated by RPLND, 42% had pathologic stage II disease, of whom 54% had pN1 disease and 16% had retroperitoneal teratoma [12]. The 5-year relapse-free probability after RPLND alone for pathologic stage I and pN1 was 90% and 86%, respectively. An estimated 28% of patients required chemotherapy as adjuvant therapy for pathologic stage II or for treatment of relapse. In contrast to the earlier reports, this study thus found that the risk for occult systemic disease in patients who had CS I with EC predominance and LVI is low and, similar to the CS I population overall, the most frequent site of metastatic disease is the retroperitoneum. In this series, RPLND in high-risk patients provided an excellent likelihood of cure without the need for additional therapy in many patients. Nonetheless, nearly one third of high-risk patients receive systemic chemotherapy at some time after RPLND and patients should be so advised when choosing their treatment.

Adjuvant chemotherapy for pathologic stage II

The role of adjuvant chemotherapy after RPLND for patients who have pathologic stage II disease is controversial. A randomized trial of adjuvant chemotherapy versus observation for pathologic stage II NSGCT showed a significant reduction in the rate of relapse (6% versus 49%), but no overall survival difference was demonstrated [28]. Most studies have found that the risk for relapse is related to the size or number of involved lymph nodes [29,30]. As a result, adjuvant chemotherapy is generally recommended for patients who have pN2–3 disease or patients who have pN1 disease who are anticipated to be noncompliant with surveillance testing. Responsible patients who have pN1 disease are safely managed with surveillance given the low (10%–20%) risk for relapse. The administration of two cycles of chemotherapy using either etoposide-cisplatin (EP) or BEP has been associated with 99% relapse-free survival [31,32]. Only patients who are completely resected and are clinically free of disease after RPLND are candidates for adjuvant chemotherapy. Patients who have incompletely resected disease or elevated serum tumor markers postoperatively should receive a full induction chemotherapy regimen.

By pathologically staging the retroperitoneum, RPLND provides more accurate information to gauge patient prognosis and thus the need for subsequent adjuvant therapy is more clearly defined. Some 70% to 80% of CS I patients are pathologic stage (PS) I and up to two thirds of PS II patients have low-volume (pN1) retroperitoneal disease. With RPLND and selective use of adjuvant chemotherapy for PS II disease, overall freedom from relapse rates after RPLND is reported in 85% to 92% of patients and adjuvant chemotherapy is administered to only 12% to 15% of CS I patients overall (40%–50% of patients who have PS II) [8,9,12,26]. If adjuvant chemotherapy is restricted to patients who have PN2–3 disease, up to 84% of patients avoid chemotherapy after RPLND as adjuvant therapy or for treatment of relapse. Many patients who have PN1 disease elect to undergo adjuvant chemotherapy, however, to reduce their relapse risk from more than 10% down to 1% [12].

Morbidity of retroperitoneal lymph node dissection

Primary RPLND is associated with negligible mortality and minimal morbidity rates when performed by experienced surgeons [33,34]. In the Indiana University experience there were no perioperative deaths, no permanent disability from complications, and 2.3% of patients required reoperation [33]. The most common long-term complications of primary RPLND are a 1% to 2% incidence of small bowel obstruction, a 0.4% incidence of lymphocele or chylous ascites, and a midline abdominal surgical scar.

The most consistent long-term sequela of RPLND is the loss of ejaculation, which in turn can compromise fertility. The postganglionic sympathetic fibers from T12–L3 mediate the neuromuscular events that are responsible for antegrade ejaculation. These fibers form the hypogastric plexus near the takeoff of the inferior mesenteric artery (IMA) just above the aortic bifurcation. Based on the improved understanding of the neuroanatomy of ejaculation, the pattern and distribution of retroperitoneal lymph node metastases for right- and left-sided tumors, and surgical mapping studies, modified RPLND templates were developed initially to minimize intraoperative injury to these structures and ejaculatory rates of 51% to 88% are reported [25,35]. In general, these modified templates attempted to minimize contralateral dissection, particularly below the level of the IMA. More recently, nerve-sparing techniques have been developed whereby the sympathetic chains, the postganglionic sympathetic fibers, and the hypogastric plexus are prospectively identified, meticulously dissected, and preserved [36]. Antegrade ejaculation rates greater than 95% have been reported with these techniques [25]. The completeness of resection should never be compromised to maintain ejaculatory function.

Modified templates of dissection

Modified RPLND remains an appropriate option for low-stage NSGCT but urologists must be diligent to extend the limits of dissection to the appropriate anatomic boundaries. Modified templates minimize contralateral dissection below the IMA. For right-sided tumors, contralateral spread to the para-aortic and left hilar regions is observed in up to 20% of patients who have low-stage NSGCT. Dissection above the IMA should thus extend to the left ureter for right-sided tumors. For left-sided tumors, contralateral spread is uncommon in low-stage disease and contralateral dissection above the IMA can safely extend to the lateral border of the IVC. Retroaortic and retrocaval dissection should never be omitted within the boundaries of a modified template. Omitting these critical areas exposes patients to the risks of retroperitoneal recurrences, which are associated with diminished survival. Alternatively, the use of nerve-sparing techniques enables a full bilateral infrahilar dissection without compromising ejaculatory dysfunction and this has replaced modified templates at several institutions.

Laparoscopic retroperitoneal lymph node dissection

To reduce the morbidity of RPLND, several investigators have evaluated the role of minimally invasive techniques [37–39]. The therapeutic efficacy of laparoscopic RPLND is largely unknown because virtually all patients who have pathologic stage II disease receive adjuvant chemotherapy regardless of the extent of retroperitoneal disease [37–40]. The routine administration of adjuvant chemotherapy to all patients who have pathologic stage II disease after laparoscopic RPLND leads to an increase in morbidity compared with standard RPLND. Moreover, the templates reported in laparoscopic series are inadequate for complete retroperitoneal clearance. Because of the technical challenge of controlling lumbar vessels, retroaortic and retrocaval tissue was not routinely removed in several of the laparoscopic series [38,39]. Some authors do not remove interaortocaval lymph nodes for left-sided tumors [38,39], nor the preaortic and para-aortic lymph nodes for right-sided tumors [38]. The risk for late relapse with an uncontrolled retroperitoneum in these patients is concerning. Laparoscopic RPLND should be considered an investigational and diagnostic procedure rather than a therapeutic operation for CS I NSGCT.

Primary chemotherapy

In distinction to adjuvant chemotherapy given to men who have PS II disease after RPLND, primary chemotherapy refers to treatment administered to men who have CS I NSGCT after orchiectomy. The goal of primary chemotherapy is to minimize the risk for relapse and to allow men to avoid RPLND and the longer course of chemotherapy administered for patients who relapse on surveillance. The rationale underlying this approach derives from the 30% relapse rate seen during surveillance and the 20% to 25% risk for needing systemic chemotherapy after RPLND given either as adjuvant therapy for PS II disease or as treatment of relapse [8,9,12,41]. Primary chemotherapy offers patients the greatest chance of being relapse-free with any single treatment modality. Only limited long-term follow-up data are available, however, and there are lingering concerns about the potential risk for late chemotherapy-refractory relapses and late chemotherapy toxicity.

Primary chemotherapy has been investigated in at least nine case series and phase II trials, almost all of which have used two cycles of BEP chemotherapy (Table 4) [42]. Primary chemotherapy using two cycles of BEP has been associated with excellent outcomes in men who have early-stage, high-risk NSGCT, but only limited long-term follow-up data are available [43,44]. In such patients, it is possible to reduce the recurrence rate from 30% to 60% down to about 2.5%. Many European institutions prefer BEP×2 to RPLND [45].

The largest three trials of primary chemotherapy were conducted in the United Kingdom (UK). The Medical Research Council (MRC) prospectively evaluated 114 patients who had CS I NSGCT who were estimated to have 50% or higher risk for relapse based on having at least three MRC risk factors [43]. MRC prognostic factors had been validated in a prospective surveillance trial and included vascular invasion, lymphatic invasion, absence of yolk sac elements,

Table 4
Published reports of primary chemotherapy for clinical stage I nonseminomatous germ cell testicular cancers

Reference	Patients	Risk factors	Chemotherapy regimen	Median follow-up (months)	Number of relapses	Relapse interval (months)	Deaths from testis cancer
Abratt et al [51]	20	≥2 MRC risk factors	2 cycles BEP (E 360)	31	0	—	0
Cullen and James [42]	114	≥3 MRC risk factors	2 cycles BEP (E 360)	48	2[a]	7, 18[a]	2[b] (1.8%)
Pont et al [52]	74	LVI	2 cycles BEP (E 500)	70	2	8, 27	1 (1.4%)
Ondrus et al [49]	18	LVI	2 cycles BEP (E 360)	36	0	—	0
Amato et al [27]	68	LVI, AFP >80, >80% EC	2 cycles CEB (E 360)	38	1	21	0
Bohlen et al [44]	58	LVI, EC, pT3–4	2 cycles BEP (E 360) 2 PVB (20 pts)	93	2	22, 90	0
Chevreau et al [50]	40	LVI EC	2 cycles BEP (E 360) 2 PVB (2 pts)	113	0	—	0
Oliver et al [48]	148	≥2 MRC risk factors	1 cycle BEP (n = 28); 2 cycles BEP (46 pts) or 2 cycles BOP (n = 74) (E 360)	33	6	Not reported	7 (1.4%)
Dearnaley et al [53]	115	LVI	2 cycles BOP	70	3[c]	3, 6, 26[c]	1 (0.9%)
Pooled data	655	—	—	N/A	16 (2.4%)		7 (0.9%)

Abbreviations: AFP, α-fetoprotein; BEP, bleomycin, etoposide, cisplatin; BOP, bleomycin, vincristine, cisplatin; CEB, carboplatin, etoposide, bleomycin; E 500, etoposide dose of 500 mg/m^2/cycle; E 360, etoposide dose of 360 mg/m^2/cycle; EC, embryonal carcinoma; LVI, lymphovascular invasion; MRC, Medical Research Council; N/A, not available; PVB, cisplatin, vinblastine, bleomycin.

[a] The original testis tumor in the patient who suffered the second relapse in this study was reclassified as adenocarcinoma of the rete testis on central pathology review blinded to outcome.

[b] One death was caused by recurrent cancer and the other resulted from an ischemic stroke during chemotherapy.

[c] It is unclear whether the third relapse in this study was a true relapse; the lesion was only biopsied after salvage chemotherapy and no neoplasm was identified. We have counted it as a relapse.

and presence of embryonal carcinoma [46,47]. With 4 years median follow-up, two men (1.7%) were reported to relapse at 7 and 18 months. The Anglian Germ Cell Tumor Group studied 382 men who had intermediate- or high-risk NSGCT who underwent either surveillance (234 men) or primary chemotherapy using either two cycles of bleomycin, vincristine, and cisplatin (BOP) or one or two cycles of BEP (n = 148). After a median follow-up of 33 months, 6 chemotherapy patients (4%) relapsed, including 6.5% after one cycle of BEP, 3.6% after two cycles of BEP, and 2.7% after BOP [48]. In contrast 30% of patients assigned to observation subsequently relapsed after a median follow-up of 83 months. The introduction of adjuvant treatment for the high-risk patients made it possible to reduce the overall relapse rate of the total cohort of patients who had CS I disease from 36% to 15.7% ($P < .001$). A second trial evaluating two cycles of BOP in 115 British and Norwegian men who had an elevated risk for relapse based on the presence of vascular invasion reported three relapses (2.6%) after a median follow-up of 70 months.

Combining data from these three trials and six other published studies, a total of 655 men received primary chemotherapy (see Table 4) [27,44,49–52]. Sixteen relapses (2.4%) were documented. Six men (0.9%) died of testis cancer. Four reports including 287 subjects had a median follow-up of at least 70 months and reported 7 (2.4%) relapses and 2 (0.7%) deaths from testis cancer [44,50,53]. In these four studies, the median time to relapse was 22 months. A lingering question is whether long-term follow-up will reveal an increased rate of late relapses after primary chemotherapy because of unresected retroperitoneal teratoma, but insufficient data exist to address that question at this time. The available data suggest that primary chemotherapy is associated with much lower relapse than RPLND (2.5% compared with 6% to 30% depending on the presence of high-risk features) with no significant difference in disease-specific survival.

Adverse effects of primary chemotherapy

Almost all men who have CS I NSGCT become long-term survivors and therefore the toxicities associated with treatment represent a prominent issue. Short- and long-term side effects from BEP and other cisplatin-based germ cell tumor regimens are well documented but the vast majority of the data comes from patients who have received a minimum of three cycles of treatment. Data from men receiving two cycles of chemotherapy are sparse. Among men receiving three or more cycles of BEP or cisplatin, vinblastine, and bleomycin (PVB), Raynaud phenomenon (30%), sensory peripheral neuropathy (20%), ototoxicity (20%), long-term renal toxicity (20% reduction in creatinine clearance, persisting hypomagnesemia or hypophosphatemia) are the most commonly reported side effects [54]. Among men receiving two cycles of BEP or BOP, 8% to 19% report long-term grade I/II neurotoxicity or ototoxicity [31,48,53]. Organ function testing after two cycles of cisplatin-based chemotherapy has documented a median 5dB hearing loss at 8 kHz ($P = .008$), a 5% reduction in DLCO ($P = .03$), and a 9% decline in glomerular filtration rate ($P = .014$) [53]. The clinical significance of these changes has not been established. The impact of two cycles of BEP or BOP chemotherapy on fertility seems to be small to nonexistent, but few data are available [53].

Long-term survivors of testicular cancer who have received three or more cycles of cisplatin-based chemotherapy are at risk for cardiac events and an unfavorable cardiovascular risk profile. The major cardiovascular issues that have been studied in connection with treatment of testicular cancer include metabolic syndrome [55–57], early atherosclerosis and coronary artery disease [58–60], Raynaud phenomenon [61,62], and thromboembolic events [63]. A large British study with a median follow-up of 10.2 years reported a relative risk of 2.59 for cardiac events with cisplatin-based chemotherapy, independent of cardiac risk factors [59]. Moreover, a recently published Dutch large series in 2512 5-year survivors of testis cancer reported a 1.9-fold and 1.5-fold increased cardiovascular disease risk with PVB and BEP regimens, respectively, after a prolonged follow-up of 18.4 years [60]. Whether such complications ensue from only two cycles of chemotherapy is unknown. We have found no reports of clinically significant pulmonary toxicity following two cycles of BEP or BOP.

Germ cell tumor chemotherapy also poses a risk for secondary malignancy. An international cancer registry study of 40,576 testis cancer patients reported that 10-year survivors who had been treated with chemotherapy had an 80% increased risk for developing non–germ cell solid tumors compared with the general population. Because this study compared chemotherapy recipients to the general population rather than to testis cancer patients who did not receive chemotherapy, however, the study was unable to distinguish the extent to which the excess cancers resulted from treatment as opposed to an inherited or acquired predisposition to cancer [64]. Cisplatin and etoposide are leukemogenic and the risk is dose related. Following a typical three- or four-cycle course of BEP, the incidence of secondary leukemia is less than 0.5% [65]. The risk associated with two cycles of chemotherapy is unknown.

Long-term side effects from chemotherapy underlie much of the opposition to primary chemotherapy in the United States. Studies of men who have received three or more cycles of germ cell tumor chemotherapy have clearly demonstrated a risk for severe late complications but future studies will need to define whether two cycles of chemotherapy poses similar dangers.

Summary

CS I NSGCT can be effectively managed with surveillance, RPLND, or primary chemotherapy. Each is associated with a roughly 1% risk for death from testis cancer and no randomized trials have been conducted to evaluate whether one approach is superior. Surveillance offers 70% of patients the benefit of avoiding any postorchiectomy therapy but is associated with a higher risk for relapse and a more burdensome follow-up schedule. The ideal surveillance patients are those who do not have risk factors for relapse because they are most likely to enjoy the benefit of avoiding chemotherapy and RPLND. It must be emphasized that patient compliance with follow-up clinical assessments and imaging studies is essential to a successful surveillance strategy to detect relapses at an early and curable stage. If questions exist regarding patient compliance, patients should be recommended to receive active treatment. RPLND lowers the risk for relapse and offers patients the best chance of avoiding chemotherapy and late relapse. Although RPLND carries a small risk for acute and chronic complications, chemotherapy seems to be associated with greater risks. One limitation to RPLND is that 15% of average-risk and up to 30% of high-risk patients end up receiving chemotherapy after RPLND either for PS II disease or for subsequent relapse. The combination of RPLND followed by adjuvant chemotherapy results in the lowest relapse rate (1%) of any treatment strategy, however. Primary chemotherapy offers the benefit of the lowest relapse rate achievable with a single postorchiectomy treatment modality. This benefit must be balanced against the potential risk for late relapse with chemoresistant disease and short- and long-term chemotherapy complications, including but not limited to secondary malignancies and cardiovascular events.

At this time, none of these three approaches can be definitely labeled as superior. Given this uncertainty and the contentious disagreement over optimal management among leading experts, it is appropriate for patients to be informed of all three options. We believe that surveillance is preferable for low-risk patients and that RPLND is supported by a larger body of long-term follow-up survival data compared with primary chemotherapy. Primary chemotherapy is best reserved for patients refusing RPLND and surveillance and for high-risk patients who do not have access to surgeons who have extensive experience performing RPLND.

References

[1] Sheinfeld J. Nonseminomatous germ cell tumors of the testis: current concepts and controversies. Urology 1994;44(1):2–14.

[2] Donohue JP, Zachary JM, Maynard BR. Distribution of nodal metastases in nonseminomatous testis cancer. J Urol 1982;128:315–20.

[3] Leibovitch L, Foster RS, Kopecky KK, et al. Improved accuracy of computerized tomography based clinical staging in low stage nonseminomatous germ cell cancer using size criteria of retroperitoneal lymph nodes. J Urol 1995;154(5):1759–63.

[4] Hilton S, Herr HW, Teitcher JB, et al. CT detection of retroperitoneal lymph node metastases in patients with clinical stage I testicular nonseminomatous germ cell cancer: assessment of size and distribution criteria. AJR Am J Roentgenol 1997;169(2):521–5.

[5] Albers P, Siener R, Kliesch S, et al. Risk factors for relapse in clinical stage I nonseminomatous testicular germ cell tumors: results of the German Testicular Cancer Study Group Trial. J Clin Oncol 2003;21(8):1505–12.

[6] Alexandre J, Fizazi K, Mahe C, et al. Stage I nonseminomatous germ-cell tumours of the testis: identification of a subgroup of patients with a very low risk of relapse. Eur J Cancer 2001;37(5):576–82.

[7] Heidenreich A, Sesterhenn IA, Mostofi FK, et al. Prognostic risk factors that identify patients with clinical stage I nonseminomatous germ cell tumors at low risk and high risk for metastasis. Cancer 1998;83(5):1002–11.

[8] Hermans BP, Sweeney CJ, Foster RS, et al. Risk of systemic metastases in clinical stage I nonseminoma germ cell testis tumor managed by retroperitoneal lymph node dissection. J Urol 2000;163(6):1721–4.

[9] Nicolai N, Miceli R, Artusi R, et al. A simple model for predicting nodal metastasis in patients with clinical stage I nonseminomatous germ cell testicular tumors undergoing retroperitoneal lymph node dissection only. J Urol 2004;171(1):172–6.

[10] Roeleveld TA, Horenblas S, Meinhardt W, et al. Surveillance can be the standard of care for stage I nonseminomatous testicular tumors and even high risk patients. J Urol 2001;166(6):2166–70.
[11] Sogani PC, Perrotti M, Herr HW, et al. Clinical stage I testis cancer: long-term outcome of patients on surveillance. J Urol 1998;159(3):855–8.
[12] Stephenson AJ, Bosl GJ, Motzer RJ, et al. Retroperitoneal lymph node dissection for nonseminomatous germ cell testicular cancer: impact of patient selection factors on outcome. J Clin Oncol 2005;23(12):2781–8.
[13] Sweeney CJ, Hermans BP, Heilman DK, et al. Results and outcome of retroperitoneal lymph node dissection for clinical stage I embryonal carcinoma–predominant testis cancer. J Clin Oncol 2000;18(2):358–62.
[14] Vergouwe Y, Steyerberg EW, Eijkemans MJ, et al. Predictors of occult metastasis in clinical stage I nonseminoma: a systematic review. J Clin Oncol 2003;21(22):4092–9.
[15] Leibovitch I, Foster RS, Kopecky KK, et al. Identification of clinical stage A nonseminomatous testis cancer patients at extremely low risk for metastatic disease: a combined approach using quantitative immunohistochemical, histopathologic, and radiologic assessment. J Clin Oncol 1998;16(1):261–8.
[16] Colls BM, Harvey VJ, Skelton L, et al. Late results of surveillance of clinical stage I nonseminoma germ cell testicular tumours: 17 years' experience in a national study in New Zealand. BJU Int 1999;83(1):76–82.
[17] Francis R, Bower M, Brunstrom G, et al. Surveillance for stage I testicular germ cell tumours: results and cost benefit analysis of management options. Eur J Cancer 2000;36(15):1925–32.
[18] Gels ME, Hoekstra HJ, Sleijfer DT, et al. Detection of recurrence in patients with clinical stage I nonseminomatous testicular germ cell tumors and consequences for further follow-up: a single-center 10-year experience. J Clin Oncol 1995;13(5):1188–94.
[19] Sharir S, Jewett MA, Sturgeon JF, et al. Progression detection of stage I nonseminomatous testis cancer on surveillance: implications for the followup protocol. J Urol 1999;161(2):472–5 [discussion: 5–6].
[20] Daugaard G, Petersen PM, Rorth M. Surveillance in stage I testicular cancer. APMIS 2003;111(1):76–85.
[21] Hao D, Seidel J, Brant R, et al. Compliance of clinical stage I nonseminomatous germ cell tumor patients with surveillance. J Urol 1998;160(3 Pt 1):768–71.
[22] Foster RS, Baniel J, Leibovitch I, et al. Teratoma in the orchiectomy specimen and volume of metastasis are predictors of retroperitoneal teratoma in low stage nonseminomatous testis cancer. J Urol 1996;155(6):1943–5.
[23] Sheinfeld J, Motzer RJ, Rabbani F, et al. Incidence and clinical outcome of patients with teratoma in the retroperitoneum following primary retroperitoneal lymph node dissection for clinical stages I and IIA nonseminomatous germ cell tumors. J Urol 2003;170(4 Pt 1):1159–62.
[24] Toner GC, Panicek DM, Heelan RT, et al. Adjunctive surgery after chemotherapy for nonseminomatous germ cell tumors: recommendations for patient selection. J Clin Oncol 1990;8(10):1683–94.
[25] Donohue JP, Foster RS. Retroperitoneal lymphadenectomy in staging and treatment. The development of nerve-sparing techniques. Urol Clin North Am 1998;25(3):461–8.
[26] Donohue JP, Thornhill JA, Foster RS, et al. Primary retroperitoneal lymph node dissection in clinical stage A non-seminomatous germ cell testis cancer. Review of the Indiana University experience 1965–1989. Br J Urol 1993;71(3):326–35.
[27] Amato RJ, Ro JY, Ayala AG, et al. Risk-adapted treatment for patients with clinical stage I nonseminomatous germ cell tumor of the testis. Urology 2004;63(1):144–8 [discussion: 8–9].
[28] Williams SD, Stablein DM, Einhorn LH, et al. Immediate adjuvant chemotherapy versus observation with treatment at relapse in pathological stage II testicular cancer. N Engl J Med 1987;317(23):1433–8.
[29] Donohue JP, Thornhill JA, Foster RS, et al. Clinical stage B non-seminomatous germ cell testis cancer: the Indiana University experience (1965–1989) using routine primary retroperitoneal lymph node dissection. Eur J Cancer 1995;31A(10):1599–604.
[30] Socinski MA, Garnick MB, Stomper PC, et al. Stage II nonseminomatous germ cell tumors of the testis: an analysis of treatment options in patients with low volume retroperitoneal disease. J Urol 1988;140(6):1437–41.
[31] Kondagunta GV, Sheinfeld J, Mazumdar M, et al. Relapse-free and overall survival in patients with pathologic stage II nonseminomatous germ cell cancer treated with etoposide and cisplatin adjuvant chemotherapy. J Clin Oncol 2004;22(3):464–7.
[32] Behnia M, Foster R, Einhorn LH, et al. Adjuvant bleomycin, etoposide and cisplatin in pathological stage II non-seminomatous testicular cancer. The Indiana University experience [see comment]. Eur J Cancer 2000;36(4):472–5.
[33] Baniel J, Foster RS, Rowland RG, et al. Complications of primary retroperitoneal lymph node dissection. J Urol 1994;152(2 Pt 1):424–7.
[34] McLeod DG, Weiss RB, Stablein DM, et al. Staging relationships and outcome in early stage testicular cancer: a report from the Testicular Cancer Intergroup Study. J Urol 1991;145(6):1178–83 [discussion: 82–3].
[35] Richie JP. Clinical stage 1 testicular cancer: the role of modified retroperitoneal lymphadenectomy. J Urol 1990;144(5):1160–3.
[36] Jewett MA. Nerve-sparing technique for retroperitoneal lymphadenectomy in testis cancer. Urol Clin North Am 1990;17(2):449–56.
[37] Bhayani SB, Ong A, Oh WK, et al. Laparoscopic retroperitoneal lymph node dissection for clinical stage I nonseminomatous germ cell testicular cancer: a long-term update. Urology 2003;62(2):324–7.

[38] Janetschek G, Hobisch A, Peschel R, et al. Laparoscopic retroperitoneal lymph node dissection for clinical stage I nonseminomatous testicular carcinoma: long-term outcome. J Urol 2000;163(6):1793–6.
[39] Nelson JB, Chen RN, Bishoff JT, et al. Laparoscopic retroperitoneal lymph node dissection for clinical stage I nonseminomatous germ cell testicular tumors. Urology 1999;54(6):1064–7.
[40] Janetschek G. Laparoscopic retroperitoneal lymph node dissection. Urol Clin North Am 2001;28(1): 107–14.
[41] Donohue JP, Thornhill JA, Foster RS, et al. Retroperitoneal lymphadenectomy for clinical stage A testis cancer (1965 to 1989): modifications of technique and impact on ejaculation. J Urol 1993;149(2): 237–43.
[42] Cullen M, James N. Adjuvant therapy for stage I testicular cancer. Cancer Treat Rev 1996;22(4):253–64.
[43] Cullen MH, Stenning SP, Parkinson MC, et al. Short-course adjuvant chemotherapy in high-risk stage I nonseminomatous germ cell tumors of the testis: a Medical Research Council report. J Clin Oncol 1996;14(4):1106–13.
[44] Bohlen D, Borner M, Sonntag RW, et al. Long-term results following adjuvant chemotherapy in patients with clinical stage I testicular nonseminomatous malignant germ cell tumors with high risk factors. J Urol 1999;161(4):1148–52.
[45] Schmoll HJ, Souchon R, Krege S, et al. European consensus on diagnosis and treatment of germ cell cancer: a report of the European Germ Cell Cancer Consensus Group (EGCCCG). Ann Oncol 2004; 15(9):1377–99.
[46] Read G, Stenning SP, Cullen MH, et al. Medical Research Council prospective study of surveillance for stage I testicular teratoma. J Clin Oncol 1992;10(11): 1762–8.
[47] Freedman LS, Parkinson MC, Jones WG, et al. Histopathology in the prediction of relapse of patients with stage I testicular teratoma treated by orchidectomy alone. Lancet 1987;2(8554):294–8.
[48] Oliver RT, Ong J, Shamash J, et al. Long-term follow-up of Anglian Germ Cell Cancer Group surveillance versus patients with Stage 1 nonseminoma treated with adjuvant chemotherapy. Urology 2004; 63(3):556–61.
[49] Ondrus D, Matoska J, Belan V, et al. Prognostic factors in clinical stage I nonseminomatous germ cell testicular tumors: rationale for different risk-adapted treatment. Eur Urol 1998;33(6):562–6.
[50] Chevreau C, Mazerolles C, Soulie M, et al. Long-term efficacy of two cycles of BEP regimen in high-risk stage I nonseminomatous testicular germ cell tumors with embryonal carcinoma and/or vascular invasion. Eur Urol 2004;46(2):209–14 [discussion: 14–5].
[51] Abratt RP, Pontin AR, Barnes RD, et al. Adjuvant chemotherapy for stage I non-seminomatous testicular cancer. S Afr Med J 1994;84(9):605–7.
[52] Pont J, De Santis M, Albrecht W, et al. Risk-adapted management for clinical stage I nonseminomatous germ cell cancer of the testis (NSGCT I) by regarding vascular invasion (VI): A-17 year experience from the Vienna Testicular Tumor Study Group. Proceedings of the American Society of Clinical Oncology 2003;22:388.
[53] Dearnaley DP, Fossa SD, Kaye SB, et al. Adjuvant bleomycin, vincristine and cisplatin (BOP) for high-risk stage I non-seminomatous germ cell tumours: a prospective trial (MRC TE17). Br J Cancer 2005; 92(12):2107–13.
[54] Kollmannsberger C, Kuzcyk M, Mayer F, et al. Late toxicity following curative treatment of testicular cancer. Semin Surg Oncol 1999;17(4):275–81.
[55] Nuver J, Smit AJ, Wolffenbuttel BHR, et al. The metabolic syndrome and disturbances in hormone levels in long-term survivors of disseminated testicular cancer [see comment]. J Clin Oncol 2005;23(16): 3718–25.
[56] Raghavan D, Cox K, Childs A, et al. Hypercholesterolemia after chemotherapy for testis cancer. J Clin Oncol 1992;10(9):1386–9.
[57] Bokemeyer C, Berger CC, Kuczyk MA, et al. Evaluation of long-term toxicity after chemotherapy for testicular cancer. J Clin Oncol 1996;14(11): 2923–32.
[58] Meinardi MT, Gietema JA, van der Graaf WT, et al. Cardiovascular morbidity in long-term survivors of metastatic testicular cancer. J Clin Oncol 2000; 18(8):1725–32.
[59] Huddart RA, Norman A, Shahidi M, et al. Cardiovascular disease as a long-term complication of treatment for testicular cancer. J Clin Oncol 2003; 21(8):1513–23.
[60] van den Belt-Dusebout AW, Nuver J, de Wit R, et al. Long-term risk of cardiovascular disease in 5-year survivors of testicular cancer. J Clin Oncol 2006; 24(3):467–75.
[61] Berger CC, Bokemeyer C, Schneider M, et al. Secondary Raynaud's phenomenon and other late vascular complications following chemotherapy for testicular cancer. Eur J Cancer 1995;31A(13–14): 2229–38.
[62] Vogelzang NJ, Bosl GJ, Johnson K, et al. Raynaud's phenomenon: a common toxicity after combination chemotherapy for testicular cancer. Ann Intern Med 1981;95(3):288–92.
[63] Weijl NI, Rutten MF, Zwinderman AH, et al. Thromboembolic events during chemotherapy for germ cell cancer: a cohort study and review of the literature. J Clin Oncol 2000;18(10):2169–78.
[64] Travis LB, Fossa SD, Schonfeld SJ, et al. Second cancers among 40,576 testicular cancer patients: focus on long-term survivors. J Natl Cancer Inst 2005;97(18):1354–65.
[65] Travis LB, Andersson M, Gospodarowicz M, et al. Treatment-associated leukemia following testicular cancer. J Natl Cancer Inst 2000;92(14):1165–71.

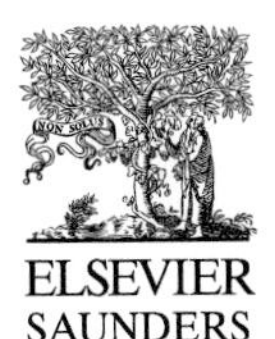
ELSEVIER
SAUNDERS

Urol Clin N Am 34 (2007) 149–158

UROLOGIC CLINICS of North America

Nerve-Sparing Retroperitoneal Lymphadenectomy

Michael A.S. Jewett, MD[a,*], Ryan J. Groll, MD[b]

[a]*Division of Urology, Department of Surgical Oncology, Princess Margaret Hospital and the University Health Network, 610 University Avenue, 3-124, Toronto, ON, Canada M5G 2C4*

[b]*Division of Urology, Department of Surgery, University of Toronto, Toronto, Ontario, Canada*

Retroperitoneal lymphadenectomy (RPL) for testicular cancer has been performed since the late 1940s [1], well before any chemotherapy was available. It was clear that patients with regional metastases could be cured. With the introduction of cisplatinum-based chemotherapy in the 1970s, the procedure was increasingly used for staging and adjuvant chemotherapy was used when the nodes removed contained metastatic tumor. More recently, patients with minimal nodal disease have been followed with salvage therapy for relapse. The trend has been to minimize morbidity while maintaining efficacy.

Historically, the major long-term morbidity of RPL was ejaculatory dysfunction and potential infertility resulting from damage to the sympathetic nerves during dissection. Specifically, injuring the lumbar sympathetic trunks, postganglionic sympathetic fibers, and/or nerves of the hypogastric plexus risked loss of seminal emission and consequently dry ejaculation. The traditional bilateral lymphadenectomy results demonstrated a 70% to 100% risk of this complication [2]. The movement to include suprahilar dissection was short lived and this approach was abandoned when no added benefit was realized [3]. The original procedures have since been further modified such that the minimal dissection is performed to spare relevant sympathetic nerves without risking an incomplete cancer resection. The initial strategy for minimizing postoperative ejaculatory dysfunction attributable to sympathetic nerve injury was the downscaling of dissection boundaries and development of unilateral resection templates so as to avoid contralateral dissection mainly in the area of the hypogastric plexus [4]. The basis for modified templates was a greater confidence in salvage results with the emergence of effective chemotherapeutic agents coupled with an improved understanding of the metastatic pattern and distribution of germ-cell tumors from surgical mapping studies [5–7]. While template surgery improved ejaculation rates in the order of 51% to 88% [8–10], success rates were increased significantly by the development of nerve-sparing techniques, referring specifically to the prospective identification, careful dissection, and preservation of relevant sympathetic nerves [11]. Nerve-sparing approaches have been adopted in other oncological surgical procedures (such as radical retropubic prostatectomy [12], radical cystectomy [13], radical hysterectomy [14], and total mesorectal excision [15], as well as retroperitoneal lymphadenectomy [11,16]) where complications related to intraoperative injury to nervous structures occur.

Currently, nerve-sparing techniques, applied to either bilateral lymphadenectomy or in conjunction with unilateral template dissections, offer carefully selected patients excellent antegrade ejaculation rates without an apparent higher risk of disease relapse.

Anatomy and neurophysiology of antegrade ejaculation

Normal antegrade ejaculation is the coordinated physiologic process involving sequential phases of seminal emission and bladder neck closure followed by expulsion of semen by

* Corresponding author.
E-mail address: m.jewett@utoronto.ca (M.A.S. Jewett).

0094-0143/07/$ - see front matter
doi:10.1016/j.ucl.2007.02.014

rhythmic contraction of the bulbocavernosus and ischiocavernosus muscles. The emission phase is under autonomic sympathetic control with afferent impulses transmitted via the pudendal nerve. Efferent impulses originate in the preganglionic fibers from T10 to L2, synapse in the ganglia of the lumbar sympathetic trunks, and exit via L1 to L4 postganglionic fibers, which decussate along the aorta bilaterally to form the hypogastric plexus. Terminal nerves from the pelvic plexus evoke seminal emission innervating the seminal vesicles, vas deferens, prostate, and bladder neck. From the surgeon's perspective, identification and careful preservation of the lumbar sympathetic trunks, the postganglionic fibers particularly at the L2 to L4 level, and the nerves of the hypogastric plexus are the objectives of the nerve-sparing approach. Dieckmann and colleagues [17] described an intraoperative test for identifying relevant lumbar sympathetic nerve fibers using direct electrostimulation. During open RPL, electrostimulation was applied to L1 to L3 sympathetic fibers while intraoperative ejaculation was observed and reproduced. These studies identified the predominance of the right-sided nerves, which are usually more prominent and easily preserved.

Anatomically, the sympathetic trunks are chains of interconnected ganglia that course between the medial aspect of the psoas major and the vertebral column in the retroperitoneum. The right sympathetic chain is situated posterior to the middle of the inferior vena cava (IVC) and the left chain is located posterolateral to the abdominal aorta with transverse rami connecting the two trunks. While they appear asymmetric to the great vessels, they are aligned with the embryonic vascular tree before regression of the left-sided venous system. Similarly, the lymphatic drainage of the testes appears asymmetric in the adult, but in both cases, if one considers the midline as the aorta, the sympathetic system as well as the vascular and lymphatic anatomy is "similar" bilaterally. The sympathetic chains are often intimately involved with lumbar vessels and the number, size, and position of paravertebral ganglia are variable. Colleselli and colleagues [18] demonstrated in a cadaver anatomical study that the L2 and L3 ganglia are close to each other and often fused. Anterior to the aortic bifurcation and extending inferiorly on the anterior surface of the fifth lumbar vertebra is the superior hypogastric plexus, which is contiguous with the inferior hypogastric plexus and pelvic plexuses connected by the right and left hypogastric nerves, which are readily identified. It is less clear if significant nerves course to the inferior plexus along the inferior mesenteric artery, which may be skeletonized or divided during lymphadenectomy.

Indications for nerve-sparing retroperitoneal lymphadenectomy

Clinical stage I nonseminomatous germ-cell tumors

Management options for Stage I nonseminomatous germ-cell tumors (NSGCTs) include surveillance, adjuvant chemotherapy, and RPL. The strategy is risk adapted depending on prognostic features, primarily the presence or absence of vascular invasion of the primary tumor. The overall relapse rate of clinical Stage I NSGCTs managed with surveillance is between 27% and 30%, but the long-term disease-free rate with chemotherapy following progression is virtually 100% [19]. Increasingly, active surveillance with delayed treatment for relapse is being recommended for low-risk cases and primary chemotherapy for high-risk cases, respectively. Primary surgery for low-risk disease subjects all patients to initial surgery and a few to subsequent chemotherapy for a stage of disease associated with an overall progression rate of 10% to 15% with modern imaging [20]. Conversely, the risk of progression without treatment in the high-risk group may be as high as 80% depending on the definition of high risk, and surgery alone may not be curative. Combination therapy with surgery and chemotherapy is therefore frequent with a high overall burden of treatment. Therefore, in many parts of the world, standard practice is surveillance or adjuvant chemotherapy after orchiectomy depending on local definition of risk and experienced rates of relapse of risk [21]. If surgery is performed, nerve sparing should be performed. It is unusual to encounter macroscopic disease in the face of negative imaging that precludes at least unilateral nerve preservation. If small-volume microscopic disease is discovered and a complete lymphadenectomy has been performed (the usual case), ongoing surveillance instead of routine adjuvant chemotherapy is an option.

Clinical stage II NSGCT

Management decisions for Stage II NSGCT depend primarily on the extent and size of the imaged retroperitoneal nodal metastases and the levels of peri-orchiectomy tumor markers [21]. For Stage IIA (mass/nodes ≤ 2 cm bidimensionally on CT), marker-negative disease, primary nerve-sparing RPL is often performed, as false-positive staging is rare today. For Stage IIA marker-positive disease, Stage IIB (mass/nodes 2–5 cm), or Stage IIC (mass/nodes > 5 cm), adjuvant chemotherapy is the usual standard of care. Reports do not always indicate the timing of preoperative markers, which should be allowed to decay after orchiectomy to find the level attributable to metastatic disease alone. As well, the vertical or Z-axis of the retroperitoneal nodes are not reported or recorded. Ovoid nodal masses may represent a significantly larger tumor burden than a relatively spherical node with similar cross-sectional bidimensional measurements. There may be a role for primary surgery in patients with relatively low but elevated markers and a small burden of nodal disease. Nerve sparing is feasible in more than 50% of Stage II cases.

Postchemotherapy residual disease

In the absence of marker elevation, RPL is indicated for residual tumor postchemotherapy in NSGCT and, occasionally, seminoma. Although the majority of residual masses contain necrosis/fibrosis or teratoma, the accuracy of preoperative prognostic factors is relatively low for necrosis/fibrosis alone. Untreated teratoma may be associated with occult cancer or growing teratoma syndrome that is extremely difficult to resect later. Finally, there is ongoing controversy about the need to resect organs that are adherent to tumor masses. It is increasingly rare to perform nephrectomy or other similar procedures despite large masses. Nerve sparing should be attempted if it does not compromise complete resection and is frequently feasible on at least one side. There is ongoing controversy regarding the need for postchemotherapy surgery when the retroperitoneum is normal on imaging. If prechemotherapy disease was imaged, some centers recommend surgery as microscopic teratoma is frequently found that may be the source of late relapse. Most centers recommend ongoing observation, as it is rare to discover active cancer in this type of case.

Surgical technique

Exposure

With the patient supine, we use a midline abdominal incision with a transperitoneal approach. The thoracoabdominal approach is a rarely performed alternative, particularly with early-stage left-sided tumors, when the planned extent of lymphadenectomy is limited to the left para-aortic and interaortocaval nodal areas.

The incision is made from the top of the xiphoid process down to the mid-lower abdomen going around the left side of the umbilicus. With retraction, the superior end of the skin incision is pulled inferiorly, which will restrict reflection of the root of the mesentery subsequently if the initial incision is not made high. The falciform ligament may be divided if there is concern about stretch injury intraoperatively. Laparotomy is then carefully performed to confirm the extent of retroperitoneal disease and to rule out other pathology, particularly in the mesentery or loops of the small bowel, which may not be imaged as accurately. The small bowel and right colon are then mobilized on their vascular attachments following a relatively avascular plane anterior to the perinephric fascia, the spermatic vessels and the retroperitoneal nodal areas using lower power cautery or sharp combined with blunt dissection. Headlamps and loop magnification are useful. The hepatic flexure can be taken down, although this may not be necessary. Care must be taken to identify the right ureter during mobilization of the colon, and the rest of the small bowel mesentery is incised cephalad to the ligament of Treitz. A vessel loop may be passed around the ureter to ensure later localization. Lymphatics that are encountered, particularly at the level of the superior border of the left renal vein, should be ligated before division to reduce the risk of chylous ascites postoperatively. The inferior mesenteric vein may be divided with its adjacent artery to allow rotation of the pancreas superiorly for better access to the retroperitoneum in the obese patient. At this point the inferior mesenteric artery is not divided. The small bowel and the right colon are then placed into a bowel bag and rotated superiorly out of the abdomen onto the chest. The center of rotation is the superior mesenteric artery, which can be easily palpated at the upper limit of dissection. Care should be taken to apply retractors lateral to this midline structure to minimize compression of venous and lymphatic drainage. The left colon may be reflected medially but this is not usually necessary. The amount of mesenteric and omental fat plus the costal angles will determine the amount of exposure, which is usually more than adequate. The operative time will in part be dictated by the exposure as well as extent of disease so it is useful to spend time on full mobilization of the bowel. An alternative approach to full mobilization as described above, is mobilization of one or both hemicolons medially. This is usually done if template surgery is planned and is faster. With the retroperitoneum now fully exposed, the limits of dissection can be defined.

Procedure

We routinely perform a bilateral lymphadenectomy with the following limits:

1. Laterally—To the ureters extending up medial to the renal hila to meet the superior limit. The distinctive yellow fat color of the renal hilum is a good landmark.
2. Superiorly—The inferior border of the superior mesenteric artery extended bilaterally at the level of the upper edge of the origin of the renal arteries. Tissue superiorly is usually pulled down during dissection including any gross disease so that, in effect, a suprahilar dissection is performed although not as formally as previously described [22].
3. Inferiorly—To at least the bifurcation of the ipsilateral common iliac arteries including the bifurcation of the aorta and inferior vena cava (IVC). Contralaterally, it is usually easier to go as far as the point that the ureter crossed the iliac vessels but this can be variable and may go to the bifurcation of the common iliac artery. The tissue inferior to the aortic bifurcation anterior to the left common iliac vein is not routinely resected as this increases the risk of nerve injury as well and venous damage, which may be difficult to repair without significant blood loss.
4. Posteriorly—The anterior spinal ligament and psoas muscle fascia. If tumor is adherent to the fascia, it is useful to dissect along the muscle fibers under the fascia, which provides an alternative plane. Lumbar vessels are preserved if possible to reduce postoperative back pain in the perioperative period.

The dissection is usually begun by incising the retroperitoneal tissue along the medial border of the IVC and inferior border of the left renal vein. The left side of the cava is exposed from the left renal vein to its origin at the left common iliac vein by peeling the adipose and lymphatic tissue medially, taking care to cauterize but usually ligate small vessels. Clips often are avulsed during retraction and are avoided. The IVC is then rolled laterally to the right with ligation and division of the left lumbar veins as required but are markers for the nerve origins. The right sympathetic chain lies posterior to the midline of the cava and can be located by following the postganglionic nerve fibers behind the IVC from the ligated proximal ends of the lumbar veins. At this point, the surgeon has a sense of the individual patient's sympathetic anatomy, which is variable. This is more apparent in slim patients. Obese patients are clearly more challenging and some oozing of blood from small vessels is inevitable but is accepted for adequate nerve identification and sparing. The aorta can now be exposed in the midline by mobilizing the left renal vein and by splitting the soft tissue over it. This has been described as the "split-and-roll" technique [22]. It is feasible even if there are enlarged nodes or masses. Dissection is carried close to the aorta. Small vessels can be encountered but are easily controlled by light cautery or suture.

Attention is then turned to the left side. The left ureter is visualized by creating a plane across the midline anterior to the retroperitoneal lymphatic tissue but behind the inferior mesenteric artery under the sigmoid mesocolon. This dissection may rarely require division of the inferior mesenteric artery, but it should be several centimeters distal to its origin and done bluntly to avoid vessels. Through the window under the sigmoid mesocolon, the left ureter can be visualized and mobilized laterally to the level of the left renal hilum. Alternatively, the left colon can be reflected medially. When the perinephric tissue is reflected laterally, the left psoas muscle can be visualized leaving the left para-aortic retroperitoneal adipose tissue containing the lymph nodes intact. This bulk of tissue is reflected medially to expose the left sympathetic chain. Gentle dissection with a pledget will help. The lumbar vessels on the left are also identified with this dissection as they course directly medially past the sympathetic chain. Again, as with the right-sided vessels, they occasionally are lateral to or bifurcate around the chain. These vessels can be sacrificed as needed. The first lumbar vein may drain into the posterior side of the left renal vein and can be injured in this dissection with bleeding. The lumbar sympathetic nerves are identified originating from the sympathetic ganglia coursing medially and anteriorly. Superiorly, there may be a branch anterior to the renal artery coming from a higher ganglion, but this may be difficult to preserve.

Accessory renal vessels may complicate the dissection but should be preserved. As each artery is exposed, topical papaverine should be applied to reduce spasm and the risk of thrombosis.

The individual sympathetic nerve branches, having been identified at their origins on both right and left sides, are seen on the anterior and lateral surfaces of the aorta just above its bifurcation. They are skeletonized as they form variable plexuses on the anterior aorta, which in turn become recognizable as the hypogastric nerves at the aortic bifurcation. This allows withdrawal of the interaortocaval lymphatic tissue and the left para-aortic tissue from between the anterior spinal ligament posteriorly and the nerves anteriorly. Identification and preservation of the two hypogastric nerves that pass over the aorta and proceed inferiorly into the pelvis allows all lymphatic tissue over the aortic bifurcation and common iliac veins down to the sacral promontory to be removed without sacrificing antegrade ejaculation. Experience is necessary to dissect what may be very fine nerves out of the adipose tissue that contains nodal tissue as well. While it does not appear necessary to spare every nerve, particularly those on the left, every attempt to spare as many as possible should be made.

The remnant of the ipsilateral spermatic cord is removed with part of the vas deferens and the spermatic vessels to their attachments in the retroperitoneum. Frequently, nodal metastases or tumor masses are immediately adjacent to or involve nerves. The surgeon should never spare nerves at the expense of an incomplete cancer resection. Moreover, it is often not necessary to preserve all postganglionic nerves to ensure antegrade ejaculation.

The retroperitoneum defined by the selected surgical margins should now be clear of all lymphatic and fatty tissue surrounding the great vessels, with the postganglionic sympathetic nerves remaining beside and on the aorta. The contents of the bowel bag are placed back into the abdomen, and the large and small bowel peritoneal reflections are closed in their normal relationships using a running absorbable suture or allowed to lie in close approximation. The abdominal incision is closed using a running #1 polyglycolic suture and interrupted figure-of-eight sutures. Drains are not routinely used. Skin may be closed with subcuticular sutures.

Postchemotherapy procedure

Patients with residual retroperitoneal disease postchemotherapy pose particular problems for the surgeon. The potentially extensive nature of the tumor may occasionally require nephrectomy en bloc, resection of part or the entire aorta, and even resection of the inferior vena cava; however, these are rare in our hands. Small lacerations or punctures of the great vessels may occur and require suturing with fine #5-0 monofilament. A full bilateral dissection remains the procedure of choice, although many patients appear to have a localized mass. Some centers advocate "lumpectomy" rather than a more extensive dissection, but this controversy is not resolved. Recently, we retrospectively reviewed the pathology of 100 postchemotherapy RPL specimens from patients with residual masses [23]. Full bilateral nerve-sparing RPL was performed in all cases; however, pathologists analyzed and recorded findings for what would have been "lumpectomy" resection of gross disease and grossly normal adjacent nodal tissue separately. In 18% of cases, grossly "normal" tissue was positive for metastatic disease (2 carcinoma, 1 seminoma, 17 teratoma), suggesting that lumpectomy in these patients would have resulted in incomplete resection.

The approach and limits of dissection are similar. Nerve sparing is still possible in at least 50% of these patients if the mass(es) is confined. The areas of greatest challenge are at the points where the masses adhere to the great vessels. A combination of sharp and blunt dissection is required with good proximal and distal control where the vessels are normal. The actual plane of dissection may appear to be under the adventitia. Because of tumor neovascularization, the locations of small vessels are difficult to predict. Distortion of normal anatomy and the frequent anomalies of retroperitoneal vessels can be challenging. Comfort with normal retroperitoneal anatomy is mandatory, and this operation requires experienced surgeons. As well, sudden blood loss may occur, so patients need close monitoring intraoperatively by an experienced anesthetist. Finally, intraoperative biopsy can be misleading and is not recommended for treatment decisions.

Template procedures

For the grossly normal retroperitoneum, some surgeons prefer to remove a template of nodes [24]. This has become more controversial as there is a swing back to bilateral lymphadenectomy for all patients, in part because an increasing percentage of cases are done after chemotherapy. Nerves are identified within the template and preserved. Surgical time is shorter and if adjuvant chemotherapy is recommended for all cases with nodal metastases, the dissection may not have to be as thorough.

For right-sided tumors, the template would include left para-aortic nodes medial to the ureter from the upper border of the renal vessels to the level of the inferior mesenteric artery below, all the inter-aortocaval nodes, the precaval and paracaval nodes, and the right common iliac nodes down to the right ureter. The sympathetic nerves can be identified and preserved within the template. It is likely that if the sympathetic chain is preserved on the left, the lower postganglionic fibers may be out of the dissected area so that antegrade ejaculation is more likely to be preserved even if nerve injury occurs within the lymphadenectomy zones. For left-sided tumors, dissection includes the same left para-aortic nodes from the renal vein to the bifurcation of the common iliac medial to the left ureter and the interaortocaval nodes from the level of the left renal vein to the inferior mesenteric artery. These limits will include the primary landing sites for nodal metastases but microscopic metastases can occur in the interaortocaval nodes so these may be removed as well. Postganglionic sympathetic nerves important for emission may be injured in this area, so dissection should include nerve identification and preservation. Any suspicious node outside these boundaries should be biopsied and, if positive, a bilateral dissection performed.

In the presence of grossly involved nodes, left para-aortic nodal involvement has been reported in up to 17%, and left iliac in up to 7% that will be missed with the template [25]. Two percent of patients might have a suprahilar node in the interaortocaval region, but that might well be grossly recognized and removed. It would seem reasonable, therefore, to omit this region for this stage of disease. It has been recommended that if one of the grossly enlarged nodes is greater than 2 cm in diameter but smaller than 5 cm, or if there are more than five nodes, a full bilateral RPL should be done. There will be no significant additional patient morbidity if more dissection is performed unless the additional dissection involves dividing further lumbar arteries.

Results

Primary nerve-sparing RPL

Early results from prospective nerve-sparing RPL data were promising in terms of both ejaculation and recurrence rates. We demonstrated that bilateral nerve identification and sparing RPL resulted in return of normal ejaculation in 90% to 97% of patients and that the number of nerves spared did not necessarily correlate with positive results [11,26]. This encouraging decrease in morbidity was not associated with retroperitoneal recurrences at 18-month follow-up. Before this report, most patients became infertile as a result of nerve damage and loss of antegrade ejaculation. Subsequently, DeBruin and colleagues [27] reported 86% and 95% 12-month antegrade ejaculation rates in clinical Stage I NSGCT patients who underwent bilateral and unilateral nerve-sparing RPL, respectively. Finally, the largest cohort reported is from the Indiana group, whose data span the evolution of RPL template modification and the adoption of prospective nerve-sparing techniques [16]. Of 2200 cases, 483 had primary nerve-sparing RPLs for clinical Stage I disease. All patients surveyed in this sample report normal ejaculation and 84% of those who have attempted pregnancy have been successful. Twenty-six percent of cases were upgraded to pathologic Stage II and the reported survival rate was 99.6%.

The German Testicular Cancer Study Group reported complications of primary nerve-sparing RPL for clinical Stage I NSGCT in 239 patients operated in a relatively large number of centers. Modified unilateral templates were used in 88.2% of cases and full bilateral RPLs in 11.8%. There was no statistically significant difference in complication rate between unilateral and bilateral procedures. Overall, minor complications such as wound infection, ileus, and lymphocele occurred in 19.7% and major complications such as chylous ascites, pulmonary embolism, and hydronephrosis occurred in 5.4% of cases. There was a 93.3% antegrade ejaculation rate but a 5.8% disease recurrence rate including three in the retroperitoneum.

Overall, the results of primary nerve-sparing RPL for low-stage NSGCT demonstrate a high rate of ejaculatory preservation and acceptable fertility with relatively few significant complications and recurrences. Results are similar for unilateral and bilateral procedures.

Postchemotherapy nerve-sparing RPL

The more challenging nature of postchemotherapy surgery prevents nerve sparing in some cases and may be associated with a slightly higher morbidity when nerve sparing is performed. Wahle and colleagues [28] reported an antegrade ejaculation rate of 89.5% and no retroperitoneal recurrences in their series of 38 postchemotherapy cases after 12-month follow-up. Full bilateral dissections were performed in 31 patients and 6 had masses greater than 6 cm in maximum diameter. In a larger cohort, Donohue and colleagues [8] report on 93 postchemotherapy RPLs in which prospective nerve-sparing techniques were used. After 2 patients died from extraperitoneal metastatic disease and 10 were lost to follow-up, the Indiana group demonstrates no retroperitoneal recurrences and 77% self-reported normal ejaculation in 81 patients with adequate follow-up. Furthermore, 11 patients have achieved pregnancy and 8 had uneventful full-term delivery. In another large series, Coogan and colleagues [29] reported results for 81 postchemotherapy nerve-sparing RPLs with a mean residual tumor size of 6.3 cm by CT scan. Antegrade ejaculation rates were 74%, 85%, and 100% for full bilateral (n = 64), left-modified template (n = 13), and right-modified template (n = 3) dissections, respectively. There were no retroperitoneal recurrences documented in this series. It appears that left-sided dissection, particularly below the level of the inferior mesenteric artery (IMA), bears the highest risk of sympathetic injury and possibly greater risk of resultant complications. Both studies underscore the importance of careful patient selection in postchemotherapy nerve-sparing RPL where low-volume unilateral disease in patients and clear desire for future fertility are favorable features. When evaluating the results of postchemotherapy RPL, one should also appreciate the potential for chemotherapy-induced azoospermia and potential subfertility that occurs in roughly 25% of these patients irrespective of surgical risk [30].

Laparoscopic nerve-sparing retroperitoneal lymphadenectomy

The laparoscopic approach to retroperitoneal lymphadenectomy is covered elsewhere in this issue. This section will focus specifically on the incorporation of nerve-sparing techniques into the retroperitoneal lymphadenectomy procedure. Laparoscopic bilateral retroperitoneal lymphadenectomy was first reported by Rukstalis and Chodak [31] in 1992 as a feasible approach to Stage I testicular cancer with potentially decreased morbidity. Throughout the mid-1990s several small series further supported the feasibility but primarily as a staging procedure using both bilateral and modified unilateral template dissections for Stage I germ-cell tumors [32–38]. The initial results revealed long procedure time and a relatively high complication rate (primarily hemorrhagic complications) that were attributed to inexperience and the recognition of an operative learning curve. In the late 1990s, the group from the University of Innsbruck, Austria, expanded the indications for laparoscopic RPL to include Stage II NSGCT and postchemotherapy masses [39] proposing that with sufficient experience, laparoscopic RPL could be a therapeutic procedure comparable to open surgery. Virtually all laparoscopic RPLs conducted by the Austrian group have used unilateral templates with the goal of preserving antegrade ejaculation [40–44]. Proponents of open surgery have contended that the boundaries of dissection are limited by a laparoscopic approach and that nerve sparing is in part the result of incomplete or no dissecting nerves on one side.

Results from the largest cohort of patients was reported by Steiner and colleagues [45] based on 185 patients over a 10-year period. The large majority of procedures were primary RPLs performed for clinical Stage I NSGCT (114 patients) and tumor marker–negative clinical Stage IIA disease (6 patients); however, post-chemotherapy RPLs were performed for tumor marker-positive Stage IIA (10 patients), Stage IIB (43 patients), and Stage IIC (15 patients) NSGCT. They reported a significant temporal decrease in operative time and an open-conversion rate of 2.6%. Pathology from clinical Stage I procedures revealed positive nodes (ie, clinical under-staging) in 19.5% of cases and mature teratoma was found in 38.2% of the postchemotherapy Stage II specimens. With a mean follow-up of 53.7 months for Stage I patients and 57.6 months for Stage II patients, the authors documented one retroperitoneal recurrence and an antegrade ejaculation rate of 98.4%. It should be noted that two cycles of adjuvant cisplatin-based chemotherapy was given in all cases of pathologic stage II disease following primary RPL.

Peschel and colleagues [44] described an explicit nerve-sparing technique for laparoscopic RPL in a series of five patients. Emphasis was placed on the prospective identification and preservation of relevant sympathetic nerves, which had not necessarily been done previously by laparoscopists in conjunction with modified unilateral template dissections. For right-sided dissections, rolling paracaval lymphatic tissue medially first identifies the sympathetic trunk and postganglionic fibers are carefully dissected and preserved to the point where they cross under the IVC. A "split-and-roll" technique [22] is used over the IVC exposing the lumbar vessels and postganglionic fibers and the nodal package is removed en bloc. The identification of postganglionic nerves in the interaortocaval region is facilitated by rotation of the IVC. The nerve-sparing approach to a left-sided dissection is described as more onerous. The left sympathetic trunk and postganglionic nerves are identified and preserved during the dissection as para-aortic lymphatic tissue is rolled medially. This procedure was performed on two patients with clinical Stage I NSGCT and three patients with clinical stage IIB disease postchemotherapy. In this small series, there were no positive histologic findings and antegrade ejaculation rate was 100%.

Intraoperative electrostimulation of sympathetic nerves has recently been applied to laparoscopic RPL in a case series by Kaiho and colleagues [46,47]. During six laparoscopic unilateral modified template RPLs, sympathetic nerves within the field of dissection were identified and preserved. While these nerves were stimulated with bipolar electrodes through a laparoscopic port, ejaculatory function was confirmed by endoscopic visualization of bladder neck closure and emission of semen into the posterior urethra.

In summary, laparoscopic RPLs are being performed by experienced surgeons in various centers with disease control and complication rates comparable to open surgery. The literature acknowledges an overall relative lack of experience with this procedure among urologists, a technical learning curve, and the need for more long-term follow-up data. With continuing efforts to minimize surgical morbidity, the laparoscopic procedure seems to be following an analogous stepwise adoption of modified resection boundaries followed by prospective identification and meticulous preservation of sympathetic nerves with the goal of maintaining ejaculatory function. However, until a sizable experience without adjuvant chemotherapy for positive nodes is reported to demonstrate that surgery alone can be complete, many will regard this procedure as a staging technique.

Summary

Surgery for retroperitoneal nodal metastases of testicular germ-cell tumors has evolved considerably since its inception. Minimizing injury to sympathetic nerves (and consequential ejaculatory dysfunction) has involved their exclusion from resection boundaries, "nerve sparing" by prospectively identifying and preserving nerves within the resection field, or a combination of both approaches. These measures have resulted in dramatic improvements in long-term procedure-related morbidity with equivalent rates of cancer control. We believe that routine nerve-sparing techniques are the standard of care and serve to enforce good principles of surgery by demanding more attention to anatomy and exposure. Experience with this procedure, good knowledge of retroperitoneal anatomy, and thoughtful clinical and surgical decision making are imperative to achieving acceptable results. It behooves urologic oncologists to offer patients maximal therapeutic benefit combined with minimal morbidity and it follows that retroperitoneal lymphadenectomy should be nerve sparing by definition.

References

[1] Cooper JF, Leadbetter WF, Chute R. The thoracoabdominal approach for retroperitoneal gland dissection: its application to testis tumors. 1950. J Urol 2002;167(2 Pt 2):920–6 [discussion: 927].

[2] Donohue JP, Rowland RG. Complications of retroperitoneal lymph node dissection. J Urol 1981; 125(3):338–40.

[3] Ray B, Hajdu SI, Whitmore WF Jr. Proceedings: distribution of retroperitoneal lymph node metastases in testicular germinal tumors. Cancer 1974;33(2): 340–8.

[4] Stephenson AJ, Sheinfeld J. The role of retroperitoneal lymph node dissection in the management of testicular cancer. Urol Oncol 2004;22(3):225–33 [discussion: 234–5].

[5] Donohue JP, Zachary JM, Maynard BR. Distribution of nodal metastases in nonseminomatous testis cancer. J Urol 1982;128(2):315–20.

[6] Weissbach L, Boedefeld EA, Oberdorster W. Modified RLND as a means to preserve ejaculation. Prog Clin Biol Res 1985;203:323–34.

[7] Weissbach L, Boedefeld EA. Localization of solitary and multiple metastases in stage II nonseminomatous testis tumor as basis for a modified staging lymph node dissection in stage I. J Urol 1987; 138(1):77–82.

[8] Donohue JP, Foster RS. Retroperitoneal lymphadenectomy in staging and treatment. The development of nerve-sparing techniques. Urol Clin North Am 1998;25(3):461–8.

[9] Fossa SD, Klepp O, Ous S, et al. Unilateral retroperitoneal lymph node dissection in patients with nonseminomatous testicular tumor in clinical stage I. Eur Urol 1984;10(1):17–23.

[10] Richie JP. Clinical stage 1 testicular cancer: the role of modified retroperitoneal lymphadenectomy. J Urol 1990;144(5):1160–3.

[11] Jewett MA, Kong YS, Goldberg SD, et al. Retroperitoneal lymphadenectomy for testis tumor with nerve sparing for ejaculation. J Urol 1988;139(6):1220–4.

[12] Walsh PC, Mostwin JL. Radical prostatectomy and cystoprostatectomy with preservation of potency. Results using a new nerve-sparing technique. Br J Urol 1984;56(6):694–7.

[13] Stenzl A, Colleselli K, Poisel S, et al. Rationale and technique of nerve sparing radical cystectomy before an orthotopic neobladder procedure in women. J Urol 1995;154(6):2044–9.

[14] Hockel M, Konerding MA, Heussel CP. Liposuction-assisted nerve-sparing extended radical hysterectomy: oncologic rationale, surgical anatomy, and feasibility study. Am J Obstet Gynecol 1998; 178(5):971–6.

[15] Maeda K, Maruta M, Utsumi T, et al. Bladder and male sexual functions after autonomic nerve-sparing TME with or without lateral node dissection for rectal cancer. Tech Coloproctol 2003;7(1):29–33.

[16] Donohue JP, Foster RS, Rowland RG, et al. Nerve-sparing retroperitoneal lymphadenectomy with preservation of ejaculation. J Urol 1990;144(2 Pt 1): 287–91 [discussion: 291–2].

[17] Dieckmann KP, Huland H, Gross AJ. A test for the identification of relevant sympathetic nerve fibers during nerve sparing retroperitoneal lymphadenectomy. J Urol 1992;148(5):1450–2.

[18] Colleselli K, Poisel S, Schachtner W, et al. Nerve-preserving bilateral retroperitoneal lymphadenectomy: anatomical study and operative approach. J Urol 1990;144(2 Pt 1):293–7 [discussion: 297–8].

[19] Spermon JR, Roeleveld TA, van der Poel HG, et al. Comparison of surveillance and retroperitoneal lymph node dissection in Stage I nonseminomatous germ cell tumors. Urology 2002;59(6):923–9.

[20] Albers P, Siener R, Krege S, et al. One course of adjuvant PEB chemotherapy versus retroperitoneal lymph node dissection in patients with stage I nonseminomatous germ-cell tumors (NSGCT). Results of the German Prospective Multicenter Trial (Association of Urological Oncology[AUO]/German testicular cancer study group [GTCSG] Trial 01-94. J Clin Oncol 2006;24:220S.

[21] Schmoll HJ, Souchon R, Krege S, et al. European consensus on diagnosis and treatment of germ cell cancer: a report of the European Germ Cell Cancer Consensus Group (EGCCCG). Ann Oncol 2004; 15(9):1377–99.

[22] Donohue JP. Retroperitoneal lymphadenectomy: the anterior approach including bilateral suprarenal hilar dissection. Urol Clin North Am 1977;4(3): 509–21.

[23] Partridge J, Sturgeon J, Moore M, et al. Surgical management of postchemotherapy residual retroperitoneal testicular germ cell tumours: complete lymphadenectomy vs. lumpectomy. Canadian Journal of Urology 2004;11:2244.

[24] Donohue JP. Nerve-sparing retroperitoneal lymphadenectomy for testis cancer. Evolution of surgical templates for low-stage disease. Eur Urol 1993; 23(Suppl 2):44–6.

[25] Donohue JP, Thornhill JA, Foster RS, et al. The role of retroperitoneal lymphadenectomy in clinical stage B testis cancer: the Indiana University experience (1965 to 1989). J Urol 1995;153(1):85–9.

[26] Jewett MA. Nerve-sparing technique for retroperitoneal lymphadenectomy in testis cancer. Urol Clin North Am 1990;17(2):449–56.

[27] de Bruin MJ, Oosterhof GO, Debruyne FM. Nerve-sparing retroperitoneal lymphadenectomy for low stage testicular cancer. Br J Urol 1993;71(3):336–9.

[28] Wahle GR, Foster RS, Bihrle R, et al. Nerve sparing retroperitoneal lymphadenectomy after primary chemotherapy for metastatic testicular carcinoma. J Urol 1994;152(2 Pt 1):428–30.

[29] Coogan CL, Hejase MJ, Wahle GR, et al. Nerve sparing post-chemotherapy retroperitoneal lymph node dissection for advanced testicular cancer. J Urol 1996;156(5):1656–8.

[30] Boyer M, Raghavan D. Toxicity of treatment of germ cell tumors. Semin Oncol 1992;19(2):128–42.

[31] Rukstalis DB, Chodak GW. Laparoscopic retroperitoneal lymph node dissection in a patient with stage 1 testicular carcinoma. J Urol 1992;148(6):1907–9 [discussion: 1909–10].

[32] Stone NN, Schlussel RN, Waterhouse RL, et al. Laparoscopic retroperitoneal lymph node dissection in stage A nonseminomatous testis cancer. Urology 1993;42(5):610–4.

[33] Gerber GS, Bissada NK, Hulbert JC, et al. Laparoscopic retroperitoneal lymphadenectomy: multi-institutional analysis. J Urol 1994;152(4):1188–91 [discussion: 1191–2].

[34] Janetschek G, Reissigl A, Peschel R, et al. Laparoscopic retroperitoneal lymph node dissection for clinical stage I nonseminomatous testicular tumor. Urology 1994;44(3):382–91.

[35] Klotz L. Laparoscopic retroperitoneal lymphadenectomy for high-risk stage 1 nonseminomatous germ cell tumor: report of four cases. Urology 1994; 43(5):752–6.

[36] Janetschek G, Reissigl A, Peschel R, et al. Diagnostic laparoscopic retroperitoneal lymph node dissection for non seminomatous testicular tumor. Ann Urol (Paris) 1995;29(2):81–90.

[37] Gerber GS, Rukstalis DB. Laparoscopic approach to retroperitoneal lymph node dissection. Semin Surg Oncol 1996;12(2):121–5.

[38] Rassweiler JJ, Seemann O, Henkel TO, et al. Laparoscopic retroperitoneal lymph node dissection for nonseminomatous germ cell tumors: indications and limitations. J Urol 1996;156(3):1108–13.

[39] Janetschek G, Hobisch A, Hittmair A, et al. Laparoscopic retroperitoneal lymphadenectomy after

chemotherapy for stage IIB nonseminomatous testicular carcinoma. J Urol 1999;161(2):477–81.

[40] Janetschek G, Hobisch A, Holtl L, et al. Retroperitoneal lymphadenectomy for clinical stage I nonseminomatous testicular tumor: laparoscopy versus open surgery and impact of learning curve. J Urol 1996;156(1):89–93 [discussion: 94].

[41] Janetschek G, Hobisch A, Peschel R, et al. Laparoscopic retroperitoneal lymph node dissection for clinical stage I nonseminomatous testicular carcinoma: long-term outcome. J Urol 2000;163(6):1793–6.

[42] Janetschek G. Laparoscopic retroperitoneal lymph node dissection. Urol Clin North Am 2001;28(1):107–14.

[43] Janetschek G, Peschel R, Hobisch A, et al. Laparoscopic retroperitoneal lymph node dissection. J Endourol 2001;15(4):449–53 [discussion: 453–5].

[44] Peschel R, Gettman MT, Neururer R, et al. Laparoscopic retroperitoneal lymph node dissection: description of the nerve-sparing technique. Urology 2002;60(2):339–43 [discussion: 343].

[45] Steiner H, Peschel R, Janetschek G, et al. Long-term results of laparoscopic retroperitoneal lymph node dissection: a single-center 10-year experience. Urology 2004;63(3):550–5.

[46] Kaiho Y, Nakagawa H, Takeuchi A, et al. Electrostimulation of sympathetic nerve fibers during nerve-sparing laparoscopic retroperitoneal lymph node dissection in testicular tumor. Int J Urol 2003;10(5):284–6.

[47] Kaiho Y, Nakagawa H, Ito A, et al. Ipsilateral seminal emission generated by electrostimulation of the lumbar sympathetic nerve during nerve sparing laparoscopic retroperitoneal lymph node dissection for testicular cancer. J Urol 2004;172(3):928–31.

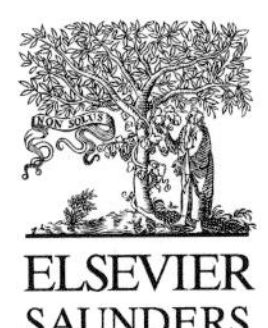

ELSEVIER
SAUNDERS

Urol Clin N Am 34 (2007) 159–169

UROLOGIC
CLINICS
of North America

Laparoscopic Retroperitoneal Lymph Node Dissection for Nonseminomatous Germ-Cell Tumors: Current Status

Robert J. Hamilton, MD, MPH[a],
Antonio Finelli, MD, MSc, FRCSC[b,*]

[a]*Division of Urology, Department of Surgery, University of Toronto, c/o University Health Network, Princess Margaret Hospital, 610 University Avenue, Toronto, Ontario, Canada M5G 2M9*
[b]*Division of Urology, Department of Surgical Oncology, University Health Network, Princess Margaret Hospital. 610 University Avenue, 3-130, Toronto, Ontario, Canada M5G 2M9*

The multimodal management of testis cancer has yielded impressive cure rates. Together, the use of accurate tumor markers, refined surgical techniques, highly effective cis-platinum–based chemotherapeutic regimens, and in the case of seminoma, radiation therapy, have brought the overall survival for this disease to greater than 90%.

Similar to the ongoing evolution of other extirpative procedures in genitourinary oncology, the introduction of technology and minimally invasive surgery has been a driving force. Since the first description of a laparoscopic approach to retroperitoneal lymph node dissection in 1992, its use has become more prevalent [1]. Yet, unlike laparoscopic nephrectomy, laparoscopic retroperitoneal lymph node dissection (LRPLND) has met considerable opposition and thus has not been widely accepted. Supporters of LRPLND refer to reduced morbidity, length of stay, time to return to normal activity, and equivalent oncologic outcome data. Those in opposition argue that oncologic equivalency has not yet been proven, the dissection is not as complete as the conventional approach, and it takes longer with greater monetary cost.

Herein, we address the current and future role of LRPLND. We review the published literature regarding the technical feasibility of a laparoscopic approach, the oncologic outcomes, the associated morbidity, and the cost-effectiveness of LRPLND.

Role of retroperitoneal lymph node dissection

The current "gold standard" to accurately stage and treat nonseminomatous germ-cell tumors (NSGCT) is a thorough dissection of retroperitoneal lymph tissue, or RPLND. With the availability of effective chemotherapy and enhanced imaging techniques used during surveillance, the indications for RPLND have been debated; however, at present, lymphadenectomy is integral to the successful management of this disease. RPLND has a clear role in the primary therapy of selected high-risk clinical stage I (CS I) patients, CS IIA (single lymph node < 2 cm), and CS IIB (single or multiple lymph nodes 2 to 5 cm) patients with normal tumor markers. Residual retroperitoneal disease postchemotherapy with normal tumor markers is also an indication for RPLND, while for patients with seminoma, there is a limited role for RPLND after chemotherapy [2,3]. The role and efficacy of RPLND is addressed elsewhere in this supplement and has been reviewed recently [4]. This review will focus on the role of LRPLND.

The retroperitoneum is often the first site of metastatic spread in 75% to 90% of cases [5] and the overall cure rate after primary RPLND is 99% [6,7]. However, 65% or more of CS I NSGCT

* Corresponding author.
E-mail address: a.finelli@utoronto.ca (A. Finelli).

doi:10.1016/j.ucl.2007.02.007

patients will not have metastatic disease in their retroperitoneum at surgery, and thus benefit little, while being exposed to the potential morbidity of surgery [6–8]. Thus, the challenge is identifying which patients will benefit from surgery. With 20% to 30% of patients inaccurately labeled as having a negative retroperitoneum by abdominal axial imaging, a niche for LRPLND was identified: a staging technique with greater sensitivity and specificity than imaging but less morbidity than open RPLND [9–11]. Some would argue that the role for LRPLND has advanced little past an expensive staging technique, while others believe it has valuable therapeutic potential.

Rationale for a laparoscopic approach

To be accepted, any new surgical technology must be compared with the current gold-standard approach. Thus, LRPLND must be proven to (1) be technically feasible, (2) provide at least equivalent oncologic outcomes to open RPLND, (3) decrease morbidity relative to RPLND, and (4) be cost-effective. The evidence for each criterion will be reviewed subsequently.

Technical feasibility

LRPLND was initially described in 1992 [1]. Since then there have been more than 100 publications on the topic. It is well established that the operation is technically feasible and morbidity may be further minimized as advances in the procedure continue. Transperitoneal [12–15] and extraperitoneal/retroperitoneoscopic [16–19] techniques have been described in detail elsewhere. However, regardless of the approach, once the retroperitoneal anatomical landmarks are exposed the dissection proceeds according to the templates established by Weissbach and Boedefeld [20].

Several groups have attempted to modify the originally described LRPLND technique in hope of further minimizing morbidity. One such technique uses radio-guided sentinel lymph node mapping to minimize the number of nodes removed and thus operative time and risk of lymphocele [21]. However, with a median follow-up of 19.5 months, 2 of 22 patients had recurrence in the retroperitoneum. Although this technique may allow shorter operative times and with higher yield, issues regarding its sensitivity need be resolved before further application. Other adjuncts used to facilitate the operation include insertion of an infrared ureteral stent to aid in identifying the ureter as the lateral border of dissection [22], use of hand-assisted techniques [23], dissection using a waterjet applicator to minimize trauma to neurovascular structures [24], use of robotic-assistance [25], and electrostimulation of the lumbar sympathetic nerves to improve nerve sparing [26,27]. These innovations have been applied in small series and have yet to amass enough evidence to warrant their recommendation during LRPLND; however, it should be recognized that the LRPLND is undergoing a constant evolution, with each modification attempting to make the procedure more feasible with less morbidity.

Oncologic equivalence

For LRPLND to be widely accepted, it must provide equivalent oncologic outcomes to the open approach. However, comparing the laparoscopic to the open technique is complicated. The extent of dissection often varies and the intraoperative algorithm may differ once a positive node is identified. Most importantly, administration of chemotherapy postoperatively to nearly all patients identified with pathologic-positive nodes makes it difficult to draw conclusions about the efficacy of LRPLND alone. As operative times, length of stay, morbidity, and oncologic outcomes vary according to stage, stage II and postchemotherapy LRPLND data are presented separately.

Stage I NSGCT

Series composed of 10 or more stage I patients, with a minimum of 24 months median follow-up and complete oncologic outcome data are reviewed here (Table 1) [12,18,24,28–30]. In cases where centers have published their experience beforehand, only the most recent publication was used. The largest series is that of the Austrian group from Innsbruck [30]. They have performed LRPLND in 103 patients with stage I NSGCT and now have a mean follow-up of 62 months. Twenty-six of the 103 patients were found to have active tumor in the nodal specimen and all went on to receive two cycles of chemotherapy. No recurrences were noted. However, of the 77 patients with negative nodes at surgery, 5 relapsed, including 1 in the retroperitoneum and 1 biochemical recurrence only. The authors note that the retroperitoneal recurrence was on the contralateral side, outside of the planned template

Table 1
Oncologic outcomes among published series of LRPLND for CS I NSGCCT

Series	No. of patients	Follow-up, mo	Yield (no. patients with N+)	No. patients receving chemotherapy	No. recurrences and location
Albqami and Janetschek, 2005 [30]	103	62	26: N+ 77: N−	26 × 2 BEP	5 (N+: 0; N−: 5) • 1 retroperitoneal: contralateral • 3 lung recurrences • 1 biochemical
Castillo et al, 2004 [28]	96	34	18: N+ 78: N−	18 × 2 BEP	4 - Location N/A
Rassweiler et al, 2000 [12]	34	40	6: N+ 28: N− 3: aborted because frozen section showed mets	6 × 3 BEP	2 Recurrences • 0 Regional • 2 Pulmonary
Bhayani et al, 2003 [29]	29	72	12: N+ 17: N−	10	3 Recurrences • N+: 1 * 1 Biochemical • N−: 2 * 1 Lung * 1 Biochemical
Leblanc et al, 2001 [18]	20	15	6: N+ 14: N−	6	0 Recurrences
Corvin et al, 2005 [24]	18	16.7	7: N+	7	0 Recurrences
TOTAL	300	—	75 N+ (25%)	73 (97% of N+)	14 (4.5% of 300)

Abbreviations: BEP = bleomycin, etoposide, cisplatin for two or three cycles; CS, clinical stage; LRPLND, laparoscopic retroperitoneal lymph node dissection; mets, metastases; NSGCT, nonseminomatous germ-cell tumors; N/A, not available; N+, node positive; N−, node negative.

dissection. Moreover, pathologic review of the resected lymph nodes from that patient demonstrated tumor that was missed on initial interpretation. If it had been detected, the patient would have received two cycles of adjuvant chemotherapy. This patient went on to have a contralateral LRPLND and two cycles of chemotherapy and remains disease free.

Other published series report similar results (see Table 1). Overall, 25% of patients are found to have positive nodes. This approximates the major open series, where 20% to 35% of patients are typically found to have positive nodes [6–8,31]. At first glance, there appears to be oncologic equivalence with open RPLND. The recurrence rate of 4.5% compares well with data from open series where typically those with negative nodes at surgery recur 10% of the time, while those with low-volume retroperitoneal disease recur between 8% and 40% of the time [6,7,32–34]. Last, relapse in the retroperitoneum was rare with one recurrence out of 300 cases (0.3%), which is on par with open series (<2%) [6,7,35]; however, comparing these data directly is inappropriate. Unlike in open series, the vast majority (97%) of patients in the LRPLND series with evidence of tumor in their retroperitoneum received two cycles or more of adjuvant chemotherapy. It is known that a complete dissection of the retroperitoneum is a predictor of relapse-free survival [35–37], and data suggest the use of adjuvant chemotherapy after RPLND does not atone for inadequate initial surgery [37,38]. In one study, 35 patients initially treated for stage I NSGCT who later relapsed (>2 years) were analyzed [38]. Nineteen of 35 patients relapsed in the retroperitoneum and 60% of these had received adjuvant chemotherapy after their primary RPLND. Most importantly, in these cases relapsing after open RPLND, the median time to disease development was more than 80 months [38]. Thus, it is possible that the LRPLND series reviewed here are too immature to appreciate the risk of late recurrence that may occur after incomplete resections treated with chemotherapy. These data underscore the importance of an initial complete lymph node dissection.

A recent retrospective study of pooled data from the United States was not included in Table 1 because of incomplete data [39]; however, if published after peer review, it may provide insight into the oncologic efficacy of LRPLND. Data from 143 clinical stage I NSGCT patients treated with LRPLND revealed only one recurrence in the pelvis, and this was outside of the template. Most importantly, this series included 10 patients with pathological stage II disease who opted for surveillance rather than adjuvant chemotherapy after LRPLND. At 35 months of follow-up, no recurrences were noted. This is the first evidence regarding the efficacy of LRPLND alone without the addition of adjuvant chemotherapy in node-positive patients.

A question of oncologic intentions

Even among those who support LRPLND, disagreement exists regarding the intentions of the operation. The limited extent of dissection and the liberal use of adjuvant chemotherapy have been cited as evidence of the nontherapeutic intentions of LRPLND. Janetschek and colleagues [30], who routinely omit dissection dorsal to the great vessels and recommend chemotherapy to all their patients with positive nodes at surgery, "consider RPLND a diagnostic measure only." In contrast, others meticulously dissect dorsal to the great vessels, but still recommend chemotherapy to all node-positive patients and follow them with serial abdominal CT scans yet feel, "[their] objectives for LRPLND evolved from a diagnostic to a therapeutic intervention" [40].

LRPLND has been criticized as an incomplete cancer operation because of the templates used. Nearly all laparoscopic series describe following the dissection templates established by Weissbach and Boedefeld [20]. However, these templates were proposed for staging the retroperitoneum, not for therapeutic purposes. Also, the template is further limited in laparoscopic series as dissection dorsal to the great vessels is commonly omitted. In support of their practice, the group from Innsbruck conducted a study of 139 NSGCT patients and showed that all solitary metastases were ventral to the lumbar vessels. Among 25 patients with multiple metastases, cancer was detected dorsal to the great vessels in 3. However, all three had concomitant ventral metastases that would have been identified with the limited dissection [41]. This finding was supported by a study examining radio-guided sentinel lymph node mapping. Of 22 patients with stage I testis cancer, 21 were found to have identifiable sentinel nodes, all of which were ventral or lateral to the great vessels [21]. Notably, in a more recent publication of postchemotherapy LRPLND, the group from Innsbruck disclose a retroperitoneal recurrence in the retrocaval area [42]. Given the reduced survival among patients with late relapse and the potential for recurrence in the uncontrolled retroperitoneum, this casts further doubt on the therapeutic efficacy of a limited dissection with the laparoscopic approach.

Last, when positive nodes are appreciated during open RPLND, a complete bilateral dissection is performed. Although bilateral LRPLND is feasible, it is performed infrequently as patient repositioning is required [40]. This adds to the surgical time and may be a disincentive to a complete dissection. In fact, many laparoscopic series either do not change their template when malignant tissue is identified intraoperatively or abort altogether, knowingly leaving residual disease. As mentioned, these patients all go on to receive adjuvant chemotherapy. Reducing or halting dissection in the presence of disease seems counter to the approach adopted for open RPLND where identification of tumor prompts bilateral RPLND. Thus, despite the varying opinions and approaches, the intentions of LRPLND remain unclear or in evolution.

How do these intentions compare in terms of oncologic outcomes? Comparing long-term results of patients in whom dorsal dissection was omitted with those who underwent dissection dorsal to the great vessels is difficult. Currently, the oncologic outcomes for the largest series of patients undergoing LRPLND with dissection dorsal to the great vessels has just been published in abstract form [39]. Only through longer follow-up and careful observation of the few patients refusing adjuvant chemotherapy will we begin to assess the issue of oncologic efficacy with LRPLND.

Morbidity

The morbidity associated with open RPLND has decreased considerably and has set the bar higher for comparisons with LRPLND. However anecdotally, those undergoing LRPLND have reduced blood loss, postoperative morbidity, and length of stay with a faster convalescence and return to normal function [43,44]. To date, no head-to-head comparisons have been conducted, but indirect comparisons of operative parameters and complications can be made.

Operative parameters

The operative results from large LRPLND series (>10 patients) have been summarized (Table 2) [12,18,24,28–30,45]. Three of the 103 patients in the Austrian series who underwent LRPLND required open conversions because of hemorrhage from vascular injuries [30]. In addition they reported four minor intraoperative complications (3.9%), of which all were vascular in etiology. In the postoperative period, three patients had lymphoceles managed conservatively, one patient had a retroperitoneal hemorrhage, and one experienced symptomatic irritation of the genitofemoral nerve. Cases were completed on average in 217 minutes with a mean estimated blood loss of 144 mL. Patients stayed in hospital a mean of 3.6 days. Of note, their reported figures exclude the first 30 cases in the learning curve when procedures took longer and were associated with greater blood loss.

Overall, among the published series, the length of operations ranged from 138 to 306 minutes and 3.1% of cases were converted to open. The estimated blood loss ranged from less than 50 mL to 390 mL and 1% of patients required transfusion. Patients' stay in hospital varied from 1.8 to 5.3 days and return to normal activities occurred between 13 and 30 days. The considerable variability in these figures may stem from some series excluding cases such as those earlier in the learning curve, or may reflect outlier cases (eg, open conversions) or local cultural norms that have been known to influence length of stay and time to return to work.

These figures compare favorably with the large open series. The German Testicular Cancer Study Group [46] published their cumulative experience of 239 patients undergoing primary open RPLND. Mean operative time was 214 minutes, mean estimated blood loss was less than 150 mL, and mean hospital stay was 8 days. Other series have similar results [47,48]; however, a recent update of the last 75 open RPLND cases at Indiana University showed that in the hands of experts the morbidity is minimal. The mean operative time was 132 minutes, mean estimated blood loss 200 mL, and the mean length of stay 2.8 days [49].

Complications

With LRPLND, major and minor intraoperative complications occurred in 4% and 2% of cases, respectively, while major and minor postoperative complications occurred in 1% and 6% of cases, respectively (see Table 2). Vascular injury was responsible for most intraoperative complications and the need to convert to open surgery, whereas the most common postoperative complication was lymphocele formation (2.3% of all cases). Antegrade ejaculation rates were between 97% and 100%. Complication rates vary considerably though. One of the larger experiences with LRPLND was recently updated, but the series also contained patients who underwent LRPLND for residual disease after chemotherapy [40]. Among 77 patients, intraoperative complications occurred in 10 (13%). Vascular injuries to the vena cava (5.4%), renal hilum (3.1%), and external iliac artery (1%) occurred most commonly.

Overall, the complication rates for LRPLND compare favorably to contemporary series of open RPLND. The reported minor and major complication rates for open RPLND are approximately 15% and 5%, respectively [35,46,50]. With nerve-sparing techniques, antegrade ejaculation is preserved in more than 90% of patients, and the most common short-term complications are wound infection (5%) and ileus (2%) [35,46,48]. The most common long-term complications are small bowel obstruction (1%–2%) and lymphocele or chylous ascites (0.4%) [48,51]. Given that nearly all patients with positive nodes after LRPLND receive adjuvant chemotherapy, the added complications of chemotherapy must be considered when comparing morbidity between LRPLND and open RPLND. Those receiving chemotherapy are at increased risk of cardiovascular events, secondary leukemia, renal dysfunction, peripheral neuropathy, hearing loss, Raynaud's phenomenon, impaired spermatogenesis, and pulmonary fibrosis [4,52–58].

Retrospective comparisons of LRPLND to open RPLND must be regarded with caution given the aforementioned differences in philosophy and operative approaches for these two procedures. However, considering the current literature, the operative parameters and morbidity for LRPLND compare favorably with open RPLND.

Stage II NSGCT and postchemotherapy RPLND

Far fewer reports of LRPLND in the context of clinical stage II NSGCT and/or residual disease

Table 2
Morbidity from reported series of LRPLND for stage I NSGCT

Series	No. cases	Mean OR time, min	No. conversions	Mean blood loss, mL	Intraoperative		Postoperative		Mean hospital stay, d	Return to normal activity, d	% Antegrade ejaculation
					Major	Minor	Major	Minor			
Albqami and Janetschek, 2005 [30]	103	217[a]	3	144[a]	3	4	0	5	3.6[a]	N/A	100
Castillo et al, 2004 [28][b]	96	138	4	120 3TSFs	8	1	1	4	1.8	N/A	100
Rassweiler et al, 2000 [12]	34	249	1	N/A	1	N/A	2	5	5.3[c]	30[c]	97.1
Bhayani et al, 2003 [29]	29	258	2	389	N/A	N/A	N/A	2	2.6[d]	17.2[d]	96.6
Porter and Lange, 2003 [45]	27	306	0	270	N/A	N/A	0	3	2.1	13	100
Leblanc et al, 2001 [18]	20	230	0	<50	0	N/A	0	N/A	1.2	15	100
Corvin et al, 2005 [24]	18	232	0	<100	0	0	0	1	N/A	N/A	100
TOTAL	327	—	10 (3.1%)	—	12 (4%)	5 (2%)	3 (1%)	20 (6%)	—	—	—

Abbreviations: LRPLND, laparoscopic retroperitoneal lymph node dissection; NSGCT, nonseminomatous germ-cell tumors; N/A, not available; TSFs, blood transfusions.

[a] Excludes first 30 "learning" cases and 1 case with a horseshoe kidney.

[b] Reported data not stratified for stage I and II disease.

[c] Excludes cases with major complications or open conversions.

[d] Excludes open conversions.

postchemotherapy exist. Six series with more than five patients have been published (Table 3) [18,24, 28,30,59,60]. Follow-up information is significantly shorter and the case-mix of patients is much greater than those series of stage I NSGCT. Despite the minimal morbidity reported by the Austrian group, which has the largest series in this setting, the conversion rate tends to be high and significant complications have been reported [30]. Rassweiler and colleagues [59] reported a conversion rate of 67% among nine patients undergoing LRPLND postchemotherapy. Palese and colleagues [60] reported a 29% conversion rate out of seven patients and a 57% overall complication rate including the need for an aortorenal bypass, an iliac bypass graft, and a nephrectomy. Clearly, differences in experience and patient selection contribute to the tremendous variance seen in the postchemotherapy LRPLND experience.

The challenge of RPLND in the postchemotherapy setting is not limited to the laparoscopic approach. The morbidity is considerably greater in open series as well [48]. This is largely a result of the coarse desmoplastic reaction that can result from chemotherapy, the often-larger volume disease, and the pulmonary effects of bleomycin

Table 3
Oncologic outcomes and morbidity among published series of LRPLND for CS II NSGCT

Series	No. patients	Follow-up, mo	Yield (no. patients with N+)	No. recurrences	Complications
Albqami and Janetschek, 2005 [30]	Postchemo: 43 IIB 16 IIC	53	IIB: • 1: Active tumor • 16: Mature teratoma • 26: No tumor IIC: • 1: Seminoma • 10: No tumor • 5: Mature teratoma	1 Recurrence (outside template)	No conversions "Higher" incidence of chylous ascites (no. not given) Ant. ejaculation: 97%
Castillo et al, 2004 [28]	20 IIA 12 IIB	34	N/A	2 IIA[a] 3 IIB[a] Location N/A	4 Conversions[a] 14 Complications[a]
Rassweiler et al, 1996 [59]	Postchemo: 2 IIB 7 IIC	29	All: Complete necrosis	0 Recurrences	6 Conversions 1 Lymphocele Ant. ejaculation: N/A
Leblanc et al, 2001 [18]	5 IIA	15	4 N+ Histology not given	0 Recurrences	0 Conversions 0 Complications Ant. ejaculation: 100%
Corvin et al, 2005 [24]	Postchemo: 1 IIA 4 IIB 2 IIC	17.2	1 Viable metastasis 3 Mature teratoma 3 Necrosis	0 Recurrences	0 Conversions 1 lymphocele Ant. ejaculation: 100%
Palese et al, 2002 [60]	Postchemo: 5 $\geq$ IIA	24	1 Viable metastasis 3 Mature teratoma 1 Necrosis	0 Recurrences	2 Conversions 3 Major complications 1 Minor complication
TOTAL	117	—	8 Tumor (6.8%) 27 Teratoma (23.1%)	6 (5.1%)	12 Conversions (10%)

Abbreviations: Ant, antegrade; CS, clinical stage; LRPLND, laparoscopic retroperitoneal lymph node dissection; NSGCT, nonseminomatous germ-cell tumors; N/A, not available; N+, node positive; N−, node negative; postchemo, postchemotherapy.

[a] Results not reported separately for stage I and II disease.

[61]. In contrast to primary series, mortalities have been reported (0.8%), and pulmonary complications comprise the largest contributor to morbidity (8%). Wound infection (4.8%), small bowel obstruction (2.3%), and chylous ascites (2%) are the next most common complications [61]. Thus, surgery for postchemotherapy residual disease is associated with greater morbidity regardless of the approach. However, in this setting, LRPLND should only be attempted by the most experienced laparoscopic surgeons, as the potential complications are significant.

Cost-effectiveness

Although efficacy and safety are paramount, monetary cost is relevant in treatment comparisons. To be accepted, LRPLND should either be more cost-effective than conventional RPLND, or require a nominal additional cost such that the health benefits to the patient justify the added expenditure. Any new surgical approach will initially take longer and be associated with more complications. Projecting long-term cost-effectiveness based on data during this learning curve is not appropriate. Janetschek and colleagues [47] quantified the learning curve early in their experience. Compared with the first 14 cases, the subsequent 15 cases had a mean operative time that was 36% shorter and a postoperative hospital stay that was 27% shorter.

There have been two reports addressing the cost-effectiveness of LRPLND. The first, published in 2002, estimated the cost per case of LRPLND at $7804 compared with $7162 for open RPLND [62]. This differential was almost entirely explained by the increased expense of equipment and the cost of longer operating times with LRPLND. In a sensitivity analysis, LRPLND became less costly when operative times were less than 216 minutes and hospital stays were shorter than 2.2 days; however, this study has several limitations. First, the investigators only used three LRPLND series totaling 136 patients, and two open series, totaling 115 patients, to model their findings. All the LRPLND series and one of two open series are from Europe and thus do not adequately represent clinical practice in North America. Second, they modeled the recurrence rate for LRPLND after data with considerably shorter follow-up time than the open series data. Thus, LRPLND would appear to have fewer relapses. Finally, they did not budget for the fact that all patients undergoing LRPLND who are identified as having positive nodes currently also incur the costs of chemotherapy and the costs of complications from the chemotherapy.

A second, more detailed, cost-effectiveness study modeled all options for treating stage I NSGCT including surveillance, primary chemotherapy, and surgery (LRPLND and open RPLND). They found that LRPLND cost $9968 per case, whereas open RPLND cost $13,212 per case [63]. Here the largest contributor to the differential costs was hospital stay, which was estimated to be twice as long for open RPLND. This study similarly did not account for the costs of chemotherapy in the LRPLND group and triple counted data from the Innsbruck group, which reported one of the shortest operative times for LRPLND.

Summary

The impressive cure rate associated with conventional RPLND is difficult to improve upon. Furthermore, contemporary series document diminished morbidity as compared with that historically associated with the procedure. However, there are clearly patients who do not require such aggressive intervention. Yet with current imaging and other prognostic modalities, a subset of patients will be understaged and consequently managed conservatively when they could have benefited from retroperitoneal dissection.

Hence, LRPLND was introduced to provide a sensitive and specific staging modality without the morbidity of conventional RPLND. With proof that it is technically feasible, several centers have become experts in this technique and morbidity appears to be less than that of open RPLND. As experience builds, operative times diminish, and patients are discharged from hospital earlier. Thus, it is likely that LRPLND will become equally if not more cost-effective than conventional RPLND. However, the oncologic outcomes, while on par with open RPLND series, are difficult to attribute to successful LRPLND alone when nearly all patients with positive nodes received chemotherapy. We must await follow-up of the rare patients who opted not to have adjuvant chemotherapy after LRPLND or look to new studies assessing the efficacy of LRPLND alone. Although uncertainties exist, LRPLND holds much future promise.

References

[1] Rukstalis DB, Chodak GW. Laparoscopic retroperitoneal lymph node dissection in a patient with stage

I testicular carcinoma. J Urol 1992;148(6):1907–9 [discussion: 1909–10].

[2] Bajorin DF, Herr H, Motzer RJ, et al. Current perspectives on the role of adjunctive surgery in combined modality treatment for patients with germ cell tumors. Semin Oncol 1992;19(2):148–58.

[3] Puc HS, Heelan R, Mazumdar M, et al. Management of residual mass in advanced seminoma: results and recommendations from the Memorial Sloan-Kettering Cancer Center. J Clin Oncol 1996;14(2):454–60.

[4] Stephenson AJ, Sheinfeld J. The role of retroperitoneal lymph node dissection in the management of testicular cancer. Urol Oncol 2004;22(3):225–33 [discussion: 234–5].

[5] Whitmore WF Jr. Surgical treatment of adult germinal testis tumors. Semin Oncol 1979;6(1):55–68.

[6] Donohue JP, Thornhill JA, Foster RS, et al. Retroperitoneal lymphadenectomy for clinical stage A testis cancer (1965 to 1989): modifications of technique and impact on ejaculation. J Urol 1993;149(2): 237–43.

[7] Hermans BP, Sweeney CJ, Foster RS, et al. Risk of systemic metastases in clinical stage I nonseminoma germ cell testis tumor managed by retroperitoneal lymph node dissection. J Urol 2000;163(6):1721–4.

[8] Nicolai N, Miceli R, Artusi R, et al. A simple model for predicting nodal metastasis in patients with clinical stage I nonseminomatous germ cell testicular tumors undergoing retroperitoneal lymph node dissection only. J Urol 2004;171(1):172–6.

[9] Richie JP. Clinical stage 1 testicular cancer: the role of modified retroperitoneal lymphadenectomy. J Urol 1990;144(5):1160–3.

[10] Hilton S, Herr HW, Teitcher JB, et al. CT detection of retroperitoneal lymph node metastases in patients with clinical stage I testicular nonseminomatous germ cell cancer: assessment of size and distribution criteria. AJR Am J Roentgenol 1997; 169(2):521–5.

[11] Fernandez EB, Moul JW, Foley JP, et al. Retroperitoneal imaging with third and fourth generation computed axial tomography in clinical stage I nonseminomatous germ cell tumors. Urology 1994;44(4): 548–52.

[12] Rassweiler JJ, Frede T, Lenz E, et al. Long-term experience with laparoscopic retroperitoneal lymph node dissection in the management of low-stage testis cancer. Eur Urol 2000;37(3):251–60.

[13] Winfield HN. Laparoscopic retroperitoneal lymphadenectomy for cancer of the testis. Urol Clin North Am 1998;25(3):469–78.

[14] Janetschek G, Reissigl A, Peschel R, et al. Laparoscopic retroperitoneal lymph node dissection for clinical stage I nonseminomatous testicular tumor. Urology 1994;44(3):382–91.

[15] Finelli A, Moinzadeh A, Singh D, et al. Critique of laparoscopic lymphadenectomy in genitourinary oncology. Urol Oncol 2004;22(3):246–54 [discussion: 254–5].

[16] Rassweiler JJ, Seemann O, Frede T, et al. Retroperitoneoscopy: experience with 200 cases. J Urol 1998; 160(4):1265–9.

[17] Hara I, Kawabata G, Yamada Y, et al. Extraperitoneal laparoscopic retroperitoneal lymph node dissection in supine position after chemotherapy for advanced testicular carcinoma. Int J Urol 2004; 11(10):934–9.

[18] LeBlanc E, Caty A, Dargent D, et al. Extraperitoneal laparoscopic para-aortic lymph node dissection for early stage nonseminomatous germ cell tumors of the testis with introduction of a nerve sparing technique: description and results. J Urol 2001; 165(1):89–92.

[19] Hsu TH, Su LM, Ong A. Anterior extraperitoneal approach to laparoscopic retroperitoneal lymph node dissection: a novel technique. J Urol 2003; 169(1):258–60.

[20] Weissbach L, Boedefeld EA. Localization of solitary and multiple metastases in stage II nonseminomatous testis tumor as basis for a modified staging lymph node dissection in stage I. J Urol 1987; 138(1):77–82.

[21] Satoh M, Ito A, Kaiho Y, et al. Intraoperative, radio-guided sentinel lymph node mapping in laparoscopic lymph node dissection for Stage I testicular carcinoma. Cancer 2005;103(10):2067–72.

[22] Kim K, Schwaitzberg S, Onel E. An infrared ureteral stent to aid in laparoscopic retroperitoneal lymph node dissection. J Urol 2001;166(5):1815–6.

[23] Tobias-Machado M, Zambon JP, Ferreira AD, et al. Retroperitoneal lymphadenectomy by videolaparoscopic transperitoneal approach in patients with non-seminomatous testicular tumor. Int Braz J Urol 2004;30(5):389–96 [discussion: 396–7].

[24] Corvin S, Sturm W, Schlatter E, et al. Laparoscopic retroperitoneal lymph-node dissection with the waterjet is technically feasible and safe in testis-cancer patient. J Endourol 2005;19(7):823–6.

[25] Davol P, Sumfest J, Rukstalis D. Robotic-assisted laparoscopic retroperitoneal lymph node dissection. Urology 2006;67(1):199.

[26] Kaiho Y, Nakagawa H, Ito A, et al. Ipsilateral seminal emission generated by electrostimulation of the lumbar sympathetic nerve during nerve sparing laparoscopic retroperitoneal lymph node dissection for testicular cancer. J Urol 2004;172(3): 928–31.

[27] Kaiho Y, Nakagawa H, Takeuchi A, et al. Electrostimulation of sympathetic nerve fibers during nerve-sparing laparoscopic retroperitoneal lymph node dissection in testicular tumor. Int J Urol 2003;10(5):284–6.

[28] Castillo OA, Urena RD, Pinto IF, et al. Laparoscopic retroperitoneal lymph node dissection for stage I and II NSGCT: 10 years' experience [abstract #933]. J Urol 2004;171(Suppl):247–8.

[29] Bhayani SB, Ong A, Oh WK, et al. Laparoscopic retroperitoneal lymph node dissection for clinical stage

I nonseminomatous germ cell testicular cancer: a long-term update. Urology 2003;62(2):324–7.
[30] Albqami N, Janetschek G. Laparoscopic retroperitoneal lymph-node dissection in the management of clinical stage I and II testicular cancer. J Endourol 2005;19(6):683–92 [discussion: 692].
[31] Albers P, Siener R, Kliesch S, et al. Risk factors for relapse in clinical stage I nonseminomatous testicular germ cell tumors: results of the German Testicular Cancer Study Group Trial. J Clin Oncol 2003; 21(8):1505–12.
[32] Rabbani F, Sheinfeld J, Farivar-Mohseni H, et al. Low-volume nodal metastases detected at retroperitoneal lymphadenectomy for testicular cancer: pattern and prognostic factors for relapse. J Clin Oncol 2001;19(7):2020–5.
[33] Richie JP, Kantoff PW. Is adjuvant chemotherapy necessary for patients with stage B1 testicular cancer? J Clin Oncol 1991;9(8):1393–6.
[34] Pizzocaro G, Monfardini S. No adjuvant chemotherapy in selected patients with pathologic stage II nonseminomatous germ cell tumors of the testis. J Urol 1984;131(4):677–80.
[35] Donohue JP, Thornhill JA, Foster RS, et al. The role of retroperitoneal lymphadenectomy in clinical stage B testis cancer: the Indiana University experience (1965 to 1989). J Urol 1995;153(1):85–9.
[36] Donohue JP, Leviovitch I, Foster RS, et al. Integration of surgery and systemic therapy: results and principles of integration. Semin Urol Oncol 1998; 16(2):65–71.
[37] McKiernan JM, Motzer RJ, Bajorin DF, et al. Reoperative retroperitoneal surgery for nonseminomatous germ cell tumor: clinical presentation, patterns of recurrence, and outcome. Urology 2003; 62(4):732–6.
[38] Baniel J, Foster RS, Einhorn LH, et al. Late relapse of clinical stage I testicular cancer. J Urol 1995; 154(4):1370–2.
[39] Lima GC, Nielson ME, Porter JR, et al. The oncological efficacy of laparoscopic retroperitoneal lymph node dissection in the treatment of clinical stage I nonseminomatous germ cell testis cancer [abstract #587]. J Urol 2006;175(4 Suppl):190.
[40] Romero FR, Wagner A, Brito FA, et al. Refining the laparoscopic retroperitoneal lymph node dissection for testicular cancer. Int Braz J Urol 2006;32(2): 196–201.
[41] Holtl L, Peschel R, Knapp R, et al. Primary lymphatic metastatic spread in testicular cancer occurs ventral to the lumbar vessels. Urology 2002;59(1):114–8.
[42] Steiner H, Peschel R, Janetschek G, et al. Long-term results of laparoscopic retroperitoneal lymph node dissection: a single-center 10-year experience. Urology 2004;63(3):550–5.
[43] Giusti G, Beltrami P, Tallarigo C, et al. Unilateral laparoscopic retroperitoneal lymphadenectomy for clinical stage I nonseminomatous testicular cancer. J Endourol 1998;12(6):561–6.
[44] Carver BS, Sheinfeld J. The current status of laparoscopic retroperitoneal lymph node dissection for non-seminomatous germ-cell tumors. Nat Clin Pract Urol 2005;2(7):330–5.
[45] Porter JR, Lange PH. Laparoscopic retroperitoneal lymph node dissection for stage I NSGCT [abstract # 302]. Presented at the American Urological Association National Meeting, Chicago, IL; April 27, 2003.
[46] Heidenreich A, Albers P, Hartmann M, et al. Complications of primary nerve sparing retroperitoneal lymph node dissection for clinical stage I nonseminomatous germ cell tumors of the testis: experience of the German Testicular Cancer Study Group. J Urol 2003;169(5):1710–4.
[47] Janetschek G, Hobisch A, Holtl L, et al. Retroperitoneal lymphadenectomy for clinical stage I nonseminomatous testicular tumor: laparoscopy versus open surgery and impact of learning curve. J Urol 1996;156(1):89–93 [discussion: 94].
[48] Baniel J, Foster RS, Rowland RG, et al. Complications of primary retroperitoneal lymph node dissection. J Urol 1994;152(2 Pt 1):424–7.
[49] Beck SD, Foster RS. Long-term outcome of retroperitoneal lymph node dissection in the management of testis cancer. World J Urol 2006;24(3):267–72.
[50] Jewett MA, Kong YS, Goldberg SD, et al. Retroperitoneal lymphadenectomy for testis tumor with nerve sparing for ejaculation. J Urol 1988;139(6): 1220–4.
[51] McLeod DG, Weiss RB, Stablein DM, et al. Staging relationships and outcome in early stage testicular cancer: a report from the Testicular Cancer Intergroup Study. J Urol 1991;145(6):1178–83 [discussion: 1182–3].
[52] Huddart RA, Norman A, Shahidi M, et al. Cardiovascular disease as a long-term complication of treatment for testicular cancer. J Clin Oncol 2003; 21(8):1513–23.
[53] Bajorin DF, Motzer RJ, Rodriguez E, et al. Acute nonlymphocytic leukemia in germ cell tumor patients treated with etoposide-containing chemotherapy. J Natl Cancer Inst 1993;85(1):60–2.
[54] Kawai K, Akaza H. Bleomycin-induced pulmonary toxicity in chemotherapy for testicular cancer. Expert Opin Drug Saf 2003;2(6):587–96.
[55] Brennemann W, Stoffel-Wagner B, Helmers A, et al. Gonadal function of patients treated with cisplatin based chemotherapy for germ cell cancer. J Urol 1997;158(3 Pt 1):844–50.
[56] Vogelzang NJ, Bosl GJ, Johnson K, et al. Raynaud's phenomenon: a common toxicity after combination chemotherapy for testicular cancer. Ann Intern Med 1981;95(3):288–92.
[57] Williams SD, Birch R, Einhorn LH, et al. Treatment of disseminated germ-cell tumors with cisplatin, bleomycin, and either vinblastine or etoposide. N Engl J Med 1987;316(23):1435–40.
[58] Bosl GJ, Motzer RJ. Testicular germ-cell cancer. N Engl J Med 1997;337(4):242–53.

[59] Rassweiler JJ, Seemann O, Henkel TO, et al. Laparoscopic retroperitoneal lymph node dissection for nonseminomatous germ cell tumors: indications and limitations. J Urol 1996;156(3): 1108–13.
[60] Palese MA, Su LM, Kavoussi LR. Laparoscopic retroperitoneal lymph node dissection after chemotherapy. Urology 2002;60(1):130–4.
[61] Baniel J, Foster RS, Rowland RG, et al. Complications of post-chemotherapy retroperitoneal lymph node dissection. J Urol 1995;153(3 Pt 2): 976–80.
[62] Ogan K, Lotan Y, Koeneman K, et al. Laparoscopic versus open retroperitoneal lymph node dissection: a cost analysis. J Urol 2002;168(5):1945–9 [discussion: 1949].
[63] Link RE, Allaf ME, Pili R, et al. Modeling the cost of management options for stage I nonseminomatous germ cell tumors: a decision tree analysis. J Clin Oncol 2005;23(24):5762–73.

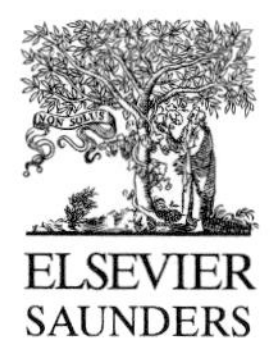
ELSEVIER
SAUNDERS

Urol Clin N Am 34 (2007) 171–177

UROLOGIC CLINICS of North America

Chemotherapy for Good-Risk Germ Cell Tumors: Current Concepts and Controversies

David J. Vaughn, MD

Division of Hematology/Oncology, Abramson Cancer Center of the University of Pennsylvania, 16 Penn Tower, 3400 Spruce Street, Philadelphia, PA 19104-4283, USA

In 2007, an estimated 7920 American men will be diagnosed with germ cell tumor (GCT), with an estimated 380 deaths [1]. The number of patients who have GCT who die each year of this disease has markedly decreased since the early 1970s because of the development of effective systemic chemotherapy and the successful incorporation of postchemotherapy surgery into treatment. Through a series of well-designed randomized clinical trials, the treatment of patients with cisplatin-based chemotherapy has evolved such that approximately 90% of patients who have good-risk metastatic GCT will be cured of their disease. This finding represents a landmark achievement in oncology. At present, first-line chemotherapy for patients who have good-risk metastatic GCT is three cycles of bleomycin/etoposide/cisplatin (BEP). An alternative to this is four cycles of etoposide/cisplatin (EP). These regimens are depicted in Box 1. This article examines the progress that has been made in the development of chemotherapy for good-risk metastatic GCT and raises questions for further consideration and investigation.

What defines good-risk disease?

As chemotherapy for metastatic GCT evolved, it was recognized that certain patient subgroups were associated with a more favorable prognosis than others. Several institutions, including Indiana University [2], Memorial Sloan Kettering Cancer Center (MSKCC) [3], and others, developed prognostic classification systems to help assess results of their respective trials and incorporated these into the design of new trials. Given the differences in the various systems (Box 2), comparison of results of clinical trials by different groups was problematic. In 1997, the International Germ Cell Cancer Collaborative Group [4], which included individuals representing these and other institutions, developed and published the International Germ Cell Cancer Consensus Classification (IGCCC) (see Box 2). The IGCCC system is widely used today and reliably differentiates patients who have varying prognoses into good-risk, intermediate-risk, and poor-risk categories. Patients who have good-risk metastatic GCT as defined by IGCCC have a 5-year overall survival of 86% for seminoma patients and 92% for nonseminomatous germ cell tumor (NSGCT) patients. The good-risk cohort thus has a favorable outcome with chemotherapy. This good-risk cohort is the focus of this article.

Caveats when reviewing germ cell tumor chemotherapy clinical trials

In reviewing clinical trials for patients who have good-risk GCT, it is important to keep in mind that each trial may have used a different prognostic classification system for eligibility. It is important to refer to the details of that system to understand what patients are being treated. These systems vary substantially in design, as demonstrated in Box 2. Some investigators have re-reported the results of prior trials using the IGCCC system. Finally, in most trials, the definition of complete response to treatment is disappearance of all clinical, radiologic, and biochemical evidence of disease, or if postchemotherapy residual masses are present, successful

E-mail address: david.vaughn@uphs.upenn.edu

0094-0143/07/$ - see front matter
doi:10.1016/j.ucl.2007.03.001

Box 1. Chemotherapy regimens for good-risk metastatic germ cell tumor

BEP
Etoposide 100 mg/m^2 IV daily for 5 days
Cisplatin 20 mg/m^2 IV daily for 5 days
Bleomycin 30 units IV once weekly for 3 weeks (eg, day 1, 8, 15; or, days 2, 9, 16)
Cycles administered every 21 days for a total of three cycles

EP
Etoposide 100 mg/m^2 IV daily for 5 days
Cisplatin 20 mg/m^2 IV daily for 5 days
Cycles administered every 21 days for a total of four cycles

resection of the residual masses containing necrotic nonviable tumor, fibrosis, or mature teratoma.

How many cycles are necessary?

As effective chemotherapy evolved for patients who had metastatic GCT, a cohort of patients emerged who had an excellent prognosis and were good risk. An important goal in the management of these patients is to minimize treatment while maximizing cure. Certainly, any compromise in the excellent cure rate of this cohort of patients in an attempt to prevent toxicity is not acceptable. One important approach to minimizing treatment is to determine what is the least number of cycles of chemotherapy necessary to maximize cure.

The Southeastern Cancer Study Group (SECSG) addressed this question in a randomized phase III trial comparing three cycles of BEP with four cycles of BEP in 184 patients who had good-risk metastatic GCT (minimal-moderate risk as defined by the Indiana University classification) [5]. The complete response rates were 98% and 97%, respectively. At a median follow-up of 19 months, 92% of patients in each arm were disease-free. Investigators from Indiana University reported long-term follow-up on the cohort of patients they treated in the SECSG trial. With a median follow-up of 10.1 years, no differences were noted in disease-free or overall survival [6].

A second randomized phase III trial performed by the European Organization for the Research and Treatment of Cancer (EORTC)/Medical Research Council (MRC) randomized 812 patients who had good-risk metastatic GCT as defined by IGCCC criteria to receive three cycles of BEP versus three cycles of BEP plus one cycle of EP [7]. The primary endpoint 2-year progression-free survival was 90.4% and 89.4%, respectively. This trial was sufficiently powered to detect ≥5% difference in 2-year progression-free survival. A second randomization compared the standard 5-day BEP regimen with a regimen used in the United Kingdom in which the same total dosages of agents were administered over 3 days. No difference in 2-year progression-free survival was demonstrated between the 5-day and 3-day schedules.

Based on these two trials, three cycles of BEP has become the standard of care for first-line chemotherapy of metastatic good-risk GCT.

Is bleomycin necessary?

Bleomycin-induced pneumonitis (BIP) is a feared complication of this agent. Studies have demonstrated that risk factors for the development of BIP include age of patient, renal function, history of smoking, underlying pulmonary disease, and total cumulative dose of bleomycin [8,9]. With three cycles of BEP, the cumulative dose of bleomycin is 270 units; with four cycles of BEP, the cumulative dose is 360 units. Although BIP is uncommon in patients who have GCT receiving three cycles of BEP, the incidence does increase with the addition of the fourth cycle. The necessity of including bleomycin in cisplatin-based combination chemotherapy has been addressed in randomized phase III trials.

The Eastern Cooperative Oncology Group randomized 171 patients who had minimal-moderate risk (as defined by the Indiana classification) metastatic GCT to three cycles of BEP versus three cycles of EP [10]. The relapse-free survival was 86% on the BEP arm versus 69% on the EP arm (P = .01). Overall survival was 95% and 86%, respectively (P = .01). No clinically significant pulmonary toxicity was observed in the BEP arm. The authors concluded that if three cycles of chemotherapy are to be administered, then bleomycin is essential.

The EORTC compared four cycles of BEP with four cycles of EP in 395 patients who had good-risk metastatic GCT [11]. The dose of etoposide in this trial was 360 mg/m^2 per cycle

Box 2. Indiana University, Memorial-Sloan Kettering Cancer Center, and International Germ Cell Cancer Consensus Risk Classification Systems for Good Risk Disease

Indiana University

Minimal risk
- Elevated markers as only evidence of disease
- Cervical nodes (± nonpalpable retroperitoneal nodes)
- Unresectable, nonpalpable retroperitoneal disease
- Minimal pulmonary metastases: <5 per lung field and largest <2 cm; (± nonpalpable retroperitoneal nodes)

Moderate risk
- Palpable abdominal mass only
- Moderate pulmonary metastases: 5–10 per lung field with largest <3 cm; or mediastinal adenopathy <50% intrathoracic diameter; or solitary pulmonary mass >2 cm (± nonpalpable retroperitoneal nodes)

Memorial-Sloan Kettering Cancer Center

NSGCT
- Gonadal origin
- Calculated probability of CR $\geq$ 0.5

Probability of CR = expH/(1 + exp H),

where H = 8.514 − 1.973 log (LDH + 1) − .530 log (β-HCG + 1) − 1.111 TOTMET

and TOTMET = total number of metastatic sites; β-HCG in ng/mL

Seminoma
- Stage IIC–III gonadal or extragonadal seminoma or relapsed after radiation therapy

International Germ Cell Cancer Consensus

NSGCT
- Testis/retroperitoneal primary and
- Nonpulmonary visceral metastases absent and
- AFP < 1000 ng/L and β-HCG < 5000 IU/L and LDH < 1.5 × ULN

Seminoma
- Any primary and
- Nonpulmonary visceral metastases absent and
- Any β-HCG and any LDH

Abbreviations: AFP, α-fetoprotein; β-HCG, β-human chorionic gonadotropin; CR, complete response; LDH, lactate dehydrogenase; ULN, upper limit of normal.

compared with 500 mg/m^2 used in most regimens. The complete response rate was 95% in the BEP arm compared with 87% in the EP arm (P = .0075). No significant difference in progression-free or overall survival was demonstrated. The lack of survival differences was attributed to successful salvage treatment. Two patients in the BEP arm died of BIP. The authors concluded that with standard treatment of good-risk metastatic GCT, bleomycin should not be omitted.

In sum, if three cycles of chemotherapy are to be administered to patients who have good-risk metastatic GCT, then bleomycin is an essential component of this treatment.

The development of the etoposide/cisplatin regimen

The EP regimen was developed by investigators at MSKCC. In an early trial of patients who had good-risk metastatic GCT, EP was compared with the VAB-6 regimen (cisplatin, vinblastine, bleomycin, dactinomycin, cyclophosphamide) [12]. Although these regimens had similar efficacy, the toxicity profile and ease of administration of the EP regimen was superior. At MSKCC, four cycles of EP became the standard for patients who had good-risk metastatic GCT.

Investigators at MSKCC recently reported a retrospective analysis of long-term follow-up on 289 patients who had good-risk metastatic GCT defined by IGCCC criteria [13]. Complete response was achieved in 98% of patients. Five-year survival for the cohort was 96% (95% CI, 94%–98%). Based on these excellent results, four cycles of EP is now considered an alternate to three cycles of BEP.

Can carboplatin be substituted for cisplatin?

Cisplatin is the cornerstone of chemotherapy regimens for advanced GCT. This agent is associated with nausea, nephrotoxicity, ototoxicity, and neurotoxicity. Carboplatin is a newer platinum analog with a better toxicity profile than cisplatin and is easier to administer. Several randomized trials have addressed the issue of whether the better tolerated carboplatin can be routinely substituted for cisplatin in combination regimens for GCT.

Investigators at MSKCC have studied the role of carboplatin in good-risk GCT as defined by the MSKCC criteria [14]. Patients were randomized to receive four cycles of standard EP versus four cycles of EC (etoposide 100 mg/m^2 IV daily for 5 days plus carboplatin 500 mg/m^2 IV on day 1 every 28 days). In 265 evaluable patients, the complete response rate was 90% for the EP arm versus 88% for the EC arm (P = .32). In the EC arm, 12% of patients relapsed compared with only 3% on the EP arm. The patients treated with EC had inferior event-free and relapse-free survival (P = .02 and P = .005, respectively). Overall survival was not significantly different between the two arms. The authors concluded that the EC regimen was inferior to EP.

The EORTC/MRC performed a randomized phase III trial in patients who had good-risk NSGCT that also addressed the issue of cisplatin versus carboplatin [15]. A total of 528 evaluable patients were randomized to receive four cycles of BEP (using the European regimen of etoposide 120 mg/m^2 on days 1, 2, 3; bleomycin 30 units day 2; cisplatin 100 mg/m^2 total over 2 or 5 days every 21 days) versus four cycles of BEC (same dose of etoposide and bleomycin, but using carboplatin AUC 5 mg/mL × min.). Complete response was 94.4% in the BEP arm and 87.3% in the BEC arm (P = .009). Failure-free survival at 1 year was 91% and 77%, respectively (P<.001). Three-year survival rate was superior for patients in the BEP arm (97% versus 90%, respectively; P = .003).

Together, these trials have demonstrated that in the treatment of patients who have good-risk metastatic GCT, carboplatin is inferior to cisplatin and should not be used.

Which regimen should be considered standard of care for good-risk metastatic germ cell tumor?

The clinician treating the patient who has good-risk metastatic GCT has an initial decision to make: should the patient be treated with BEP for three cycles or EP for four cycles? At the 2003 meeting of the American Society of Clinical Oncology (ASCO), Culine and colleagues [16] presented a randomized trial comparing three cycles of BEP to four cycles of EP in patients who had good-risk metastatic GCT. The primary endpoint of the trial was a "favorable response rate" (FRR), defined as chemotherapy complete response, surgical complete response, or marker-negative partial response. The trial was designed to demonstrate less than 10% difference in FRR between the two arms. A total of 270 patients were randomized and 258 patients were eligible. The FRR was 92% for the BEP arm versus 91% for the EP arm (P = .6). No statistically significant differences in 4-year event-free survival or 4-year overall survival were reported. The final results of this trial have not been published in a peer-reviewed journal. In this author's opinion, either three cycles of BEP or four cycles of EP should be considered standard of care in the management of good-risk metastatic GCT.

Which of these two regimens should be preferred? The treating physician and patient need to individualize the choice of treatment and discuss the relative pros and cons of each. Given that risk factors for BIP in patients who have GCT include age greater than 40 years, renal dysfunction, underlying pulmonary disease, smoking, and cumulative bleomycin dose, there may be reason to choose four cycles of EP and avoid bleomycin. It should be remembered, however, that the overall risk for BIP with 270 units of bleomycin is low, so avoidance of bleomycin in young individuals who have normal renal and pulmonary function is not warranted. In patients who have underlying peripheral neuropathy or hearing loss in whom minimizing cisplatin exposure might be advantageous, three cycles of BEP may be preferred to avoid the extra cycle of cisplatin.

Guideline recommendations: what is the standard of care?

Based on the evidence discussed above, the National Comprehensive Cancer Network in their Testicular Cancer guideline (Version 1.2006) writes "Presently, two regimens are considered standard treatment programs in the United States for good-risk germ cell tumors: 4 cycles of EP, or 3 cycles of BEP" [17]. In their consensus statement, the European Germ Cell Cancer Consensus Group states that "For patients with 'good' prognosis disease, according to IGCCCG criteria, standard treatment is three cycles of BEP. In cases of contraindications against bleomycin four cycles of cisplatin and etoposide (PE) can be given" [18].

Late effects of cisplatin-based chemotherapy

For many patients who have GCT, cisplatin-based chemotherapy is required for cure. Because patients who have GCT are usually young and are likely to become long-term survivors, issues related to long-term complications of this treatment are important. Cisplatin-based chemotherapy for patients who have GCT may be associated with long-term consequences that may affect several organ systems (Box 3). A review concerning the medical management of the long-term GCT survivor has recently been published [19].

The most studied late effect of cisplatin-based chemotherapy in patients who have GCT is cardiovascular risk. Raynaud phenomenon has been reported in patients who have GCT treated with cisplatin-based chemotherapy [20]. Serious vascular complications (eg, myocardial infarction, stroke, thromboembolic disease) have been reported in patients who had GCT treated with cisplatin-based chemotherapy [21–23]. Larger series have examined the risk for cardiovascular events in patients who have been treated with chemotherapy. In a study of patients who have GCT treated with surgery or surgery plus chemotherapy (intergroup adjuvant trial), Nichols and colleagues [24] reported no increased risk for cardiovascular events in the chemotherapy group at a median follow-up of 5 years. Meinardi and colleagues [25] have demonstrated a relative risk for cardiovascular events of 7.1 (95% CI, 1.9–18.3) in patients less than 50 years old who had GCT who had received cisplatin-based chemotherapy and were in remission for 10 years or more compared with a general male population. Huddart and colleagues [26] also recently reported on cardiovascular risk in a large cohort of long-term GCT. Among 992 patients who had GCT at a median of 10.2 years of follow-up, 68 cardiovascular events were reported, including 18 deaths. Increased risk for cardiovascular events was seen in patients who had GCT who had received chemotherapy, radiation therapy, or chemotherapy/radiation compared with those treated only with surveillance. Most recently, van den Belt-Dusebout and colleagues [27] have reported on long-term cardiovascular disease in 2512 long-term survivors of GCT. With a median follow-up of 18.4 years, the standardized incidence ratio for coronary heart

Box 3. Potential late effects of cisplatin-based chemotherapy in germ cell tumor survivors

Vascular/cardiovascular
Raynaud phenomenon
Hyperlipidemia
Hypertension
Metabolic syndrome
Coronary heart disease

Renal
Impaired glomerular filtration rate
Hypomagnesemia
Increased plasma renin and aldosterone

Otologic
Tinnitus
Hearing loss

Reproductive
Impaired spermatogenesis

Neurologic
Peripheral neuropathy

disease was 1.17 (95% CI, 1.04–1.31). Cisplatin-based chemotherapy was associated with a 1.9-fold (95% CI, 1.7- to 2.0-fold) increased risk for myocardial infarction.

The underlying mechanism for the increased cardiovascular risk associated with cisplatin-based chemotherapy is not clear. Patients who have GCT treated with cisplatin-based chemotherapy may prematurely develop hyperlipidemia, hypertension, increased body mass index, and metabolic syndrome [25,28,29]. This point underscores that long-term survivors of GCT should have lifelong medical follow-up, especially if treated with cisplatin-based chemotherapy.

Second malignancies

Acute myelogenous leukemia with specific abnormalities in chromosome 11q23 may occur 2 to 3 years after treatment with etoposide [30]. The risk for leukemia seems to be cumulative and dose-dependent. Studies generally report the risk break point is a cumulative etoposide dose less than or equal to 2 g/m^2 versus greater than 2 g/m^2. Fortunately, the risk for leukemia for most patients who have GCT is low, with a cumulative incidence at 5 years of less than 0.6%.

Travis and colleagues [31] have recently reported a population-based registry study examining the risk for secondary solid malignancies in long-term survivors of GCT. Based on 14 registries, 40,576 1-year survivors of GCT were identified with a median follow-up of 11.3 years. In this cohort, 2285 second solid cancers were identified for an observed-to-expected ratio of 1.41 (95% CI, 1.35–1.47). The risk increased with increasing age of the patient at diagnosis of GCT and continued for 35 years. Increased risk for second solid cancers was observed in patients treated with radiation therapy alone (relative risk [RR] = 2.0; 95% CI, 1.9–2.2), chemotherapy alone (RR = 1.8; 95% CI, 1.3–2.5), and both (RR = 2.9; 95% CI, 1.9–4.2). The finding that patients treated with chemotherapy alone are at statistically increased risk for second solid cancers has not previously been demonstrated. The underlying mechanism associated with this risk is unknown.

Summary

The excellent outcome for patients who have GCT who have good-risk metastatic disease is a major medical advance. Through well-designed cooperative group studies, standard therapies are in place to maximize cure while minimizing toxicity. Future investigation of the late effects of cisplatin-based chemotherapy in patients who have GCT will lead to interventions to keep long-term GCT survivors healthy for decades to come.

References

[1] American Cancer Society. Cancer Facts and figures, 2007. Atlanta: American Cancer Society; 2007.

[2] Birch R, Williams S, Cone A, et al. Prognostic factors for favorable outcome in disseminated germ cell tumors. J Clin Oncol 1986;4:400–7.

[3] Bosl GJ, Geller NL, Cirrincione C, et al. Multivariate analysis of prognostic variables in patients with metastatic testicular cancer. Cancer Res 1983;43: 3403–7.

[4] International Germ Cell Cancer Collaborative Group. International germ cell consensus classification: a prognostic factor-based staging system for metastatic germ cell cancers. J Clin Oncol 1997;15: 594–603.

[5] Einhorn LH, Williams SD, Loehrer PJ, et al. Evaluation of optimal duration of chemotherapy in favorable-prognosis disseminated germ cell tumors: a Southeastern Cancer Study Group Protocol. J Clin Oncol 1989;7:387–91.

[6] Saxman SB, Finch D, Gonin R, et al. Long-term follow-up of a phase III study of three versus four cycles of bleomycin, etoposide, and cisplatin in favorable-prognosis germ cell tumors: the Indiana University experience. J Clin Oncol 1998;16:702–6.

[7] De Wit R, Roberts JT, Wilkinson PM, et al. Equivalence of three or four cycles of bleomycin, etoposide, and cisplatin chemotherapy and of a 3- or 5-day schedule in good-prognosis germ cell cancer: a randomized study of the European Organization for the Research and Treatment of Cancer Genitourinary Tract Cancer Cooperative Group and the Medical Research Council. J Clin Oncol 2001;19:1629–40.

[8] Sleijfer S. Bleomycin-induced pneumonitis. Chest 2001;120:617–24.

[9] O'Sullivan JM, Huddart RA, Norman AR, et al. Predicting the risk of bleomycin lung toxicity in patients with germ-cell tumours. Ann Oncol 2003;14:91–6.

[10] Loehrer PJ, Johnson D, Elson P, et al. Importance of bleomycin in favorable-prognosis disseminated germ cell tumors: an Eastern Cooperative Oncology Group trial. J Clin Oncol 1995;13:470–6.

[11] deWit R, Stoter G, Kaye SB, et al. Importance of bleomycin in combination chemotherapy for good-prognosis testicular nonseminoma: a randomized trial of the European Organization for the Research and Treatment of Cancer Genitourinary Tract Cancer Cooperative Group. J Clin Oncol 1997;15: 1837–43.

[12] Bosl GJ, Geller NL, Bajorin D, et al. A randomized trial of etoposide + cisplatin versus vinblastine + bleomycin + cisplatin + cyclophosphamide + dactinomycin in patients with good-prognosis germ cell tumors. J Clin Oncol 1988;6:1231–8.
[13] Kondagunta GV, Bacik J, Bajorin D, et al. Etoposide and cisplatin for metastatic good-risk germ cell tumors. J Clin Oncol 2005;23:9290–4.
[14] Bajorin DF, Sarosdy MF, Pfister DG, et al. Randomized trial of etoposide and cisplatin versus etoposide and carboplatin in patients with good-risk germ cell tumors: a multiinstitutional study. J Clin Oncol 1993;11:598–606.
[15] Horwich A, Sleijfer DT, Fossa SD, et al. Randomized trial of bleomycin, etoposide, and cisplatin compared with bleomycin, etoposide, and carboplatin in good-prognosis metastatic nonseminomatous germ cell cancer: a multiinstitutional Medical Research Council/European Organization for the Research and Treatment of Cancer Trial. J Clin Oncol 1997; 15:1844–55.
[16] Culine S, Kerbrat P, Bouzy J, et al. The optimal chemotherapy regimen for good-risk metastatic nonseminomatous germ cell tumors (MNSGCT) is 3 cycles of bleomycin, etoposide, and cisplatin: mature results of a randomized trial [abstract # 1536]. Proc Amer Soc Clin Oncol 2003;22:383.
[17] Motzer RJ, Bolger GB, Boston B, et al. Testicular cancer. J Natl Compr Canc Netw 2006;4(10):1038–58. Available at: http://www.nccn.org/professionals/physician_gls/PDF/testicular.pdf.
[18] Schmoll HJ, Souchon R, Krege S, et al. European consensus on diagnosis and treatment of germ cell cancer: a report of the European Germ Cell Cancer Consensus Group (EGCCCG). Annals of Oncology 2004;15:1377–99.
[19] Vaughn DJ, Gignac GA, Meadows AT. Long-term medical care of testicular cancer survivors. Ann Intern Med 2002;136(6):463–70.
[20] Vogelzang NJ, Bosl GJ, Johnson K, et al. Raynaud's phenomenon: a common toxicity after combination chemotherapy for testicular cancer. Ann Intern Med 1981;95:288–92.
[21] Vogelzang NJ, Frenning DH, Kennedy BJ. Coronary artery disease after treatment with bleomycin and vinblastine. Cancer Treat Rep 1980;64: 1159–60.
[22] Doll DC, List AF, Greco FA, et al. Acute vascular ischemic events after cisplatin-related combination chemotherapy for germ cell tumors of the testis. Ann Intern Med 1986;105:48–51.
[23] Lederman GS, Garnick MB. Pulmonary emboli as a complication of germ cell cancer treatment. J Urol 1987;137:1236–7.
[24] Nichols CR, Roth BJ, Williams SD, et al. No evidence of acute cardiovascular complications of chemotherapy for testicular cancer: an analysis of the Testicular Cancer Intergroup Study. J Clin Oncol 1992;10:760–5.
[25] Meinardi MT, Gietema J, Van der Graaf WT, et al. Cardiovascular morbidity in long-term survivors of metastatic testicular cancer. J Clin Oncol 2000;18: 1725–32.
[26] Huddart RA, Norman M, Shahidi M, et al. Cardiovascular disease as a long term complication of treatment for testicular cancer. J Clin Oncol 2003;21: 1513–23.
[27] van den Belt-Dusebout AW, Nuver J, deWit R, et al. Long-term risk of cardiovascular disease in 5-year survivors of testicular cancer. J Clin Oncol 2006; 20:467–75.
[28] Nuver J, Smit AJ, Wolffenbuttel BH, et al. The metabolic syndrome and disturbances in hormone levels in long-term survivors of disseminated testicular cancer. J Clin Oncol 2005;23:3718–25.
[29] Sagstuen H, Aass N, Fossa SD, et al. Blood pressure and body mass index in long-term survivors of testicular cancer. J Clin Oncol 2005;23: 4980–90.
[30] Bokemeyer C, Schmoll HJ. Treatment of testicular cancer and the development of secondary malignancies. J Clin Oncol 1995;13:283–92.
[31] Travis LB, Fossa SD, Schonfeld SJ, et al. Second cancers among 40576 testicular cancer patients: focus on long-term survivors. J Natl Cancer Inst 2005;97:1361–5.

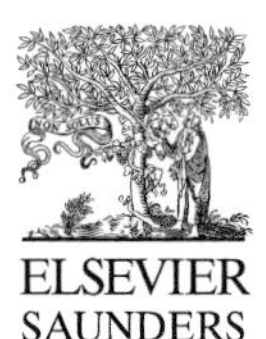
ELSEVIER
SAUNDERS

Urol Clin N Am 34 (2007) 179–185

UROLOGIC CLINICS of North America

Adjuvant Chemotherapy for Stage II Nonseminomatous Germ Cell Tumors

G. Varuni Kondagunta, MD[a,b,*], Robert J. Motzer, MD[a,b]

[a]*Genitourinary Oncology Service, Division of Solid Tumor Oncology, Department of Medicine, Memorial Sloan-Kettering Cancer Center, 1275 York Avenue, New York, NY 10021, USA*
[b]*Department of Medicine, Joan and Sanford I. Weill Medical College of Cornell University, 1275 York Avenue, New York, NY 10021, USA*

Almost all patients who have non-bulky stage II nonseminomatous germ cell tumors (NSGCT) can be cured with a cisplatin-based regimen following retroperitoneal lymph node dissection (RPLND). The study of adjuvant therapy in this clinical setting has included risk stratification of patients and a search for the most effective and least toxic chemotherapeutic regimen.

Chemotherapy programs in advanced disease

Germ cell tumors (GCT) are considered a model for curable cancer based on the successful treatment of metastatic disease with cisplatin-containing chemotherapy (More than 90% of newly diagnosed GCT patients are cured.) [1]. Accumulated data from phase II and III trials show that treatment with cisplatin, vinblastine, and bleomycin (VAB series, PVB) achieves a durable response in 70% to 80% of patients who have metastatic GCT [2–5]. Treatment-related toxicity was substantial in these regimens, however, including hematologic, gastrointestinal, neurologic, dermatologic, and pulmonary toxicities [3].

In an effort to decrease toxicity while maintaining a high rate of cure, patients are stratified into "good-risk" and "poor-risk" groups by using prognostic criteria based on primary site, extent of disease, and serum tumor markers. The goal with good-risk patients is to maintain the high cure rate but minimize the toxicity of the treatment regimen. Standard good-risk regimens (three cycles of cisplatin, etoposide, and bleomycin [BEP]; and four cycles of etoposide and cisplatin [EP]) were established in randomized trials [6–10]. These regimens were shown to result in a durable complete response in approximately 90% of good-risk patients. The high cure rate achieved in patients who had metastatic disease led to the use of good-risk regimens in the postoperative (adjuvant) setting, following RPLND as primary treatment. In contrast, only half of all patients who had poor-risk features achieved a durable complete response to four cycles of BEP [3,11]. The goal in this poor-risk population is to increase the cure rate, with reduction of toxicity as a secondary objective.

Retroperitoneal lymph node dissection and pathologic staging for low-volume stage II nonseminoma

The American Joint Committee on Cancer and the Union Internationale Contre le Cancer revised the tumor, nodes, metastasis (TNM) classification of testicular GCT to include serum concentrations of α-fetoprotein, human chorionic gonadotropin, and lactate dehydrogenase into staging of advanced disease. Findings of vascular or lymphatic invasion were incorporated in the staging of the primary testicular tumor, and the pathologic staging for stage II disease was modified [1].

* Corresponding author. Genitourinary Oncology Service, Division of Solid Tumor Oncology, Department of Medicine, Memorial Sloan-Kettering Cancer Center, 1275 York Avenue, New York, NY 10021.

E-mail address: kondaguv@mskcc.org (G.V. Kondagunta).

doi:10.1016/j.ucl.2007.02.005

RPLND is used as the primary curative treatment for selected patients who have clinical stage I and stage II disease. A recent retrospective analysis by Stephenson and colleagues [12] demonstrated that primary RPLND in selected patients can circumvent the toxicity associated with chemotherapy by excluding patients who have elevated serum tumor markers and clinical stage IIb disease or greater, thus minimizing chemotherapy toxicity for the other carefully selected patients. For others who have more advanced disease, adjuvant chemotherapy is indicated to maintain the high rate of cure. At RPLND, pathologic TNM staging is assessed based on four staging groups (Table 1), and treatment is planned according to staging. For example, because 90% or more of patients who have pN0 disease usually experience a disease-free survival with surgery alone, adjuvant chemotherapy is not offered to these patients [13,14].

Early trials of adjuvant chemotherapy

Before the advent of cisplatin-based chemotherapy, patients who had completely resected node-positive disease (pN1 and pN2) were offered either no adjuvant chemotherapy, minimally effective chemotherapy, or postoperative radiotherapy [15,16]. The relapse rate in this patient population was 20% to 70%, with most studies showing a relapse rate of 50% to 60% [17]. As cisplatin-based chemotherapeutic regimens were found to be effective in stage III GCT, these regimens were studied in the adjuvant setting. The hope was to decrease the proportion of patients who relapsed after RPLND and to increase the proportion of patients who were cured. These early trials of adjuvant chemotherapy are summarized in Table 2. The regimens, which included cisplatin, vinblastine, and bleomycin, were superior to prior trials of non–platinum-based chemotherapy.

Table 1
Pathologic staging of regional lymph nodes after retroperitoneal lymph node dissection

Stage	Lymph node status
pN0	No regional lymph node metastases
pN1	Lymph node mass ≤2 cm at greatest dimension; or multiple lymph nodes, none >2 cm in greatest dimension
pN2	Lymph node mass >2 cm but not >5 cm in greatest dimension; or multiple lymph nodes, any one mass >2 cm but not >5 cm in greatest dimension; or any evidence of extranodal extension
pN3	Lymph node mass >5 cm in greatest dimension

One non–platinum-containing regimen studied at Memorial Sloan-Kettering Cancer Center (MSKCC) was "mini-VAB," which consisted of vinblastine, dactinomycin, bleomycin, and chlorambucil. This regimen proved ineffective because of the lack of cisplatin, but the experience with mini-VAB was useful in defining the relapse pattern for patients who had completely resected stage II disease. The patients were retrospectively grouped, using the older classification system, into stage IIA (microscopically positive or grossly positive with <6 nodes, all nodes ≤2 cm in diameter) and stage IIB disease (≥6 nodes involved, and/or any node >2 cm, or extranodal extension) [18]. No patient who had stage IIA disease relapsed, whereas a relapse proportion of 34% was seen in patients who had stage IIB disease [18]. Since this trial, therefore, adjuvant therapy has not been routinely offered to compliant patients who have low-volume nodal involvement (pN1), and cisplatin-based chemotherapy has been administered to patients who have high-volume disease (pN2).

Cisplatin-, bleomycin-, and vinblastine-containing regimens (PVB) have resulted in a disease-free survival of greater than 90% in patients who have advanced-stage disease [18–20]. Consistent with the treatment of patients who have advanced GCT, efforts in the management of completely resected stage II nonseminoma focused on maintaining efficacy while decreasing treatment-related morbidity.

One randomized study involving 225 patients compared two versus four cycles of adjuvant PVB. This trial showed that both groups had an equally high survival rate after a median follow-up of 43 months [21]. Patients treated with four cycles of therapy had more toxicity, but no appreciable improvement in survival. The trial established two cycles of therapy as standard in patients who had completely resected stage II nonseminomatous germ cell tumor after RPLND. This study also focused on the use of surveillance, with chemotherapy withheld until relapse, and better-tolerated cisplatin-based adjuvant regimens, in an effort to decrease toxicity and maintain a high cure rate.

Surveillance

The surveillance approach entails close monitoring of patients after RPLND, with

Table 2
Early trials of adjuvant chemotherapy after relapse from retroperitoneal lymph node dissection

Regimen (author/reference)	No. of patients	Relapse-free (%)	Median follow-up (mo.)
Vinblastine-containing regimens			
VAB-3 (Vugrin et al, 1981 [18])	29	100	24
VAB-6 (Vugrin et al, 1983 [20])	42	98	24
PVB (Vogelzang et al, 1983 [17])	11	100	36
PVB (Pizzocaro et al, 1984 [32])	14	100	29
PVB, VAB-4 (Williams et al, 1987 [30])	92	99	>48
PVB (Weissbach and Hartlapp, 1991 [21])	225	97	43
Etoposide-containing regimens			
EP (Motzer et al, 1995 [31])	50	100	42
BEP (Behnia et al, 2000 [35])	86	99	47

Abbreviations: VAB 3, VAB 4, VAB 6, cisplatin + vinblastine plus bleomycin + actinomycin D + cyclophosphamide; PVB, cisplatin, vinblastine, and bleomycin; EP, etoposide, cisplatin; BEP, bleomycin, etoposide, and cisplatin.

chemotherapy reserved for patients who relapse. The benefit of this approach is that it spares some patients from chemotherapeutic treatment, although even more chemotherapy, and possibly additional surgery, is required for patients who do relapse. The surveillance approach is particularly amenable for patients who have low-volume disease (pN1), as the proportion of relapse in these patients is low [5,17,22–24].

The impact of surveillance on survival for patients who have pathologic stage II GCT was addressed in a randomized trial [24]. A total of 195 patients were randomized to surveillance (98 patients) or to routine adjuvant chemotherapy with two cycles of cisplatin-, vinblastine-, and bleomycin-containing chemotherapy (97 patients). Those on the surveillance arm who relapsed (49% of 98 observed patients) were treated with three or four cycles of systemic chemotherapy for disseminated disease. One of the 97 patients assigned to the adjuvant therapy group relapsed after completing adjuvant chemotherapy. Three patients died of GCT with observation alone, whereas 1 patient died of GCT in the adjuvant therapy group. The proportion of patients who remained alive was no different between the two treatment groups (96% overall) at a median follow-up of more than 4 years. The conclusion of the study was that two courses of cisplatin-based adjuvant chemotherapy almost always prevents relapse in patients who have pathologic stage II disease who have had RPLND, and in this trial, close surveillance led to an equivalent outcome [24].

It is important to note that 51% of the patients on the surveillance arm had low-volume disease, and only 5% of the surveillance arm had extranodal extension. Because low-volume disease is associated with a low likelihood of relapse [5,20,25–27], the population of patients treated on the observation arm had a favorable prognosis when compared with the other patients on observation alone. Patients who had low-volume disease have been shown by other studies to have a low likelihood of relapse (one third or less) on surveillance. In contrast, the relapse proportion for patients who have high-volume disease exceeds 50%, and has been reported to be as high as 90% for patients who have extranodal disease when no adjuvant chemotherapy is given [28]. The differences in makeup of the two randomized groups may have resulted in a disproportionately high number of patients on surveillance alone who did not relapse.

Another important point to consider in interpreting the results of the surveillance study is that that those patients who do relapse after observation alone require a longer course of chemotherapy, consisting of three or four cycles of cisplatin-based chemotherapy as opposed to just two cycles of adjuvant chemotherapy. In addition, 25% of patients on the surveillance arm failed to present for at least half of the required monthly follow-up visits during the first year. Patients who have node-positive GCT (pN1) following RPLND who are unwilling to adhere to the rigorous follow-up schedule associated with the surveillance approach should be treated with adjuvant chemotherapy.

Etoposide and cisplatin adjuvant chemotherapy

In patients who have high-volume metastases, the use of well-tolerated adjuvant chemotherapy should be strongly considered. Substitution of etoposide for vinblastine in two randomized studies of standard therapy for good- and poor-risk patients who had disseminated NSGCT showed less toxicity and equivalent or superior efficacy [7,29,30].

Based on the efficacy and tolerability of four cycles of EP in patients who had disseminated GCT, a prospective trial of two cycles of EP was conducted in the adjuvant setting [31]. Eligibility for the study was restricted to patients who had pN2 disease at RPLND, representing a group of patients who have an otherwise 50% or greater probability of relapse in surveillance. Fifty evaluable patients were treated in the study (Table 3) [31]. None of the 50 patients had relapsed at a median follow-up of 35 months (range 12–72 months) [31]. The stomatitis, dermatologic toxicity, and ileus reported with vinblastine-based adjuvant chemotherapy were not present in the etoposide-based chemotherapy [5,20,26,32]. No pulmonary or renal toxicity was noted, and neurotoxicity was minimal. The efficacy and tolerability of this regimen led the authors to regard two cycles of EP as the standard adjuvant regimen for patients who have pathologic stage N_2 NSGCT.

A retrospective analysis was conducted of these 50 patients plus an additional 37 patients who were identified from a surgical database of patients undergoing RPLND who had been treated at MSKCC with two cycles of EP as adjuvant therapy for node-positive disease [33]. Ten patients (11%) had pN1 disease, 73 (84%) had pN2 disease, and 4 (5%) had pN3 disease. Eighty-six patients received two cycles of EP, and 1 patient received an additional two cycles of EP following a transient marker increase after the first cycle. Eighty-seven patients are alive; 86 (98%) remain relapse-free at a median follow-up of 8 years (range 0.9–13.5 years) [33].

Table 3
Effective, low-toxicity adjuvant regimens in patients who have nonseminomatous germ cell tumors and high-volume metastases

Drug	Cycles	Dose	Days
Adjuvant etoposide and cisplatin (EP)[a] [33]			
Cisplatin	2 cycles Within 4 wks of RPLND; no later than 8 wks after surgery	20 mg/m^2	1–5
Etoposide		100 mg/m^2	
Adjuvant bleomycin, etoposide, and cisplatin (BEP)[b] [35]			
Cisplatin	2 cycles (given every 28 days)	20 mg/m^2	1–5
Etoposide		100 mg/m^2	
Bleomycin	Weekly for 8 wks	30 IU	

Abbreviation: RPLND, retroperitoneal lymph node dissection.
[a] Relapse-free survival (8 yr) >98% (n = 87).
[b] n = 86.

This analysis shows that two cycles of adjuvant etoposide plus cisplatin is effective adjuvant therapy for patients who have pathologic stage II disease. Of the 87 NSGCT patients in our series, 89% had pathologic stage N2 or higher. Treatment was well tolerated [10,33], and long-term toxicity was uncommon.

Past efforts to reduce chemotherapy-related toxicity in the management of advanced GCT also included replacement of vinblastine with etoposide, elimination or reduction of bleomycin, and reduction of treatment cycles. At our Center, we studied four cycles of cisplatin plus etoposide with elimination of bleomycin in patients who had good-risk metastatic GCT [34]. Our trial involving two cycles of etoposide plus cisplatin (EP) evolved as part of that effort (see Table 3).

In a retrospective series, two cycles of BEP have also been reported as an effective adjuvant regimen [35]. In a study of 86 patients, 49 (57%) had pathologic stage IIA disease on RPLND, whereas 37 (43%) had pathologic stage IIB disease on RPLND [35]. After RPLND, patients received two cycles of BEP (see Table 3). After a median follow-up of 85 months, 82 patients were evaluable, and 4 were lost to follow-up. Only 1 patient experienced relapse of a cervical node with teratoma; this patient is relapse-free after resection of disease. Toxicity was limited to 12% who suffered neutropenic fever during the course of therapy, although pulmonary function tests were not formally assessed [35].

Although two cycles of either EP or BEP may be considered for adjuvant therapy, we prefer EP because it avoids the use of bleomycin, and our data show more than 98% relapse-free survival with this regimen [33].

Primary management for patients who have clinical stage II disease often involves cisplatin combination chemotherapy before consideration of RPLND. Based on efficacy with the use of chemotherapy in the primary management of stage II NSGCT, patients who have clinical stage N2 or higher generally receive full-course chemotherapy before RPLND. In the rare instance in which pN3 disease is present at RPLND, our preference is full treatment with four cycles of EP or three cycles of BEP.

There is a higher risk for relapse in patients who have pN2 disease, and these patients are offered adjuvant chemotherapy after RPLND. Also, patients who have pN1 disease may choose adjuvant chemotherapy over observation. Adjuvant chemotherapy for noncompliant patients remains mandatory, however, and patients who have more advanced nodal disease (pN3) or unresected disease should receive full-course chemotherapy.

Serum markers as a prognostic factor in low-volume nodal metastases

Rabbani and colleagues [36] recently reviewed reports of NSGCT patients who had low-volume nodal metastases at RPLND (pN1) to determine predictive factors for relapse. Of the 50 patients studied, 11 patients relapsed. The most common pattern of relapse arose from marker elevation [36]. Persistent marker elevation before RPLND was a significant predictor of relapse, with a relative risk of 8.0. Patients who have clinical stage I and IIA disease with persistent marker elevation after orchiectomy thus have a high rate of relapse. In this group, primary RPLND may not be adequate, and these patients should be treated with primary chemotherapy followed by consideration of RPLND for residual disease [36].

Current recommendations

RPLND as primary therapy is potentially curative. In addition, it defines the pathologic stage and directs management of patients who have clinical stage I or stage IIA disease and negative markers. Nodal involvement is categorized as low-volume (pN1) or high-volume (pN2) nodal disease.

The recommended treatment for patients who do not have nodal involvement (pN0) is observation alone. In patients who have pN1 disease who are compliant observation is acceptable, whereas in patients who are not compliant adjuvant therapy with two cycles of EP or BEP is suggested. Patients who have pN2 disease have a 50% to 90% risk for relapse, so adjuvant therapy with two cycles of EP or BEP is strongly favored. The preference at MSKCC for two cycles of adjuvant EP is based on tolerability of the treatment programs and the near assurance of relapse-free survival in a group of patients who otherwise have a greater than 50% chance of relapse. In the rare instance that a resected mass from RPLND is found to be greater than 5 cm (pN3) or disease is unresectable, then four cycles of EP or three cycles of BEP are warranted.

Acknowlegements

The authors thank Carol Pearce for her editing assistance.

References

[1] DeVita VT, Hellman S, Rosenberg SA, editors. Cancer: principles and practice of oncology. 7th edition. Philadelphia: Williams and Wilkins; 2005.

[2] Cheng E, Cvitkovic E, Wittes RE, et al. Germ cell tumors (II): VAB II in metastatic testicular cancer. Cancer 1978;42:2162–8.

[3] Einhorn LH, Donohue J. Cis-diamminedichloroplatinum, vinblastine, and bleomycin combination chemotherapy in disseminated testicular cancer. Ann Intern Med 1977;87:293–8.

[4] Reynolds TF, Vugrin D, Cvitkovic E, et al. VAB-3 combination chemotherapy of metastatic testicular cancer. Cancer 1981;48:888–98.

[5] Vugrin D, Whitmore WF, Cvitkovic E, et al. Adjuvant chemotherapy combination of vinblastine, actinomycin D, Bleomycin, and Chlorambucil following retroperitoneal lymph node dissection for stage II testis tumor. Cancer 1981;47:840–4.

[6] Bajorin DF, Sarosdy MF, Pfister DG, et al. Randomized trial of etoposide and cisplatin versus etoposide and carboplatin in patients with good-risk germ cell tumors: a multi-institutional study. J Clin Oncol 1993;11:598–606.

[7] Bosl GJ, Geller NL, Bajorin D, et al. A randomized trial of etoposide + cisplatin versus vinblastine + bleomycin + cisplatin + cyclophosphamide + dactinomycin in patients with good-prognosis germ cell tumors. J Clin Oncol 1988;6:1231–8.

[8] Einhorn LH, Williams SD, Loehrer PJ, et al. Evaluation of optimal duration of chemotherapy in favorable-prognosis disseminated germ cell tumors: a Southeastern Cancer Study Group protocol. J Clin Oncol 1989;7:387–91.

[9] Loehrer PJ Sr, Johnson D, Elson P, et al. Importance of bleomycin in favorable-prognosis disseminated germ cell tumors: an Eastern Cooperative Oncology Group trial. J Clin Oncol 1995;13:470–6.

[10] Xiao H, Mazumdar M, Bajorin DF, et al. Long-term follow-up of patients with good-risk germ cell tumors treated with etoposide and cisplatin. J Clin Oncol 1997;15:2553–8.

[11] Donohue JP, Einhorn LH, Perez JM. Improved management of nonseminomatous testis tumors. Cancer 1978;42:2903–8.

[12] Stephenson AJ, Bosl GJ, Motzer RJ, et al. Retroperitoneal lymph node dissection for nonseminomatous germ cell testicular cancer: impact of patient selection factors on outcome. J Clin Oncol 2005;23:2781–8.

[13] Foster RS, Roth BJ. Clinical stage I nonseminoma: surgery versus surveillance. Semin Oncol 1998;25:145–53.

[14] Johnson DE, Bracken RB, Blight EM. Prognosis for pathologic stage I non-seminomatous germ cell tumors of the testis managed by retroperitoneal lymphadenectomy. J Urol 1976;116:63–5.

[15] Bredael JJ, Vugrin D, Whitmore WF Jr. Selected experience with surgery and combination chemotherapy in the treatment of nonseminomatous testis tumors. J Urol 1983;129:985–8.

[16] Jacobs EM, Muggia FM. Testicular cancer: risk factors and the role of adjuvant chemotherapy. Cancer 1980;45:1782–90.

[17] Vogelzang NJ, Fraley EE, Lange PH, et al. Stage II nonseminomatous testicular cancer: a 10-year experience. J Clin Oncol 1983;1:171–8.

[18] Vugrin D, Whitmore W, Cvitkovic E, et al. Adjuvant chemotherapy with VAB-3 of stage II-B testicular cancer. Cancer 1981;48:233–7.

[19] Vugrin D, Cvitkovic E, Whitmore WF Jr, et al. VAB-4 combination chemotherapy in the treatment of metastatic testis tumors. Cancer 1981;47:833–9.

[20] Vugrin D, Whitmore WF Jr, Herr HW, et al. VAB-6 combination chemotherapy in resected stage II-B testis cancer. Cancer 1983;51:5–8.

[21] Weissbach L, Hartlapp JH. Adjuvant chemotherapy of metastatic stage II nonseminomatous testis tumor. J Urol 1991;146:1295–8.

[22] Richie JP, Kantoff PW. Is adjuvant chemotherapy necessary for patients with stage B1 testicular cancer? J Clin Oncol 1991;9:1393–6.

[23] Skinner DG, Scardino PT. Relevance of biochemical tumor markers and lymphadenectomy in management of non-seminomatous testis tumors: current perspective. J Urol 1980;123:378–82.

[24] Williams SD, Stablein DM, Einhorn LH, et al. Immediate adjuvant chemotherapy versus observation with treatment at relapse in pathological stage II testicular cancer. N Engl J Med 1987;317:1433–8.

[25] Vugrin D, Whitmore WF Jr, Herr H, et al. Adjuvant vinblastine, actinomycin D, bleomycin, cyclophosphamide and cis-platinum chemotherapy regimen with and without maintenance in patients with resected stage IIB testis cancer. J Urol 1982;128:715–7.

[26] Hartlapp JH, Weissbach L, Bussar-Maatz R. Adjuvant chemotherapy in nonseminomatous testicular tumour stage II. Int J Androl 1987;10:277–84.

[27] Pizzocaro G, Monfardini S. No adjuvant chemotherapy in selected patients with pathologic stage II nonseminomatous germ cell tumors of the testis. J Urol 1984;131:677–80.

[28] Fraley EE, Narayan P, Vogelzang NJ, et al. Surgical treatment of patients with stages I and II nonseminomatous testicular cancer. J Urol 1985;134:70–3.

[29] Bajorin DF, Geller NL, Weisen SF, et al. Two-drug therapy in patients with metastatic germ cell tumors. Cancer 1991;67:28–32.

[30] Williams SD, Birch R, Einhorn LH, et al. Treatment of disseminated germ-cell tumors with cisplatin, bleomycin, and either vinblastine or etoposide. N Engl J Med 1987;316:1435–40.

[31] Motzer RJ, Sheinfeld J, Mazumdar M, et al. Etoposide and cisplatin adjuvant therapy for patients with pathologic stage II germ cell tumors. J Clin Oncol 1995;13:2700–4.

[32] Pizzocaro G, Piva L, Salvioni R, et al. Adjuvant chemotherapy in resected stage-II nonseminomatous germ cell tumors of testis. In which cases is it necessary? Eur Urol 1984;10:151–8.

[33] Kondagunta GV, Sheinfeld J, Mazumdar M, et al. Relapse-free and overall survival in patients with pathologic stage II nonseminomatous germ cell cancer treated with etoposide and cisplatin adjuvant chemotherapy. J Clin Oncol 2004;22(3): 464–7.

[34] Kondagunta GV, Bacik J, Bajorin D, et al. Etoposide and cisplatin chemotherapy for metastatic good-risk germ cell tumors. J Clin Oncol 2005; 23(36):9290–4.

[35] Behnia M, Foster R, Einhorn LH, et al. Adjuvant bleomycin, etoposide and cisplatin in pathological stage II non-seminomatous testicular cancer: the Indiana University experience. Eur J Cancer 2000; 36:472–5.

[36] Rabbani F, Sheinfeld J, Farivar-Mohseni H, et al. Low-volume nodal metastases detected at retroperitoneal lymphadenectomy for testicular cancer: pattern and prognostic factors for relapse. J Clin Oncol 2001;19:2020–5.

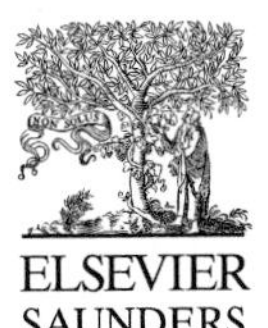
ELSEVIER
SAUNDERS

Urol Clin N Am 34 (2007) 187–197

UROLOGIC CLINICS of North America

The Challenge of Poor-Prognosis Germ Cell Tumors

Guy C. Toner, MBBS, MD, FRACP[a,b,*]

[a] *University of Melbourne, Melbourne, Australia*
[b] *Department of Medical Oncology, Peter MacCallum Cancer Centre, 7 St Andrews Place, East Melbourne, VIC 3002, Australia*

Chemotherapy and surgery as first-line treatment for patients who have metastatic germ cell tumors produce cure in 70% to 80% of cases [1]. Despite the excellent outcome in most cases, 20% to 30% of patients treated for metastatic disease currently die as a result of the malignancy or its treatment. Most of those destined to fail can be identified before treatment based on specific clinical characteristics.

Effective treatment for patients relapsing or failing to achieve an adequate response has been developed, but its success is limited. Only a minority of patients receiving salvage therapy achieve prolonged survival and those failing to respond to initial chemotherapy have a worse outlook [2]. The limited success of salvage therapy dictates that treatment choices and their skilled implementation by a multidisciplinary team are vital. The treating clinicians should have an understanding of the results of available treatment, be able to identify patients likely to fail initial therapy, and have considerable experience in their challenging management.

Prognostic factors

Determination of treatment based on pretreatment clinical characteristics was proposed early in the development of effective chemotherapy [3]. In the 1980s, several major groups identified factors predictive of a poor outcome, including tumor marker elevation, extent or bulk of metastatic disease, visceral organ involvement, histopathology, and primary site [4–9]. The most common finding was that tumor bulk and levels of tumor markers were the most important prognostic variables. Extragonadal primary site was also identified as an adverse prognostic factor, particularly for mediastinal primary nonseminomatous germ cell tumors, which seem to have distinct clinical characteristics and respond poorly to treatment [10,11]. Although most analyses identified similar factors, unfortunately many trial groups or individual centers produced their own prognostic classification systems and used them exclusively in the design and reporting of clinical trials. All of these analyses and classifications were open to criticism for their small numbers, exclusion of certain variables found important by other groups, and lack of consensus.

The impact of the variability in prognostic classification between different centers was demonstrated by Bajorin and colleagues [12]. This study showed that patient selection criteria could make the results of a treatment seem better than an equally effective alternative used in a more stringently selected patient population. This study demonstrated the need for uniform criteria for prognostic classification in clinical trial design and demonstrated clearly the problems of comparison of small phase II trials using differing patient selection criteria.

The International Germ Cell Consensus Classification

An international group pooled data from more than 6000 cases of germ cell tumors undergoing

* Department of Medical Oncology, Peter MacCallum Cancer Centre, 7 St Andrews Place, East Melbourne, VIC 3002, Australia.
E-mail address: guy.toner@petermac.org

0094-0143/07/$ - see front matter
doi:10.1016/j.ucl.2007.02.016

chemotherapy and published a prognostic factor–based staging system in 1997 [13]. The IGCCC identifies three groups with good, intermediate, and poor prognoses. The classification includes seminomas and nonseminomas along with testicular and extragonadal primary sites. The intermediate- and poor-prognosis categories are described in Table 1. The intermediate-prognosis category included 26% of germ cell tumors and achieved 79% overall survival at 5 years. The poor-prognosis group made up 14% of germ cell tumors and had a 48% survival at 5 years.

Since it was published in 1997, the IGCCC classification has been widely accepted. The IGCCC groupings should be used to select the most appropriate treatment for patients requiring chemotherapy. Recently reported clinical trials have successfully used the classification to determine eligibility [14]. This use promises to allow better analysis of results and comparability with other studies. Unless an improved and widely accepted classification is developed, all clinical trial results should be reported using the IGCCC criteria.

Several studies have assessed prognostic factors within the poor-prognosis group [15] or in groups that commonly have a poor prognosis, such as those with an extragonadal primary site [10,16]. Within the IGCCC poor-prognosis group, patients who had a mediastinal primary nonseminoma with metastases had the worst outlook, whereas those who had a testis or retroperitoneal primary site and no visceral metastases other than lung metastases had the best prognosis [15]. A recent evaluation of the international experience with extragonadal germ cell tumors confirmed the findings of the IGCCC with extragonadal seminomas having a good prognosis and mediastinal nonseminoma clearly having the worst outcomes [16].

Serum tumor marker decline during chemotherapy

Investigators at Memorial Sloan Kettering Cancer Center (MSKCC) retrospectively reviewed serum tumor marker data and found that a slower-than-expected decline in either human chorionic gonadotropin (HCG) or α-fetoprotein (AFP) allowed early prediction of subsequent failure in patients who had both good- and poor-prognosis tumors [17]. Similar results were found in the salvage setting [18]. Slow decline of markers has been used in clinical trials at MSKCC to identify patients for early crossover to high-dose chemotherapy with bone marrow transplant [19]. The initial surge in tumor marker levels after initiation of chemotherapy was also found to be prognostic in one study [20]. Assessment of marker decline has been assessed by other investigators with variable results [21], including a recent large study that suggested particular value in poor-prognosis IGCCC patients [22]. The latter approach is being studied prospectively by the French in a randomized trial for poor-prognosis patients to assess the value of changing chemotherapy in those cases with a predicted slow marker normalization [22]. Although there is increasing evidence of the potential value of assessing the pattern of change of serum tumor markers, there remains no consensus as to the most appropriate methodology. At present, it should remain an investigational tool and awaits confirmation by prospective data [21].

Systemic therapy

Investigators at Indiana University performed a randomized trial in unselected patients who had germ cell tumors comparing bleomycin, vinblastine, and cisplatin (PVB) with cisplatin, etoposide,

Table 1
International Germ Cell Collaborative Group Consensus Classification of intermediate and poor prognosis groups [13]

	Intermediate Prognosis	Poor Prognosis
Non-Seminoma	Testis/retroperitoneal primary site, AND No non-pulmonary visceral metastases, AND Intermediate markers–ANY OF: AFP $\geq$ 1000 and $\leq$ 10,000 ng/mL or HCG $\geq$ 5000 iu/l and $\leq$ 50,000 iu/l or LDH $\geq$ 1.5× and $\leq$ 10× upper limit of normal	Mediastinal primary site, OR Non-pulmonary visceral metastases (e.g. brain, bone or liver metastases), OR Poor markers–ANY OF: AFP > 10,000 ng/mL or HCG > 50,000 iu/l (10,000 ng/mL) or LDH > 10× upper limit of normal
Seminoma	Any primary site, AND Non-pulmonary visceral metastases, AND Normal AFP, any HCG, any LDH	No patients with pure seminoma classified as having a poor prognosis

and bleomycin (BEP) [23,24]. In the subgroup of patients considered to have a poor prognosis by Indiana University criteria, 37 were randomized to PVB and 35 to BEP. Some 63% of these patients receiving BEP achieved disease-free status compared with only 38% of patients receiving PVB. The etoposide arm also produced less toxicity. As a result of this trial, four cycles of BEP chemotherapy has been the standard therapy for patients who have poor prognosis germ cell tumors since the mid-1980s.

Multiple studies have been performed attempting to improve on the results with standard BEP. These have generally focused on increased dose intensity, the use of alternate or additional cytotoxic agents, strategies of alternating or sequential chemotherapy regimens, and high-dose chemotherapy with autologous hemopoietic stem cell support. Only some of these strategies have been tested adequately in randomized trials. The results of completed randomized trials are summarized in Table 2 and are discussed below. Selected promising results from nonrandomized studies are also discussed.

Cisplatin dose

Preclinical models and clinical trials [25] suggest a dose–response relationship for cisplatin. Ozols and colleagues [26] at the National Cancer Institute investigated double-dose cisplatin (200 mg/m^2/cycle) with vinblastine, etoposide, and bleomycin compared with standard-dose PVB (100 mg/m^2/cycle of cisplatin). In a small group of patients there was a higher response rate and less frequent relapses with the more aggressive therapy. The apparent superiority of the more aggressive regimen may have been due to factors other than the cisplatin dose, including the addition of etoposide.

The importance of cisplatin dose was clarified by a clinical trial performed by the Southeastern Cancer Study Group. In this study, patients were randomized to receive standard BEP or the same treatment but with double-dose cisplatin [27]. A total of 159 patients entered the study, of which 153 were evaluable for toxicity and response. There was no significant difference between the two groups in relation to response or disease-free survival (see Table 2). Not unexpectedly, the

Table 2
Randomized trials in patients who have poor-risk germ cell tumors

Study	Treatment arm	No. of patients	Complete response rate (%)	Durable response rate (%)	Benefit over control arm
Williams et al [23]	PVB	37	38	NS	Yes[a]
	BEP	35	63	NS	
Ozols et al [26]	PVB	18	67	33	Yes
	P(200)VBE	34	88	68	
Nichols et al [27]	BEP	77	73	61	No
	BEP(200)	76	68	63	
Nichols et al [29]	BEP	141	60	57	No
	VIP	145	63	56	
Wozniak et al [30]	PVB	52	73	NS	No[a]
	PEV	62	65	NS	
de Wit et al [31]	BEP	118	72	58	No
	BEP/PVB	116	76	64	
Kaye et al [33]	BEP	185	57	48	No
	BOP/VIP	186	54	46	
Droz et al [49]	P(200)VBE	49	61	59	No[b]
	P(200)VBE + ABMT	53	41	37	
Bajorin et al [50]	4BEP	111	55	48	No[b]
	2BEP + 2CEC	108	56	52	

Abbreviations: ABMT, autologous bone marrow transplant; B, bleomycin; CEC, high dose carboplatin, etoposide, and cyclophosphamide with stem cell support; E, etoposide; I, ifosfamide; NS, not stated; O, vincristine; P, cisplatin 100 mg/m^2; P(200), cisplatin 200 mg/m^2; V, vinblastine.

[a] Description of poor-prognosis group as a subset analysis of a larger trial.

[b] Published in Abstract form only.

high-dose arm was associated with significantly greater toxicity, including ototoxicity, neurotoxicity, and myelosuppression. This trial demonstrated that there was no advantage to doubling the standard dose of cisplatin.

Alternative or additional drugs and alternating chemotherapy regimens

Ifosfamide is one of only a few drugs that have shown activity in relapsed germ cell tumors. Its inclusion in the VIP regimen of cisplatin, etoposide, and ifosfamide demonstrated significant activity after failure of first-line therapy [28]. The VIP regimen was compared with BEP in a study performed by the Eastern Cooperative Oncology Group [29]. The aim of the study was to assess whether ifosfamide, when substituted for bleomycin, was more active in combination therapy. A total of 304 patients who had Indiana University advanced-stage germ cell cancer were randomized between 1987 and 1992. There was not a statistically significant advantage for the ifosfamide-containing arm (see Table 2), the VIP arm was more toxic, and therefore BEP was recommended as standard therapy.

The Southwest Oncology Group compared a standard PVB regimen with cisplatin, etoposide, and vinblastine (PEV) in a randomized trial for a broad group of germ cell tumor patients [30]. The doses of etoposide and vinblastine were reduced in the experimental arm. There was no benefit for the PEV arm and a trend for a worse outcome in the subgroup of patients who had maximal disease (see Table 2).

The Genitourinary Tract Cancer Cooperative Group of the European Organization for the Research and Treatment of Cancer (EORTC) compared four cycles of BEP to four alternating cycles of BEP plus PVB [31]. There was no advantage to the alternating regimen (see Table 2). Investigators of the Medical Research Council (MRC) and EORTC developed a novel regimen termed BOP-VIP composed of initial intensive therapy with cisplatin, bleomycin, and vincristine followed sequentially by three cycles of a modified VIP regimen. Initial results in a large phase II study were encouraging [32]. A randomized comparison to a BEP regimen failed to demonstrate any benefit, however (see Table 2) [33].

Older nonrandomized trials are not discussed here because many of the issues considered have subsequently been addressed in randomized trials. In other reports, variation in patient selection, small patient numbers, variable treatment policies, or outcome measures all limit the interpretability of the data.

Some nonrandomized published trial data are relevant. Since the publication of the IGCCC classification, some groups have retrospectively reanalyzed their results [34–39]. Selected results are summarized in Table 3. Patients who had a poor prognosis treated with the POMB-ACE regimen developed at Charing Cross Hospital [34,35] and the C-BOP-BEP regimen reported by Horwich and colleagues [37,38] had better survival than predicted in the report describing the classification. These results cannot be considered to indicate the superiority of these regimens over standard therapy because there are other potential explanations for a difference in outcome, including era of treatment, expertise of the treatment center, referral bias, and stage migration within the poor-prognosis subgroup.

Table 3
Selected nonrandomized series for International Germ Cell Consensus Classification poor-prognosis patients

Study	Treatment arm	Number of patients	Complete response rate (%)	Durable response rate (%)
Bower et al [34]	POMB-ACE	92	NS	5-year OS 75%
Germa-Lluch et al [36]	BOMP-EPI	38	60	53
Decatris et al [39]	BEP-CEC$_{(y)}$	20	70	50
Fizazi et al [40]	BOP-CisC$_{(y)}$A-POMB-A$_{(c)}$C$_{(y)}$E	38	NS	3-year PFS 65%
Christian et al [38]	C-BOP-BEP	54	30	3-year RFS 83%
Fossa et al [41]	C-BOP-BEP	29	56	2-year PFS 56%
Schmoll et al [42]	High-dose VIP	182	66	2-year PFS 69%

Abbreviations: A, doxorubicin; A$_{(c)}$, actinomycin D; B, bleomycin; C, carboplatin; Cis, cisplatin; C$_{(y)}$, cyclophosphamide; E, etoposide; I, ifosfamide; M, methotrexate; NS, not stated; OS, overall survival; P, cisplatin; PFS, progression-free survival; RFS, relapse-free survival; V, vinblastine.

Several nonrandomized studies have been reported that have prospectively used the IGCCC poor-prognosis criteria [40–42]. The results are summarized in Table 3. Although the results have generally been promising compared with historical data, these data are inadequate to determine a change in treatment outside a clinical trial. Rather, the most promising regimens should be considered for phase III assessment. Of those regimens assessing additional drugs and alternating chemotherapy regimens, one of the most promising is the C-BOP-BEP regimen. It has been studied prospectively by several groups [38,41], with encouraging results, and is currently the subject of a randomized trial in the United Kingdom.

High-dose chemotherapy supported by hemopoietic progenitor cells

Reinfusion of autologous hemopoietic stem cells has enabled the administration of much higher doses of myelosuppressive chemotherapy. This technique has been investigated in the last 2 decades and continues to develop. Recent advances include the use of harvested, mobilized progenitor cells from the peripheral circulation [43]. Technological improvements and increased physician expertise have reduced the morbidity and mortality. Initial use in patients who have germ cell tumors has been in the salvage setting in which a proportion of patients refractory to conventional chemotherapy achieve prolonged survival [44,45]. Success in the salvage setting has led to investigation in the initial therapy of patients who have a poor prognosis, because less toxicity is expected and greater potential for benefit exists [19,46–48]. The high-dose regimens have generally incorporated carboplatin and etoposide with or without cyclophosphamide or ifosfamide.

An early randomized study of high-dose chemotherapy as initial therapy was performed by Droz and colleagues [49]. A total of 115 previously untreated patients who had poor prognosis germ cell tumors, according to the Institut Gustave-Roussy prognostic model, were randomized to receive intensive, standard-dose chemotherapy or two cycles of standard-dose chemotherapy followed by a single high-dose treatment with autologous bone marrow transplant support. There was no evidence of benefit to the bone marrow transplant arm in this study (see Table 2). There was a lower dose intensity of cisplatin in the high-dose arm, however, and delays before the high-dose therapy was implemented. Many investigators believed that the role of high-dose chemotherapy was not answered by this trial given these criticisms and subsequent improvements in techniques for high-dose chemotherapy and support.

Investigators at MSKCC have studied the role of high-dose therapy in a subset of poor-prognosis patients predicted to be at high risk for failure. Initial treatment was composed of two cycles of conventional chemotherapy. Those who had a slower-than-expected decline of either AFP or HCG received two cycles of high-dose carboplatin, etoposide, and cyclophosphamide. Two sequential studies demonstrated feasibility, improved survival compared with historical controls, and that more intensive therapy can be given initially than in the salvage setting [19,46]. These promising results led to a randomized trial comparing four cycles of BEP to two cycles of BEP followed by two cycles of high-dose carboplatin, etoposide, and cyclophosphamide supported by peripheral blood progenitor cells. The trial was performed as an Intergroup study and IGCCC intermediate (if LDH $>3\times$ normal) and poor-prognosis patients were eligible. The study was designed to detect a 20% improvement in response proportion at 1 year. The initial results were recently presented at the American Society of Clinical Oncology 2006 Annual Meeting and showed no advantage for the more intensive therapy (see Table 2) [50]. The investigators reported that a subgroup analysis of those patients who had a slow marker decline showed a better outcome with the high-dose chemotherapy. This conclusion was controversial, however, and should not alter routine clinical practice without more careful consideration of the data and the appropriateness of the analysis.

The most important nonrandomized data considering high-dose chemotherapy comes from the German Testicular Cancer Study Group, which has investigated escalating doses of initial chemotherapy with hemopoietic growth factor and peripheral blood progenitor cell support [42]. They have demonstrated the feasibility of administering four cycles of escalated dose cisplatin (150 mg/m^2/cycle), etoposide (1250 mg/m^2/cycle), and ifosfamide (10 g/m^2/cycle). In contrast to the use of high-dose therapy as consolidation after standard chemotherapy, this approach potentially allows increased dose and dose-intensity from an earlier stage in treatment. The benefit of treatment in this study may be limited by the inclusion of cisplatin rather than carboplatin, however. The dose-limiting toxicities of cisplatin are nonhematologic and dose escalation within the range considered did not improve results when studied in a randomized trial [27]. Nevertheless, their promising results have led to an EORTC phase III trial in poor-prognosis patients.

Management issues

The IGCCC classification of prognosis should be used to determine prognosis for selection of treatment and in reporting the results of therapy in the medical literature. Four cycles of bleomycin, etoposide, and cisplatin (BEP), in the regimen developed at Indiana University [23,24], followed by surgical resection of residual masses, remains the standard of care for patients who have poor-prognosis germ cell tumors. No other chemotherapy regimen has been demonstrated to be superior in randomized trials. The VIP regimen, composed of ifosfamide, etoposide, and cisplatin, had similar efficacy but was more toxic in a randomized comparison to BEP. Many clinicians and patients have heard of the choice of a famous sportsman to receive VIP rather than BEP to avoid the potential pulmonary toxicity of bleomycin. This decision should not change the standard approach for most patients, however, because VIP is associated with greater short- and long-term toxicity. The unsatisfactory results of current therapy stress the need for participation in clinical trials. All eligible patients should be encouraged to enter studies of new approaches that hold promise to improve outcomes.

The clinician must ensure that an uncompromised course of chemotherapy is delivered. In general, the doses of chemotherapy agents should be calculated according to actual body weight and not adjusted down by artificially capping body weight or body surface area. Every attempt should be made to deliver chemotherapy according to the planned dose and schedule. The use of hemopoietic growth factor support can facilitate effective delivery of chemotherapy [51] by allowing avoidance of dose reductions or delays. Dose adjustments for toxicity should rarely be required, other than the potential need to cease bleomycin for pulmonary toxicity. In this situation, it is reasonable to substitute ifosfamide for the bleomycin, given the results of a randomized trial demonstrating equivalent efficacy [29].

Surgical resection of residual masses at sites of metastatic disease is part of the standard management for patients who have nonseminoma. In patients who have a poor prognosis, however, surgery probably plays a more important role in attaining cure. Patients who have a poor prognosis are more likely to have persistent neoplasia in residual masses. The results of surgery in the salvage setting emphasize that resection of viable malignancy and teratoma is curative in some cases [52]. An additional advantage of an aggressive surgical approach is that it allows identification of those patients who have persisting malignancy, who may benefit from further chemotherapy. The indications and type of retroperitoneal lymph node dissection vary considerably internationally. In the group of patients who have poor-prognosis nonseminoma, a bilateral template dissection should be performed after chemotherapy and the threshold for undertaking surgery at any site should be low.

Primary mediastinal nonseminomas

Primary mediastinal nonseminomas have been identified as having a poor prognosis by many groups [10], and are included as such in the IGCCC classification. They also have features that are unique, however, including a different frequency of histologic components [10] and associations with various hematologic abnormalities [53,54] and Klinefelter syndrome [55,56]. More importantly for treatment, mediastinal nonseminomas have demonstrated resistance to initial treatment and also to salvage therapy, including high-dose chemotherapy and hemopoietic stem cell support [57,58].

Novel approaches to therapy for mediastinal nonseminomatous germ cell tumors may be required to improve survival. In most patients who have nonseminomatous germ cell tumors, if serum tumor markers are elevated after initial chemotherapy, further chemotherapy is recommended rather than surgical resection [59]. In view of the poor results with chemotherapy for mediastinal nonseminomas, however, complete surgical resection of residual disease, if technically feasible, should be considered in responding patients even if markers remain elevated after chemotherapy [60]. Additional salvage chemotherapy could then follow. This concept is supported by the findings of some authors that all long-term survivors had undergone surgical resection at some stage in their treatment [61,62] and the results of surgery as a final attempt at salvage for patients who have refractory germ cell tumors and resectable disease [52].

Cerebral metastases

A multi-institutional study reported cerebral lesions in 1.2% of all cases of metastatic germ cell tumors [63]. Cases were subdivided into two groups: those who had cerebral lesions found at diagnosis and those who developed lesions after induction chemotherapy. In the former group, all patients had lesions elsewhere in the body and 82% had associated pulmonary metastases. Chemotherapy was the principal treatment of patients in this group and in selected cases was supplemented with surgery. Cerebral radiotherapy did not seem to confer a benefit but should be considered in those cases who fail to achieve a complete response to chemotherapy and surgery. Overall cause-specific survival at 5 years was 45%. Patients fared worse if they had liver or bone metastases, had more than one cerebral lesion, and did not have surgery. Six of seven patients who had a solitary metastasis who underwent a surgical resection followed by chemotherapy survived as opposed to only 9/19 who had a solitary lesion and received chemotherapy alone.

Liver metastases

A recent report reviewed the multimodality management of patients who had liver metastases and again stressed the value of surgery after chemotherapy [64]. Of 37 cases, 35 had complete resection of the residual mass. Twelve patients had residual malignancy, 7 had mature teratoma, and 18 had only necrosis. Prognostic factors for poor outcome in univariate analysis were the presence of pure embryonal carcinoma in the primary tumor, liver metastases measuring greater than 30 mm at the time of surgery, and the finding of viable malignancy in the resected mass.

Impact of the treating institution on outcome

Several studies have focused on the role of the institution in the management of poor-prognosis testicular cancer patients. The EORTC found that the risk for death from cancer was approximately doubled in those institutions that recruited fewer than five patients for the EORTC/MRC trial 30895/TE13, as opposed to the larger institutions who recruited more than five 5 patients [65]. Improved 2-year overall (77% versus 62%, $P = .006$) and progression-free survivals (73% versus 55%, $P = .006$) for those treated in larger institutions was demonstrated with reduced postoperative mortality (2% versus 9%). The authors concluded that specialist centers demonstrate superior results to nonspecialist centers [65]. This conclusion is echoed by MSKCC data showing their results to be superior at all stages of the disease to the SEER database results [66]. The Swedish Norwegian testicular cancer project also demonstrated an 84% versus 60% 3-year survival ($P = .01$) for those patients who had large-volume testicular cancer treated at large oncology centers versus nonspecialist centers, respectively [66]. These figures need to be interpreted with some caution because the results are subject to many biases. However, it is appropriate to recommend referral to specialist units for treatment of germ cell tumors, particularly for patients who have a poor prognosis at presentation.

Summary

Interpretation of literature published in the 1980s and 1990s was difficult because of the small numbers of patients studied and wide variation in patient selection criteria, treatment policies, and reporting criteria. The publication and acceptance of the IGCCC [13] has led to greater standardization in the description of patient groups. International trial groups are now using the IGCCC classification to determine eligibility for trials and to report their results.

Randomized comparisons performed to date have failed to identify any systemic therapy approach that is clearly superior to four cycles of cisplatin, etoposide, and bleomycin, which was first described in the mid-1980s. The recently reported results of the Intergroup trial that showed no benefit with high-dose chemotherapy and stem cell support add to a sense of frustration at the lack of progress, despite the extensive effort put into developmental and phase III trials. These results also suggest that other attempts to improve outcomes by intensifying therapy are unlikely to result in major improvement. Future opportunities for significantly improving therapy for poor-prognosis patients include the development of new therapeutic agents, particularly approaches targeting molecular mechanisms of resistance. The study of biologic markers to predict outcome and influence the choice of therapy is also warranted.

In the shorter term, three randomized trials are currently underway in Europe. The German Testicular Cancer Study Group has shown that the dose intensity of repetitive cycles of chemotherapy can be escalated significantly [42]. In contrast to the approach used in the Intergroup study, this approach introduces high-dose chemotherapy earlier and dose intensity is ensured by recycling the chemotherapy every 3 weeks. This approach is the subject of a phase III trial being performed by the EORTC group. The C-BOP-BEP regimen has been extensively studied in nonrandomized trials and is currently being compared with standard BEP in a phase III trial in the United Kingdom. Finally, the Genitourinary Group of the French Federation of Cancer Centers will assess the value of changing treatment for those patients who have a slow predicted time to serum tumor marker normalization, according to the paradigm that they have described [22].

The role of surgery and the impact of the treating institution are often underemphasized in discussions of therapy, because they are not the subject of large trials or of the evidence base. Despite this, the surgical resection of residual masses from multiple sites is a vital component of optimal care. Surgery also is potentially effective as a salvage procedure for patients who subsequently relapse. There is convincing evidence that patients who have poor-prognosis germ cell tumors have better outcomes if they are managed at centers that manage a large number of similar cases. It is likely that at least some of this improvement is attributable to the expertise of the surgeons at these centers and their willingness and ability to tackle difficult cases.

The failure to define clear advances in the management of poor-prognosis germ cell tumors in the last 10 years emphasizes the need for well-conceived and carefully conducted randomized studies using standard patient selection and reporting criteria. All patients presenting with poor-prognosis tumors should be encouraged to participate in clinical trials. The expertise and experience of the treating clinicians is likely to be one of the most important factors in determining outcome for this group of patients. Referral to a specialist center is warranted. Attempts to intensify therapy may improve outcomes modestly but the major challenges currently are the identification of molecular mechanisms of resistance and the development of novel molecularly targeted therapeutic approaches.

References

[1] Bosl GJ, Motzer RJ. Testicular germ-cell cancer. N Engl J Med 1997;337(4):242–53.

[2] Motzer RJ, Geller NL, Tan CC, et al. Salvage chemotherapy for patients with germ cell tumors. The Memorial Sloan-Kettering Cancer Center experience (1979–1989). Cancer 1991;67(5):1305–10.

[3] Germa-Lluch JR, Begent RH, Bagshawe KD. Tumour-marker levels and prognosis in malignant teratoma of the testis. Br J Cancer 1980;42(6):850–5.

[4] Bosl GJ, Geller NL, Cirrincione C, et al. Multivariate analysis of prognostic variables in patients with metastatic testicular cancer. Cancer Res 1983;43(7): 3403–7.

[5] Stoter G, Sylvester R, Sleijfer DT, et al. Multivariate analysis of prognostic factors in patients with disseminated nonseminomatous testicular cancer: results from a European Organization for Research on Treatment of Cancer Multi-institutional Phase III Study. Cancer Res 1987;47(10):2714–8.

[6] Birch R, Williams S, Cone A, et al. Prognostic factors for favorable outcome in disseminated germ cell tumors. J Clin Oncol 1986;4(3):400–7.

[7] Prognostic factors in advanced non-seminomatous germ-cell testicular tumours: results of a multicentre study. Report from the Medical Research Council Working Party on Testicular Tumours. Lancet 1985;1(8419):8–11.

[8] Droz JP, Kramar A, Ghosn M, et al. Prognostic factors in advanced nonseminomatous testicular cancer. A multivariate logistic regression analysis. Cancer 1988;62(3):564–8.

[9] Mead GM, Stenning SP, Parkinson MC, et al. The Second Medical Research Council study of prognostic factors in nonseminomatous germ cell tumors. Medical Research Council Testicular Tumour Working Party. J Clin Oncol 1992;10(1):85–94.

[10] Toner GC, Geller NL, Lin SY, et al. Extragonadal and poor risk nonseminomatous germ cell tumors. Survival and prognostic features. Cancer 1991; 67(8):2049–57.

[11] Nichols CR, Saxman S, Williams SD, et al. Primary mediastinal nonseminomatous germ cell tumors. A modern single institution experience. Cancer 1990; 65(7):1641–6.

[12] Bajorin D, Katz A, Chan E, et al. Comparison of criteria for assigning germ cell tumor patients to "good risk" and "poor risk" studies. J Clin Oncol 1988; 6(5):786–92.

[13] International Germ Cell Cancer Collaborative Group. International germ cell consensus classification: a prognostic factor-based staging system for metastatic germ cell cancers. J Clin Oncol 1997; 15(2):594–603.

[14] de Wit R, Roberts JT, Wilkinson PM, et al. Equivalence of three or four cycles of bleomycin, etoposide, and cisplatin chemotherapy and of a 3- or 5-day schedule in good-prognosis germ cell cancer: a randomized study of the European Organization for Research and Treatment of Cancer Genitourinary Tract Cancer Cooperative Group and the Medical Research Council. J Clin Oncol 2001;19(6):1629–40.

[15] Kollmannsberger C, Nichols C, Meisner C, et al. Identification of prognostic subgroups among

patients with metastatic 'IGCCCG poor-prognosis' germ-cell cancer: an explorative analysis using cart modeling. Ann Oncol 2000;11(9):1115–20.

[16] Bokemeyer C, Nichols CR, Droz JP, et al. Extragonadal germ cell tumors of the mediastinum and retroperitoneum: results from an international analysis. J Clin Oncol 2002;20(7):1864–73.

[17] Toner GC, Geller NL, Tan C, et al. Serum tumor marker half-life during chemotherapy allows early prediction of complete response and survival in nonseminomatous germ cell tumors. Cancer Res 1990; 50(18):5904–10.

[18] Murphy BA, Motzer RJ, Mazumdar M, et al. Serum tumor marker decline is an early predictor of treatment outcome in germ cell tumor patients treated with cisplatin and ifosfamide salvage chemotherapy. Cancer 1994;73(10):2520–6.

[19] Motzer RJ, Mazumdar M, Gulati SC, et al. Phase II trial of high-dose carboplatin and etoposide with autologous bone marrow transplantation in first-line therapy for patients with poor-risk germ cell tumors. J Natl Cancer Inst 1993;85(22):1828–35.

[20] de Wit R, Collette L, Sylvester R, et al. Serum alphafetoprotein surge after the initiation of chemotherapy for non-seminomatous testicular cancer has an adverse prognostic significance. Br J Cancer 1998; 78(10):1350–5.

[21] Toner GC. Early identification of therapeutic failure in nonseminomatous germ cell tumors by assessing serum tumor marker decline during chemotherapy: still not ready for routine clinical use. J Clin Oncol 2004;22(19):3842–5.

[22] Fizazi K, Culine S, Kramar A, et al. Early predicted time to normalization of tumor markers predicts outcome in poor-prognosis nonseminomatous germ cell tumors. J Clin Oncol 2004;22(19): 3868–76.

[23] Williams SD, Birch R, Einhorn LH, et al. Treatment of disseminated germ-cell tumors with cisplatin, bleomycin, and either vinblastine or etoposide. N Engl J Med 1987;316(23):1435–40.

[24] Williams SD, Birch R, Greco FA, et al. Comparison of cisplatin + bleomycin + either vinblastine or VP-16 in disseminated testicular cancer: a preliminary report. Prog Clin Biol Res 1984;153:219–23.

[25] Samson MK, Rivkin SE, Jones SE, et al. Dose-response and dose-survival advantage for high versus low-dose cisplatin combined with vinblastine and bleomycin in disseminated testicular cancer. A Southwest Oncology Group study. Cancer 1984; 53(5):1029–35.

[26] Ozols RF, Ihde DC, Linehan WM, et al. A randomized trial of standard chemotherapy versus a high-dose chemotherapy regimen in the treatment of poor prognosis nonseminomatous germ-cell tumors. J Clin Oncol 1988;6(6):1031–40.

[27] Nichols CR, Williams SD, Loehrer PJ, et al. Randomized study of cisplatin dose intensity in poor-risk germ cell tumors: a Southeastern Cancer Study Group and Southwest Oncology Group protocol. J Clin Oncol 1991;9(7):1163–72.

[28] Loehrer PJ Sr., Lauer R, Roth BJ, et al. Salvage therapy in recurrent germ cell cancer: ifosfamide and cisplatin plus either vinblastine or etoposide. Ann Intern Med 1988;109(7):540–6.

[29] Nichols CR, Catalano PJ, Crawford ED, et al. Randomized comparison of cisplatin and etoposide and either bleomycin or ifosfamide in treatment of advanced disseminated germ cell tumors: an Eastern Cooperative Oncology Group, Southwest Oncology Group, and Cancer and Leukemia Group B Study. J Clin Oncol 1998;16(4):1287–93.

[30] Wozniak AJ, Samson MK, Shah NT, et al. A randomized trial of cisplatin, vinblastine, and bleomycin versus vinblastine, cisplatin, and etoposide in the treatment of advanced germ cell tumors of the testis: a Southwest Oncology Group study. J Clin Oncol 1991;9(1):70–6.

[31] de Wit R, Stoter G, Sleijfer DT, et al. Four cycles of BEP versus an alternating regime of PVB and BEP in patients with poor-prognosis metastatic testicular non- seminoma; a randomised study of the EORTC Genitourinary Tract Cancer Cooperative Group. Br J Cancer 1995;71(6):1311–4.

[32] Lewis CR, Fossa SD, Mead G, et al. BOP/VIP—a new platinum-intensive chemotherapy regimen for poor prognosis germ cell tumours. Ann Oncol 1991;2(3):203–11.

[33] Kaye SB, Mead GM, Fossa S, et al. Intensive induction-sequential chemotherapy with BOP/VIP-B compared with treatment with BEP/EP for poor-prognosis metastatic nonseminomatous germ cell tumor: a Randomized Medical Research Council/European Organization for Research and Treatment of Cancer study. J Clin Oncol 1998;16(2):692–701.

[34] Bower M, Newlands ES, Holden L, et al. Treatment of men with metastatic non-seminomatous germ cell tumours with cyclical POMB/ACE chemotherapy. Ann Oncol 1997;8(5):477–83.

[35] Bower M, Brock C, Holden L, et al. POMB/ACE chemotherapy for mediastinal germ cell tumours. Eur J Cancer 1997;33(6):838–42.

[36] Germa-Lluch JR, Garcia del Muro X, Tabernero JM, et al. BOMP/EPI intensive alternating chemotherapy for IGCCC poor-prognosis germ-cell tumors: the Spanish Germ-Cell Cancer Group experience. Ann Oncol 1999;10(3):289–93.

[37] Horwich A, Mason M, Fossa SD, et al. Accelerated induction chemotherapy (C-BOP-BEP) for poor and intermediate prognosis metastatic germ cell tumours. Proc Am Soc Clin Oncol 1997;16:319a.

[38] Christian JA, Huddart RA, Norman A, et al. Intensive induction chemotherapy with CBOP/BEP in patients with poor prognosis germ cell tumors. J Clin Oncol 2003;21(5):871–7.

[39] Decatris MP, Wilkinson PM, Welch RS, et al. High-dose chemotherapy and autologous haematopoietic support in poor risk non-seminomatous germ-cell

tumours: an effective first-line therapy with minimal toxicity. Ann Oncol 2000;11(4):427–34.
[40] Fizazi K, Prow DM, Do KA, et al. Alternating dose-dense chemotherapy in patients with high volume disseminated non-seminomatous germ cell tumours. Br J Cancer 2002;86(10):1555–60.
[41] Fossa SD, Paluchowska B, Horwich A, et al. Intensive induction chemotherapy with C-BOP/BEP for intermediate- and poor-risk metastatic germ cell tumours (EORTC trial 30948). Br J Cancer 2005; 93(11):1209–14.
[42] Schmoll HJ, Kollmannsberger C, Metzner B, et al. Long-term results of first-line sequential high-dose etoposide, ifosfamide, and cisplatin chemotherapy plus autologous stem cell support for patients with advanced metastatic germ cell cancer: an extended phase I/II study of the German Testicular Cancer Study Group. J Clin Oncol 2003;21(22): 4083–91.
[43] Beyer J, Schwella N, Zingsem J, et al. Hematopoietic rescue after high-dose chemotherapy using autologous peripheral-blood progenitor cells or bone marrow: a randomized comparison. J Clin Oncol 1995; 13(6):1328–35.
[44] Motzer RJ, Mazumdar M, Bosl GJ, et al. High-dose carboplatin, etoposide, and cyclophosphamide for patients with refractory germ cell tumors: treatment results and prognostic factors for survival and toxicity. J Clin Oncol 1996;14(4):1098–105.
[45] Broun ER, Nichols CR, Turns M, et al. Early salvage therapy for germ cell cancer using high dose chemotherapy with autologous bone marrow support. Cancer 1994;73(6):1716–20.
[46] Motzer RJ, Mazumdar M, Bajorin DF, et al. High-dose carboplatin, etoposide and cyclophosphamide with autologous bone marrow transplantation in first-line therapy for patients with poor-risk germ cell tumors. J Clin Oncol 1997;15(7):2546–52.
[47] Droz JP, Pico JL, Ghosn M, et al. A phase II trial of early intensive chemotherapy with autologous bone marrow transplantation in the treatment of poor prognosis non seminomatous germ cell tumors. Bull Cancer 1992;79(5):497–507.
[48] Barnett MJ, Coppin CM, Murray N, et al. High-dose chemotherapy and autologous bone marrow transplantation for patients with poor prognosis nonseminomatous germ cell tumours. Br J Cancer 1993;68(3):594–8.
[49] Droz JP, Pico JL, Biron P, et al. No evidence of a benefit of early intensified chemotherapy with autologous bone marrow transplantation in first line treatment of poor risk non seminomatous germ cell tumors: preliminary results of a randomized trial. Proc Am Soc Clin Oncol 1992;11:197.
[50] Bajorin DF, Nichols CR, Margolin KA, et al. Phase III trial of conventional-dose chemotherapy alone or with high-dose chemotherapy for metastatic germ cell tumors patients: a cooperative group trial by Memorial Sloan-Kettering Cancer Center, ECOG, SWOG, and CALGB. Proc Am Soc Clin Oncol 2006;24:4510A.
[51] Fossa SD, Kaye SB, Mead GM, et al. Filgrastim during combination chemotherapy of patients with poor-prognosis metastatic germ cell malignancy. European Organization for Research and Treatment of Cancer, Genito-Urinary Group, and the Medical Research Council Testicular Cancer Working Party, Cambridge, United Kingdom. J Clin Oncol 1998; 16(2):716–24.
[52] Murphy BR, Breeden ES, Donohue JP, et al. Surgical salvage of chemorefractory germ cell tumors. J Clin Oncol 1993;11(2):324–9.
[53] deMent SH, Eggleston JC, Spivak JL. Association between mediastinal germ cell tumors and hematologic malignancies. Report of two cases and review of the literature. Am J Surg Pathol 1985;9(1):23–30.
[54] Nichols CR, Hoffman R, Einhorn LH, et al. Hematologic malignancies associated with primary mediastinal germ-cell tumors. Ann Intern Med 1985;102(5): 603–9.
[55] Nichols CR, Heerema NA, Palmer C, et al. Klinefelter's syndrome associated with mediastinal germ cell neoplasms. J Clin Oncol 1987;5(8):1290–4.
[56] Dexeus FH, Logothetis CJ, Chong C, et al. Genetic abnormalities in men with germ cell tumors. J Urol 1988;140(1):80–4.
[57] Saxman SB, Nichols CR, Einhorn LH. Salvage chemotherapy in patients with extragonadal nonseminomatous germ cell tumors: the Indiana university experience. J Clin Oncol 1994;12(7):1390–3.
[58] Beyer J, Kramar A, Mandanas R, et al. High-dose chemotherapy as salvage treatment in germ cell tumors: a multivariate analysis of prognostic variables. J Clin Oncol 1996;14(10):2638–45.
[59] Motzer RJ, Bosl GJ. Chemotherapy for germ cell tumors. Urol Clin North Am 1987;14(2):389–98.
[60] Vuky J, Bains M, Bacik J, et al. Role of postchemotherapy adjunctive surgery in the management of patients with nonseminoma arising from the mediastinum. J Clin Oncol 2001;19(3):682–8.
[61] Kay PH, Wells FC, Goldstraw P. A multidisciplinary approach to primary nonseminomatous germ cell tumors of the mediastinum. Ann Thorac Surg 1987;44(6):578–82.
[62] Vogelzang NJ, Raghavan D, Anderson RW, et al. Mediastinal nonseminomatous germ cell tumors: the role of combined modality therapy. Ann Thorac Surg 1982;33(4):333–9.
[63] Fossa SD, Bokemeyer C, Gerl A, et al. Treatment outcome of patients with brain metastases from malignant germ cell tumors. Cancer 1999;85(4):988–97.
[64] Rivoire M, Elias D, De Cian F, et al. Multimodality treatment of patients with liver metastases from germ cell tumors: the role of surgery. Cancer 2001; 92(3):578–87.
[65] Collette L, Sylvester RJ, Stenning SP, et al. Impact of the treating institution on survival of patients with "poor-prognosis" metastatic nonseminoma.

European Organization for Research and Treatment of Cancer Genito-Urinary Tract Cancer Collaborative Group and the Medical Research Council Testicular Cancer Working Party. J Natl Cancer Inst 1999;91(10):839–46.

[66] Feuer EJ, Sheinfeld J, Bosl GJ. Does size matter? Association between number of patients treated and patient outcome in metastatic testicular cancer. J Natl Cancer Inst 1999;91(10): 816–8.

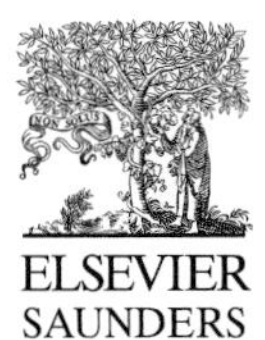
ELSEVIER
SAUNDERS

Urol Clin N Am 34 (2007) 199–217

UROLOGIC
CLINICS
of North America

Role of Post-Chemotherapy Surgery in Germ Cell Tumors

Hong Gee Sim, MBBS, MRCSEd, MMED, FAMS, Paul H. Lange, MD, FACS, Daniel W. Lin, MD*

Department of Urology, University of Washington, Box 356510, 1959 NE Pacific Street, Seattle, WA 98195, USA

Improvements in combination chemotherapy regimens, supportive care, and surgical techniques over the last 2 decades have dramatically altered the treatment of patients who have metastatic testicular cancer. In the late 1970s, chemotherapeutic regimens for testicular cancer included the use of actinomycin, vinblastine, methotrexate, and bleomycin and were hampered by significant adverse effects and limited efficacy. Surgery in the form of bilateral retroperitoneal lymph node dissection (RPLND) was similarly associated with substantial complication rates and significant functional consequences [1]. The subsequent discovery, introduction, and integration of improved cisplatin-based chemotherapy regimens and nerve-sparing surgical techniques have resulted in not only markedly improved disease-specific mortality but also decreased morbidities and improved quality of life [2].

Although the emergence of effective chemotherapy for advanced germ cell tumor (GCT) yielded remarkable advancements in overall patient survival, a significant proportion of men who initially presented with metastatic germ cell tumor have persistent residual masses after chemotherapy. These masses are primarily retroperitoneal in location; however, they also may be present in multiple non-retroperitoneal locations, such as the neck, lung, and mediastinum. This article focuses on the rationale, approach, outcome, and morbidity of post-chemotherapy surgery in advanced testicular cancer.

Rationale for surgery after chemotherapy

The rationale for post-chemotherapy RPLND is based on (1) the established diagnostic role, (2) the therapeutic efficacy of the procedure, (3) the natural history of residual masses, and (4) the decreasing morbidity of these surgical procedures.

With regard to the diagnostic role of RPLND, surgical resection after chemotherapy yields one of the following histologic findings: (1) pure necrosis or fibrosis, (2) teratoma with or without necrosis/fibrosis, (3) viable germ cell carcinoma to any degree, or (4) non–germ cell carcinoma to any degree. The frequencies of these histologies vary in the literature and are summarized in Table 1 [3–17]. In general, necrosis/fibrosis is found in 50%, teratoma in 35%, and viable germ cell tumor in 15%. The rare finding of non–germ cell elements (ie, malignant transformation) is addressed in another article in this issue. There is no established instrument, parameter, or nomogram to accurately predict the histology of the residual mass preoperatively. Because precise determination of the histology is crucial in dictating further therapy and follow-up, surgical excision is usually necessary. For instance, in the setting of negative serum tumor markers (STM) after chemotherapy, one cannot discern if the residual mass is necrosis/fibrosis only (destined never to harm the patient in long term follow-up without surgery) or if the mass harbors viable germ cell tumor. Proposed predictive models are discussed in a later section of this article.

Another rationale for post-chemotherapy RPLND is the established therapeutic benefit to complete removal of the residual mass,

* Corresponding author.
E-mail address: dlin@u.washington.edu (D.W. Lin).

doi:10.1016/j.ucl.2007.02.010

Table 1
Histologic findings for standard post-chemotherapy retroperitoneal lymph node dissection studies in relation to tumor size

Study	Year	N	Clinical stage	Chemotherapy	Tumor marker levels	Residual masses (cm)	Necrosis N (%)	Teratoma N (%)	Carcinoma N (%)	Median follow-up (months)	Survival (%)
Donohue et al [3]	1982	51	II–IV	Induction	Normal	NS	16 (31%)	16 (31%)	19 (37%)	NS	Fibrosis: 15/16 NED; Teratoma: 15/16 NED; cancer: 10/19 NED
Bracken et al [4]	1983	45	III	Induction	Normal	22 not palpable, 23 palpable	14 (64%) 8 (35%)	3 (14%) 7 (30%)	5 (23%) 7 (30%)	60 (24–105) 33 (30–41)	13/22 (59%) NED18/23 (78%) NED
Freiha et al [5]	1984	40	IIc = 10, III = 30	Induction	Normal	NS	21 (52%)	18 (45%)	1 (3%)	36	37 NED, 3 relapse
Pizzocaro et al [6]	1985	36	II–III	Induction	Normal	NS	16 (44%)	10 (28%)	10 (28%)	36 (28–52)	11/18 (61%) NED
Fossa et al [7]	1989	101	II–IV	Induction	Normal	NS	52 (51%)	37 (37%)	12 (12%)	55	Fibrosis/ teratoma: 83/89 (93%) NED; cancer: 7/12 (58%) NED
Gelderman et al [84]	1988	35	III–IV	Induction	Normal	NS	17 (49%)	14 (40%)	4 (11%)	65 (36–99)	25/35 (66%) NED
Williams et al [8]	1989	29	II	Induction, 4; 2nd line, 3 RT	23 normal, 6 elevated	NS	13 (52%)	9 (36%)	3 (12%)	33 (1–93)	29/29 (100%) NED
Mulders et al [9]	1990	55	IIc–IV	Induction	Normal	>1	31 (56%)	12 (22%)	12 (22%)	36 (5–96)	Fibrosis 93% (3 y); teratoma 92% (3 y); cancer: 27% (3 y)

Harding et al [10]	1989	42	IIb–IV	Induction	Normal	>1.5	19 (45%)	14 (33%)	9 (21%)	36 (6–95)	36/42 (86%) NED
Aass et al [11]	1991	173	II–IV	Induction	Normal	None, 30; <2, 6; 2–5, 107; >5, 57	85 (49%)	50 (25%)	38 (29%)	75 (49–107)	160/173 (92%) NED, 82% CSS
Kulkarni et al [12]	1991	67	IIb–IV	Induction	Normal, 63%; elevated, 37%	NS	18 (27%)	29 (43%)	20 (30%)	50 (2–121)	55/67 (82%) NED
Aprikian et al [67]	1994	40	IIb–III	Induction, 5 2nd line	Normal	Stage II: <5, 2 (5%); >5, 17 (42%); Stage II: NS	18 (45%)	17 (43%)	5 (13%)	36 (24–60)	32/40 (80%) NED; 8/40 (20%) relapse
Steyerberg et al [26]	1995	556	II–IV	Induction	Normal	NS	250 (45%)	236 (42%)	70 (13%)	NS	NS
Brenner et al [13]	1996	24	II–IV	Induction, 21 salvage, 5 BM transplant	22 normal, 2 elevated	2–20	13 (54%)	8 (33%)	3 (13%)	NS	79% 5-y overall survival
Coogan et al (nerve sparing) [74]	1996	81	B = 31, C = 50	Induction, 6 2nd line, 3 BM transplant	Normal	6.3 (1–19)	23 (28%)	54 (66%)	4 (5%)	35.5 (12–87)	79 NED, 1 relapse, 1 death
Rabbani et al [36]	1998	50	II & III	Induction, 9 2nd line	Normal	>1.5	27/76 (36%)	38/76 (50%)	11/76 (14%)	Right-sided lesions: 60 (12–126), left-sided lesions: 49 (1–122)	Right: 20/22 (91%) NED; Left: 15/17 (88%) NED
Stenning et al [14]	1998	153	II–III	Induction	Normal	≥2	45 (29%)	85 (56%)	23 (15%)	84 (24–120)	Fibrosis: 90% 2-y NED; teratoma: 88% 2-y NED; cancer: 43% 2-y NED

(*continued on next page*)

Table 1 (*continued*)

Study	Year	N	Clinical stage	Chemotherapy	Tumor marker levels	Residual masses (cm)	Necrosis N (%)	Teratoma N (%)	Carcinoma N (%)	Median follow-up (months)	Survival (%)
Donohue et al [33]	1998	414	II–IV	Induction	Normal	NS	25%	52%	23%	108	Relapse rate 11.8%, CSS 95%
Napier et al [15]	2000	48	II–IV	Induction	Normal	NS	15 (31%)	24 (50%)	9 (19%)	66 (12–153)	37/48 (77%) NED
Hendry et al [16]	2002	330	II–IV	Induction	46% normal, 54% elevated	≥1	84 (25%)	218 (66%)	28 (8%)	77	83% 5-y NED, 89% 5-y overall survival
Oldenburg et al [40]	2003	87	II	Induction	19 elevated, 68 normal	1 (0–2)	58 (67)	23 (26%)	6 (7)	80 (15–148)	94% 5-y NED, 96% 5-y overall survival
Albers et al [45]	2004	193	II–III	Induction	Normal	NS	35%	34%	31%	NS	NS
Muramaki et al [17]	2004	24	II–III	Induction, 12 2nd line	Normal	≤3, 62.5%; >3, 37.5%	15 (63%)	6 (25%)	3 (12%)	NS	Complete resection: 100% 3-y CSS; incomplete resection: 50% 3-y CSS

Abbreviations: BM, bone marrow; CSS, cancer-specific survival; NED, no evidence of disease; NS, not specified; RT, radiotherapy.

particularly in the setting of residual viable GCT and teratoma. Fox and associates [18] from Indiana University reported on the results of 580 men who underwent post-chemotherapy RPLND, 417 after primary chemotherapy and 163 after salvage chemotherapy. Forty-three (10%) patients after primary chemotherapy and 90 (55%) after salvage chemotherapy had viable germ cell tumor in the resection specimens. Overall, in patients who had viable tumor in the post-chemotherapy mass, incomplete resection was associated with a significantly higher rate of death from testis cancer (88% in incomplete resections versus 40% in complete resections). The survival advantage of complete resection of viable germ cell tumor was even significant in the group of patients who did not receive further chemotherapy after RPLND, further supporting the therapeutic role of post-chemotherapy RPLND. In addition to the therapeutic benefit, surgical resection for remnant viable germ cell also confers staging benefits because the surgery removes the residual cancer, and patients who received only primary chemotherapy can then benefit from additional chemotherapy [18].

Perhaps as important as the diagnostic and therapeutic roles of post-chemotherapy RPLND for the patient who harbors viable GCT is the role of surgery in influencing the well-recognized natural history of teratoma and its impact on patient survival and morbidity. The finding of teratoma in the resected specimen confers a therapeutic benefit to the patient because surgery is the definitive treatment modality for teratomas that are not chemosensitive. Left alone, masses containing teratoma can remain stable, locally grow and potentially compromise vital adjacent organ function by compression (eg, growing teratoma syndrome [19]), or undergo malignant transformation or degeneration into other types of cancer, which are generally resistant to chemotherapy [20–22].

A final rationale for post-chemotherapy surgery is its now acceptable morbidity. This advance came about in part by refinements in surgical approaches, brought by a better understanding of the primary landing zones for metastatic spread in testis cancer and the anatomic relations of the hypogastric nerves that control ejaculation. These refinements include obviating the need for suprahilar dissection, using modified unilateral surgical templates, and applying nerve-sparing techniques in selected cases. Another reason for the decreased morbidity is enhanced perioperative medical care [23,24]. This topic is discussed further later in this article.

In summary, surgical resection of retroperitoneal lymph nodes after chemotherapy has the advantage of accurate determination of the retroperitoneal histology and staging of the disease, factors that dictate the need for additional therapy and allow for improved prognostication. More importantly, complete resection of residual retroperitoneal masses results in therapeutic control over any masses that may cause late relapse of GCT. In particular, teratoma may undergo malignant transformation, a deadly result of an uncontrolled retroperitoneum. The natural history and biology of late relapses are covered in a separate article in this issue. Lastly, the morbidities of the procedure do not outweigh the benefits of the diagnostic and therapeutic gains.

Classification of post-chemotherapy retroperitoneal lymph node dissection

RPLND constitutes most surgical resection after systemic chemotherapy for advanced testicular carcinoma. The Indiana classification of RPLND categorizes different types of RPLND to facilitate assessment of the outcome in this setting [25]. Standard RPLND refers to patients after induction chemotherapy who have disseminated testicular cancer and present with residual radiographic disease in the retroperitoneum and normalized STM. Salvage RPLND refers to cases that are status post second-line salvage chemotherapy (additional courses of cisplatin-based or high-dose chemotherapy with bone marrow support) with normalized tumor markers. Desperation RPLND refers to cases that are post–second-line salvage chemotherapy with elevated markers. Redo RPLND refers to surgery for patients who had previous RPLND with in-field recurrence. Unresectable RPLND denotes extensive unresectable tumor at the time of surgery.

Patient selection and indications for post-chemotherapy retroperitoneal lymph node dissection

The current indications for surgery after initial systemic chemotherapy depend on several factors, including (1) histology of primary tumor, (2) the presence and size of residual radiographic masses, and (3) the known distributions and natural history of the various post-chemotherapy mass histologies. Others have used predictive models to calculate the likelihood of viable GCT, using these models to guide therapeutic decision-making [26–29].

Histology of primary tumor

The approach to residual masses after chemotherapy in the setting of pure seminoma differs substantially from the residual masses in the setting of nonseminomatous GCT (NSGCT) for several reasons. First, the post-chemotherapy seminoma masses tend to be more desmoplastic in nature and consequently are more intimately associated with the great vessels. The result of this desmoplastic response to chemotherapy is an obliteration of tissue planes, more difficult resection, and resulting increased morbidity. Second, teratoma is rare in a pure seminoma mass after chemotherapy. The aforementioned dangerous biologic potential of teratoma is thus avoided.

Lastly, there is evidence that some post-chemotherapy seminoma masses do not require resection. In a study of 55 patients who had advanced seminoma treated with chemotherapy, Herr and colleagues [30] showed that residual retroperitoneal masses greater than 3 cm harbored viable seminoma in 30%, but all masses less than 3 cm were found to have necrosis/fibrosis only. Others have found viable tumor in 13% to 22% of residual masses larger than 3 cm but none in masses smaller than 3 cm [31,32].

The remainder of this article focuses on post-chemotherapy surgery in the setting of NSGCT. In NSGCT, the finding of teratoma in the primary tumor has been associated with teratoma in the post-chemotherapy mass, and also has been incorporated into the multiple predictive models discussed later in this chapter. In general, the finding of teratoma in the primary tumor as a single variable correlates poorly with teratoma in the post-chemotherapy mass, and the authors support removal of all post-chemotherapy residual masses in NSGCT.

Persistent residual radiographic masses

Patients who have good-risk advanced disease experience disappearance of all radiographic tumor in 70% of cases but persistence of radiographic lesions in 30% [33]. The presence of persistent radiographic masses in the setting of normalized STM still poses the risk for residual teratoma or germ cell tumor as previously discussed, and surgery to remove these masses is recommended. Two clinical situations remain controversial, however: (1) the radiologic criteria of abnormal lesions, and (2) the need for surgery in radiologic complete responses to chemotherapy. With regard to radiologic criteria, the cutoff for a significant radiographic lesion varies with different institutions and different definitions of normality are used for CT scans. In some centers, lesions less than 20 mm are considered normal, whereas others classify lesions only less than 15 mm or 10 mm as normal [34–36]. Several investigators have found up to 35% and 44% false-negative rates when the cutoff for normal CT scans was 20 mm and 30 mm, respectively [34,37,38]. Toner and colleagues [39] reviewed their data in 39 patients who had residual masses less than 15 mm and found that 3 patients (8%) had remnant germ cell tumor and 5 (13%) had teratoma. Oldenberg and colleagues [40] confirmed this observation in 87 patients from Norway and found that 33% of lesions less than 20 mm contained teratoma or germ cell tumor. This finding was supported by data from Steyerberg and colleagues [41] who found teratoma or viable germ cell tumor in 29% of lesions between 0 to 10 mm and 44% of lesions between 11 to 20 mm. In this study, even lesions less than 10 mm, clearly within the definition of normal at most institutions, still harbored unfavorable histology in almost one third of cases. Size of the residual mass alone in patients who have minimal radiographic lesions after chemotherapy is therefore a poor predictor of histology, and the authors recommend the removal of all detectable masses.

With regard to the need for surgery in patients who initially present with retroperitoneal disease and experience a complete response to chemotherapy, multiple investigators have addressed the outcome of surgery in this setting. Fossa and colleagues [42] examined the retroperitoneal histology in men who had previously metastatic NSGCT with normal post-chemotherapy CT scans. In this series 67% of men had necrosis in the retroperitoneal dissection specimen, 30% had teratoma, and 3% had viable germ cell tumor. In a recent Memorial Sloan-Kettering Cancer Center study, 23% of men who had normal post-chemotherapy CT scans had teratoma in the RPLND specimen [43]. The need for surgery in chemotherapy complete responders thus remains controversial. This uncertainty has led many to attempt to develop instruments to predict retroperitoneal histology and thus theoretically avoid or tailor their surgery.

Predictors of retroperitoneal histology

Models to predict retroperitoneal histology have been developed by several investigators [26–29]. The goal of most models is to avoid surgery in patients who harbor necrosis or fibrosis, thus in those for whom surgery is associated with no therapeutic benefit and may cause unnecessary morbidity. Others have constructed models to predict teratoma in the post-chemotherapy residual mass [43]. These models use various parameters, including primary tumor histology, pre-chemotherapy STM status, post-chemotherapy mass size, and mass size change during chemotherapy. An examination of the sensitivity, specificity, and accuracy of these models is central to their usefulness in the management of residual masses following chemotherapy.

Proponents of predictive models for the probability of necrosis or fibrosis posit such factors as the lack of teratomatous elements in the primary tumor, more than 90% decrease in size of mass, low pre-chemotherapy STM, and serologic complete response as the determinants of whether or not to proceed with surgical removal of the residual mass following induction chemotherapy. For example, Donohue and colleagues [44] studied the change in volume and computerized tomographic density of retroperitoneal disease before and after chemotherapy, the presence of teratoma in the primary testis tumor, and the histologic findings at retroperitoneal lymphadenectomy in 80 patients who had stage B3 or B2/C germ cell tumors. Of the patients who had no teratomatous elements in the original tumor and a greater than 90% decrease in the volume of retroperitoneal masses, no teratoma or viable germ cell tumor was found in the surgical specimen. In contrast, 7 of 9 patients (78%) who had teratomatous elements in the original specimen had either teratoma or carcinoma in the retroperitoneal lymphadenectomy specimens despite having a greater than 90% decrease in tumor volume ($P < .05$). These data suggest that patients who have no teratomatous elements in the original specimen and a greater than 90% decrease in the volume of retroperitoneal masses in response to chemotherapy may be closely observed and thus avoid surgery. This series was updated by Debono and colleagues [35] who examined 295 patients placed into five groups based on response to primary chemotherapy and the presence or absence of teratoma in the primary tumor: group A (complete remission [CR]), group B (unresectable), group C (serologic CR, teratoma-positive primary tumor, resectable partial remission [PR]), group D (serologic CR, teratoma-negative primary tumor, <90% radiographic PR), and group E (serologic CR, teratoma-negative primary tumor, ≥90% radiographic PR). Group A, B, and E patients were routinely observed after chemotherapy, whereas group C and D patients were routinely taken to surgery after chemotherapy. The investigators found that patients had no evidence of disease in 92% of group A, 40% of group B, 87% of group C, 86% of group D, and 74% of group E. They concluded that patients who have NSGCT who achieve a serologic and radiographic CR with primary chemotherapy (group A) can be safely observed without surgical intervention, regardless of initial tumor bulk. Patients who had a teratoma-negative primary tumor who achieve a serologic CR and 90% or greater radiographic remission were still found to be of significantly greater risk for relapse on surveillance, and the study concluded that these patients could be either observed or undergo RPLND.

Other groups have performed similar analyses, confirming the Indiana findings. In a small study of 48 patients, Stomper and colleagues [38] found no significant correlation between the combined features of absence of teratoma in a histologic specimen of the primary testicular tumor and CT findings (residual mass size, attenuation, and greater than 90% shrinkage of masses during chemotherapy) and the absence of malignancy or teratoma in residual masses. The German Testicular Cancer Study Group [45] also studied percentage shrinkage during chemotherapy in 193 patients who had nonseminomatous germ cell tumor but found that α-fetoprotein (AFP) values before chemotherapy less than 20 ng/mL and a high percentage of shrinkage during chemotherapy reliably predicted only 19% of cases of necrosis with a test accuracy of 75%, a sensitivity to predict necrosis of 52%, and a specificity of 87%. Furthermore, with regard to the issue of teratoma in the orchiectomy specimen as a primary determinant of teratoma in the retroperitoneum, several series have shown that even in the absence of teratoma in the orchiectomy specimen, teratoma is present in 28% to 41% of the post-chemotherapy retroperitoneal masses [35,43]. Even in the setting of post-chemotherapy masses of less than 1 cm and no teratoma in orchiectomy specimen, teratoma was still found in 19% of the retroperitoneal lymph nodes [43].

Finally, multiple logistic regression analyses incorporating all variables with more sophisticated modeling have been performed by others.

Steyerberg and associates [46] incorporated several patient characteristics in a statistical model, including the presence of teratomatous elements in the primary testis tumor, pre-chemotherapy STM levels, size of residual mass, and reduction in size after chemotherapy. These investigators validated the model in a study of 172 patients and found that this model could predict the probability of necrosis in more than 90% of cases (goodness-of-fit tests, $P > .20$); however, cancer could not be reliably discriminated from mature teratoma. In an external validation study using this model, Vergouwe and colleagues [27] compared the observed histology with the predicted probability in 105 patients who had good-prognosis germ cell cancer who underwent RPLND between 1995 and 1998, finding that nearly all predicted probabilities ($n = 101$) were less than 70%, and that 35% of patients currently under surveillance (84 out of 241) had predicted probabilities less than 70%, thus concluding that use of the model would change the policy from RPLND to surveillance in relatively few patients.

In summary, extensive modeling has sought to define appropriate post-chemotherapy surgical candidates based on various clinical and pathologic parameters. These investigations have certainly provided insight into predictive factors for necrosis/fibrosis and teratoma in the retroperitoneal specimen. In large single- and multi-institutional series, the combination of factors seemed to more accurately predict histology than the known histologic distributions. Controversy remains about not only whether these models can predict histology with acceptable accuracy and thus stratify patients by need for surgery but also whether these models will ultimately affect disease-specific survival.

Role of imaging

Multiple groups have examined the role of positron emission tomography (PET) in post-chemotherapy testis cancer masses. In NSGCT, the usefulness of PET has been hampered by the limited accuracy for predicting viable germ cell tumor as opposed to teratoma, because teratoma can also be 2-^{18}fluoro-deoxy-D-glucose avid, and thus PET positive. Furthermore, inflammation in necrotic masses may mimic viable GCT on PET scans, and timing of PET in relation to chemotherapy is a crucial issue. Most recently, the largest series of PET in post-chemotherapy NSGCT examined 140 patients who had post-chemotherapy masses following various chemotherapy regimens. The test sensitivity and specificity of PET were 73% and 44%, respectively, with an accuracy of 56%. As in other studies, these authors concluded that FDG-PET for germ cell tumor following chemotherapy has a higher accuracy than CT, but the sensitivity is still too low to avoid subsequent resections in patients who have NSGCT [47–51].

Conversely, the role of PET in seminoma is more encouraging. This clinical promise is largely due to the aforementioned rare teratomatous differentiation of seminoma during chemotherapy. Consequently, the binary outcome of viable tumor versus necrosis/fibrosis increases the accuracy of PET. In the largest prospective trial, involving 51 patients who had pure seminoma, De Santis and colleagues [52] reported that a positive 2-^{18}fluoro-deoxy-D-glucose positron emission tomography (FDG PET) scan reliably predicts the presence of viable residual tumor in post-chemotherapy seminoma residual masses. The specificity, sensitivity, positive predictive value, and negative predictive value of FDG PET were 100% (95% CI, 92%–100%), 80% (95% CI, 44%–95%), 100%, and 96%, respectively, versus 74% (95% CI, 58%–85%), 70% (95% CI, 34%–90%), 37%, and 92%, respectively, for CT discrimination of the residual tumor by size. The efficacy of FDG PET is further supported by the findings of Putra and colleagues [53] in a group of Australian men. In a smaller study by Ganjoo and colleagues [54], however, FDG PET was less efficacious in detecting viable residual seminoma in the post-chemotherapy setting. Although these studies were limited by incomplete pathologic confirmation (ie, some patients did not undergo surgical resection), the improvements in PET accuracy and relative accuracy to CT supports the use of PET in post-chemotherapy seminoma masses. Still, until larger prospective trials are completed, the general 3 cm cutoff rule previously discussed has largely remained standard of care.

Increasing serum tumor markers after chemotherapy

Persistently elevated STMs after chemotherapy present a unique and difficult clinical scenario. Traditionally, elevated tumor markers after primary induction chemotherapy mandates second-line chemotherapy, and persistence of elevated tumor markers following second-line therapy portends a poor prognosis. There is, however, a subset of patients who have elevated STMs after primary chemotherapy who are curable with surgery, particularly those who have normalization of markers following salvage or second-line chemotherapy. Most notable in these situations is the histologic distribution in the retroperitoneal masses, a distribution distinctly different from the more common situation of normalization of tumor markers after induction chemotherapy. For example, Beck and colleagues [55] reviewed 114 patients who had elevated STMs after first-line (50 patients) or second-line chemotherapy (64 patients) who underwent salvage or desperation RPLND between 1977 and 2000 with a minimum follow-up of 2 years. The 5-year overall survival was 53.9%. Sixty-one patients (53.5%) are alive with a median follow-up of 72 months. Fifty-three patients died of disease, with a median time to death of 8.0 months. Histopathology revealed germ cell cancer in 53.5% of patients, teratoma in 34.2% of patients, and fibrosis in 12.2% of patients, with 5-year survival rates of 31.4%, 77.5%, and 85.7%, respectively ($P<.0001$). The prognostic factors predictive of outcome in this analysis include an increasing β-HCG, serum AFP level, redo RPLND, and germ cell cancer in the resected specimen. Albers and colleagues [56] evaluated 30 patients who had persistent marker elevation after chemotherapy for metastatic germ cell tumors who underwent salvage RPLND with a mean follow-up of 120.3 months (range 1 to 228). Overall persistent viable cancer and teratomatous elements were identified in 64% and 11% of cases, respectively. Seventeen patients (57%) had no evidence of disease after salvage surgery. Those who had worse outcome included poor-risk patients according to International Germ Cell Cancer Collaborative Group (IGCCCG) guidelines [57], viable residual germ cell tumor with predominant embryonal histology, multiple site involvement, and incomplete resection.

Not all patients who had elevated serum markers post-chemotherapy may require second-line chemotherapy. Beck and colleagues [58] reported 11 cases of primary testicular teratoma with post-chemotherapy cystic masses. Fluid from these lesions contained elevated levels of HCG and AFP, and the authors postulated that they may have slow leak of fluid into the serum, resulting in elevated serum markers. Two of the patients who subsequently underwent RPLND had marker normalization postoperatively.

In summary, patients who undergo induction chemotherapy, have increasing STMs, and undergo second-line salvage chemotherapy or high-dose chemotherapy with bone marrow support with subsequent normalization of STMs are offered surgery to remove significant residual masses (salvage RPLND). Patients who have clinically localized retroperitoneal disease with increasing STMs despite second-line combination chemotherapy may be offered surgical resection (desperation RPLND), and patients who had previous RPLND with in-field recurrence may be offered a redo RPLND. Their outcomes are described in Table 2 [59–62] and discussed later in this article.

Extent of surgery after chemotherapy

Historically, RPLND encompassed a full bilateral suprahilar dissection from ureter to ureter, from the crus of the diaphragm to the bifurcation of the common iliac arteries [63]. In the early 1980s it was shown that right testicular tumors were more likely to have metastatic tumor deposits in the interaortocaval zone, just below the left renal vein. Left-sided primary testicular tumors were more likely to have tumor spread in the preaortic and left para-aortic areas. The right and left suprahilar zones were rarely involved in low-stage disease [64]. Surgical techniques were modified to omit routine suprahilar dissection for low-volume disease [65]. Earlier treatment of lower-stage, low-volume disease with smaller residual masses led to an increase in the role of template dissections and nerve-sparing techniques, which improved the chance of retaining antegrade ejaculation [2,66]. These template approaches are balanced with the risk for residual germ cell tumor or teratoma outside the field of resection, however.

Multiple institutions have examined the role of limited RPLND in the post-chemotherapy setting. Aprikian and colleagues [67] from Memorial Sloan-Kettering Cancer Center studied the use of intraoperative frozen section analysis to dictate the extent of surgery in 40 patients who had metastatic NSGCT. If frozen section revealed necrosis, then a modified template RPLND was performed; however, if teratoma or viable tumor was found, then a bilateral RPLND was attempted. Twenty-one patients (53%) had necrosis

Table 2
Complicated retroperitoneal lymph node dissection after chemotherapy

Study	Year	N	Clinical stage	Tumor marker levels	Residual masses (cm)	Necrosis N (%)	Teratoma N (%)	Carcinoma N (%)	Median follow-up (months)	Survival (%)
Salvage										
Donohue et al [33]	1998	80	II–III	Normal	NS	NS	NS	NS	108	99/180 (60%) NED, 3/180 (2%) AWD, 64/180 (39%) DOD
Hendry et al [16]	2002	112	II–IV	46% normal, 54%elevated	≥1	14 (13%)	43 (38%)	55 (49%)	77	62% 5-y NED, 56% 5-y overall survival
Fox et al [18]	1993	163	II–IV	Normal and elevated	NS	NS	NS	90 (55%)	36	28/90 (31%) NED, 5/90 (6%) AWD, 55/90 (61%) DOD, 2 postoperative deaths
Desperation										
Wood et al [59]	1992	15	NS	Elevated	NS	2/15	1/15	12/15	3–127	11/15 (73%) NED, 1/15 (7%) AWD, 3/15 (20%) DOD
Eastham et al [60]	1994	16	B3	Elevated	NS	NS	NS	NS	64 (20–145)	5/10 (50%) NED
Coogan et al [61]	1997	15	B = 7, C = 8	Elevated	NS	2 (13%)	7 (47%)	6 (40%)	32 (9–66)	11 (73%) NED, 1 (0.05%) relapse, 3 (20%) deaths

Donohue et al [33]	1998	152	II–III	Elevated	NS	NS	NS	NS	108	87/152 (58%) NED, 12/152 (8%) AWD, 51/152 (34%) DOD
Albers et al [56]	2000	30	II–IV	Elevated	NS	7/28 (25%)	3/28 (11%)	18/28 (64%)	120 (1–228)	17/30 (57%) NED
Redo										
Waples and Messing [62]	1993	9	Interval 12	NS	NS	NS	NS	NS	32	6/9 (67%) NED
Donohue et al [33]	1998	202	II–III, Interval NS	Normal	NS	NS	NS	NS	108	104/202 (55%) NED, 14/202 (7.5%) AWD, 70/202 (37%) DOD
McKiernan et al [81]	2003	56	Interval 17 (2–324)	NS	NS	9/34 (%)	13/34 (%)	14/34 (%)	29.5	Complication rate 27%, 5-y cancer-specific 56%
Heidenreich et al [82]	2005	18	Interval 18 (2–30)	Normal	7.8 (3.5–25)	8 (44%)	6 (33%)	4 (22%)	22 (1–45)	Complication rate 38.8%, cancer-specific 89%, necrosis 100%, teratoma 85%, cancer 50%

Abbreviations: AWD, alive with disease; DOD, died of disease; NED, no evidence of disease; NS, not specified.

identified in frozen section analysis of the residual masses, with 18 (85.7%) confirmed in permanent section. Two patients had microscopic viable germ cell tumor unrecognized on frozen section, and 1 had microscopic teratoma in the residual mass. Of these 21 patients, 3 (14.3%) experienced recurrences, 2 had germ cell tumors in the chest, and 1 had liver metastasis. The remaining 18 (85.7%) patients had no evidence of disease, with a mean follow-up of 33 months (range, 24–60 months). The authors concluded that limited RPLND if frozen section analysis shows only necrosis is a safe alternative to bilateral dissection. Similarly, Rabbani and colleagues [36] studied 50 patients who had metastatic NSGCT after chemotherapy in Vancouver, British Columbia; 39 patients (78%) had bilateral dissection, 9 patients (22%) underwent resection of residual masses and modified-template dissection, and 2 patients had resection of residual masses only. Of the 9 patients who had resection of residual masses and modified-template dissection, all were relapse-free at a median follow-up of 55 months. One of 2 patients undergoing resection of residual mass alone had two recurrences arising from incomplete resection.

There is, however, emerging evidence that a substantial proportion of patients harbor disease, usually teratoma, outside the proposed modified templates. This disease could potentially account for the late recurrence, a formidable and often fatal outcome of the uncontrolled retroperitoneum. Furthermore, the boundaries of template dissections in the literature vary significantly [68–72]. Carver and associates [73] recently examined 532 men undergoing post-chemotherapy RPLND and found that of the 269 patients who had viable germ cell tumor or teratoma, 7% to 32% had evidence of disease outside the boundaries of a modified template, depending on the definition of the template boundaries. In this study, disease outside the template was associated with a decreased disease-free survival. The incidence of late recurrence is increasing, possibly as a result of these incomplete or inadequate resections, and the authors support the traditional bilateral dissection. These surgeries can often be accomplished with nerve-sparing techniques, even in the post-chemotherapy retroperitoneum.

Coogan and colleagues [74] evaluated 81 patients who underwent nerve-sparing procedure after chemotherapy. At a median follow-up of 35 months, 6 had disease recurrence but none of the recurrences were in-field. Antegrade ejaculation was maintained in 76.5% of the patients. Nonomura and colleagues [75] also showed that nerve-sparing RPLND after chemotherapy could still preserve antegrade ejaculation in 84.6% (22/26) of patients while maintaining disease-free status of 96% (25/26) with a mean follow-up of 25.8 months (range 6–76 months). The study cohorts in these nerve-sparing studies included a mixed group of patients, although NSGCT was the predominant pathology.

In summary, retroperitoneal surgery for testis tumor has evolved over the past 3 decades with increasing knowledge of neuroanatomy and tumor distributions. Some authors have advocated more limited dissections to limit the morbidities of the procedure, whereas others cite the inadequate resections of potentially harmful histologies. As surgical series of limited dissections continue to mature, the extent of post-chemotherapy RPLND still remains controversial.

Outcome and management after surgery

The outcome following surgery after chemotherapy for advance testicular cancer depends on (1) the pathology of retroperitoneal resection, (2) completeness of resection, and (3) subsequent adjuvant treatment.

The management of viable germ cell tumor in the retroperitoneal specimen after induction chemotherapy dictates additional chemotherapy, usually in the form of two additional cycles of the induction chemotherapy regimen [18]. Fizazi and associates [76] challenged the need for additional chemotherapy in their examination of 238 patients who had viable germ cell tumor in the retroperitoneal specimens following chemotherapy. These investigators stratified patients based on three risk factors: complete resection, greater than 10% viable tumor in specimen, and IGCCCG risk group. Good-, intermediate-, and poor-prognostic groups were assigned to patients who had 0, 1, or 2 or more risk factors, respectively. Postoperative chemotherapy was not associated with statistically significant improved overall survival in the good- or poor-prognostic groups, yet seemed beneficial only in the intermediate-prognostic group. The authors concluded that complete resection of disease may be more critical than postoperative chemotherapy in the setting of post-chemotherapy viable NSGCT. Others have validated the significance of these three risk factors; however, they did not validate that the effects of adjuvant chemotherapy differ by prognostic group [77]. In summary, although the Fizazi and colleagues findings are provocative, the standard of care remains additional chemotherapy if viable tumor is found in the post-chemotherapy residual mass [78].

Table 1 gives the comparison of residual tumor mass, histologic findings, and oncologic outcome of patients who have standard RPLND after induction chemotherapy. The trends evident in Table 1 include (1) a gradual decrease in proportion of germ cell tumor in the residual masses, (2) a gradual increase in proportion of residual teratoma, (3) favorable survival in those who have histology showing necrosis or teratoma, (4) disease-free status of 80% to 94%, and (5) 5-year overall survival rate of 83% to 96%.

Table 2 gives the outcome following complicated RPLND after standard and salvage chemotherapy. In the complicated RPLND group (see Table 2), the outcome depends heavily on (1) the presence of viable germ cell in the residual tumor, and (2) the completeness of resection. The proportion of viable germ cell tumor is much higher, from 22% to 49%, and the cancer-specific survival and overall survival are correspondingly much lower. Current concepts and clinical outcomes in these difficult scenarios are presented in detail in other articles of this issue.

Morbidity of retroperitoneal lymph node dissection after chemotherapy

RPLND after induction chemotherapy is a challenging operation because of the complexity of the procedure and the severe desmoplastic reaction from prior exposure to chemotherapeutic agents. The morbidity of post-chemotherapy RPLND ranges from 18% to 29% in the standard group [23,79,80] and up to 39% in the complicated RPLND group [81,82]. Perioperative complications may be subdivided into pulmonary, infectious, lymphatic, vascular, neurologic, and gastrointestinal complications.

Pulmonary-related complications occur in up to 8% of cases and include atelectasis, pneumonia, adult respiratory distress syndrome, and pulmonary embolism [23]. Aggressive chest physiotherapy, adequate analgesia, and early mobilization may reduce the incidence. Wound infections occur in 5% of cases and urinary tract infections in 0.8% of cases [23].

Injury to lymphatic channels, resulting in chylous ascites, occurs in 2% of cases [23]. Factors that predispose to this complication include suprahilar dissection, liver resection, or resection of the inferior vena cava. Dietary manipulation with medium-chain triglycerides and diuretic therapy are the mainstays of management. Lymphoceles may also result from the lymphatic injury, and percutaneous drainage is necessary if there is superimposed infection, hydronephrosis, or prolonged ileus. Injury to the inferior vena cava or aorta may necessitate primary repair or the use of interposition grafts, and injury to renal vessels may occur, resulting in renal infarction and loss of the kidney. Spinal cord ischemia is rare and is usually associated with advancing age and dissection around the anterior spinal artery near the T8 level. Small bowel obstruction is present in 2% and often responds to conservative measures [23]. Prolonged ileus may mask underlying pancreatitis, retroperitoneal hematoma, urinary extravasation, or bowel ischemia. Hemorrhage after RPLND necessitating transfusion is rare in tertiary centers, ranging from 0.3% to 1% in large studies [23,79,80]. Adjunctive procedures, including en bloc nephrectomy, inferior vena cava resection, orchiectomy, bowel resection, hepatic resection arterial graft, caval thrombectomy, adrenalectomy, and cholecystectomy, occur in 29% to 52% of cases [23,79]. Long-term morbidity and fertility issues are covered in a separate chapter of this edition.

Mediastinal, neck and hepatic resections

Extra-retroperitoneal spread of advanced testicular cancer may involve the cervical nodes, lung, mediastinum, liver, and brain. Resection of pulmonary nodules is the most common extra-retroperitoneal procedure, whereas resection of cervical nodes and hepatic resection occur less frequently [33,39,83,84]. Table 3 [85–95] gives a summary of the histologic profile and outcome following extra-retroperitoneal surgery. There is significant discordance of histology between the extra-retroperitoneal mass and retroperitoneal mass with different studies citing a 25% to 64% discordance rate. There is adequate justification for surgery to resect the extra-retroperitoneal mass, therefore, even if the initial retroperitoneal resection yielded necrosis or teratoma. Further review of this topic is the subject of another article in this issue.

Table 3
Metastases outside of the retroperitoneum after chemotherapy for advanced testicular cancer

Study	Year	N	Site	Intervention	Size (cm)	Necrosis N (%)	Teratoma N (%)	Carcinoma N (%)	Discordance[a]	Median follow-up (months)	Survival (%)
Mandelbaum et al [85]	1983	72	Chest	Thoracotomy, median sternotomy	NS	22 (31%)	28 (39%)	22 (31%)	29%	36	74% overall survival,83% with RPLND
Tiffany et al [86]	1986	15	Chest neck	Thoracotomy neck dissection	NS	6 (40%)	5 (33%)	4 (27%)	35%	29 (1–58)	73% recurrence-free
Gerl et al [87]	1994	38	Chest neck liver	Thoracotomy neck dissection hepatectomy	NS	15 (39%)	19 (50%)	4 (11%)	39%	84 (5–146)	66% recurrence-free
Brenner et al [13]	1996	24	Chestneck	Thoracotomyneck dissection	NS	18	5	1	25%	60	79% overall survival
See et al [88]	1996	7	Neck	Neck dissection	NS	3 (42%)	2 (29%)	2 (29%)	NS	42 (6–82)	5/7 NED
Hartmann et al [89]	1997	27	Chest liver neck brain	21 thoracotomies 4 hepatectomies 3 neck dissections 1 craniotomy	NS	15 (71%) 4 (100%) 1 (33%)	2 (10%)	4 (19%) 2 (66%) 1 (100%)	30%	33 (1–167)	18/27 NED, 67% recurrence-free, 73% overall survival
Gels et al [90]	1997	31	Chest	Thoracotomy	1.5 (0.2–6)	11 (36%)	16 (52%)	4 (13%)	50%	80 (2.5–203)	87% 5-y survival, 82% 10-y survival

Steyerberg et al [91]	1997	215	Chest	Thoracotomy	40% ≤2, 60% >2	116 (54%)	70 (33%)	29 (13%)	36%	NS	NS
Weisberger and McBride [92]	1999	45	Neck	Neck dissection	NS	8 (17%)	29 (64%)	8 (17%)	NS	32	72% recurrence-free
Hahn et al [93]	1999	57	Liver	Hepatectomies	NS	9 (16%)	29 (51%)	19 (33%)	47	—	97% 2-y survival
McGuire et al [94]	2003	105	Chest	130 thoracotomies	NS	57 (44%)	49 (38%)	14 (11%)	Synchronous 28%, asynchronous 57%	24 (1–89)	68/105 NED, necrosis 96% NED, teratoma 82% NED, cancer 25% NED
Eskicorapci et al [95]	2004	19	Chest	Thoracotomy	NS	7 (37%)	7 (37%)	5 (26%)	64%	30 (15–212)	14/19 NED, necrosis/teratoma 85% NED, cancer 40% NED

Abbreviations: NED, no evidence of disease; NS, not specified.

[a] Discordance in histology of non-retroperitoneal mass compared with retroperitoneal residual mass.

Summary

Surgery after systemic chemotherapy for advanced testicular cancer has maintained its role in staging and therapeutic management. The clinical outcome is strongly influenced by patient selection and extent of extirpative surgery. Although extensive predictive modeling has attempted to define appropriate post-chemotherapy surgical candidates based on various clinical and pathologic parameters, the accuracy of these models remains controversial. Complete removal of all post-chemotherapy residual masses in NSGCT remains the standard of care and allows for improved prognostication of the long-term oncologic and functional outcome.

References

[1] Foster RS, Beck S, Bihrle R. Secondary surgery in germ cell tumors—when and how extensively should it be performed? World J Urol 2004;22(1):37–40.
[2] Donohue JP, Foster RS. Retroperitoneal lymphadenectomy in staging and treatment. The development of nerve-sparing techniques. Urol Clin North Am 1998;25(3):461–8.
[3] Donohue JP, Roth LM, Zachary JM, et al. Cytoreductive surgery for metastatic testis cancer: tissue analysis of retroperitoneal masses after chemotherapy. J Urol 1982;127(6):1111–4.
[4] Bracken RB, Johnson DE, Frazier OH, et al. The role of surgery following chemotherapy in stage III germ cell neoplasms. J Urol 1983;129(1):39–43.
[5] Freiha FS, Shortliffe LD, Rouse RV, et al. The extent of surgery after chemotherapy for advanced germ cell tumors. J Urol 1984;132(5):915–7.
[6] Pizzocaro G, Salvioni R, Pasi M, et al. Early resection of residual tumor during cisplatin, vinblastine, bleomycin combination chemotherapy in stage III and bulky stage II nonseminomatous testicular cancer. Cancer 1985;56(2):249–55.
[7] Fossa SD, Aass N, Ous S, et al. Histology of tumor residuals following chemotherapy in patients with advanced nonseminomatous testicular cancer. J Urol 1989;142(5):1239–42.
[8] Williams SN, Jenkins BJ, Baithun SI, et al. Radical retroperitoneal node dissection after chemotherapy for testicular tumours. Br J Urol 1989;63(6):641–3.
[9] Mulders PF, Oosterhof GO, Boetes C, et al. The importance of prognostic factors in the individual treatment of patients with disseminated germ cell tumours. Br J Urol 1990;66(4):425–9.
[10] Harding MJ, Brown IL, MacPherson SG, et al. Excision of residual masses after platinum based chemotherapy for non-seminomatous germ cell tumours. Eur J Cancer Clin Oncol 1989;25(12):1689–94.
[11] Aass N, Klepp O, Cavallin-Stahl E, et al. Prognostic factors in unselected patients with nonseminomatous metastatic testicular cancer: a multicenter experience. J Clin Oncol 1991;9(5):818–26.
[12] Kulkarni RP, Reynolds KW, Newlands ES, et al. Cytoreductive surgery in disseminated non-seminomatous germ cell tumours of testis. Br J Surg 1991;78(2):226–9.
[13] Brenner PC, Herr HW, Morse MJ, et al. Simultaneous retroperitoneal, thoracic, and cervical resection of postchemotherapy residual masses in patients with metastatic nonseminomatous germ cell tumors of the testis. J Clin Oncol 1996;14(6):1765–9.
[14] Stenning SP, Parkinson MC, Fisher C, et al. Postchemotherapy residual masses in germ cell tumor patients: content, clinical features, and prognosis. Medical Research Council Testicular Tumour Working Party. Cancer 1998;83(7):1409–19.
[15] Napier MP, Naraghi A, Christmas TJ, et al. Long-term follow-up of residual masses after chemotherapy in patients with non-seminomatous germ cell tumours. Br J Cancer 2000;83(10):1274–80.
[16] Hendry WF, Norman AR, Dearnaley DP, et al. Metastatic nonseminomatous germ cell tumors of the testis: results of elective and salvage surgery for patients with residual retroperitoneal masses. Cancer 2002;94(6):1668–76.
[17] Muramaki M, Hara I, Miyake H, et al. Clinical outcome of retroperitoneal lymph node dissection after induction chemotherapy for metastatic non-seminomatous germ cell tumors. Int J Urol 2004;11(9):763–7.
[18] Fox EP, Weathers TD, Williams SD, et al. Outcome analysis for patients with persistent nonteratomatous germ cell tumor in postchemotherapy retroperitoneal lymph node dissections. J Clin Oncol 1993;11(7):1294–9.
[19] Logothetis CJ, Samuels ML, Trindade A, et al. The growing teratoma syndrome. Cancer 1982;50(8):1629–35.
[20] Motzer RJ, Amsterdam A, Prieto V, et al. Teratoma with malignant transformation: diverse malignant histologies arising in men with germ cell tumors. J Urol 1998;159(1):133–8.
[21] Ahmed T, Bosl GJ, Hajdu SI. Teratoma with malignant transformation in germ cell tumors in men. Cancer 1985;56(4):860–3.
[22] Donadio AC, Motzer RJ, Bajorin DF, et al. Chemotherapy for teratoma with malignant transformation. J Clin Oncol 2003;21(23):4285–91.
[23] Baniel J, Foster RS, Rowland RG, et al. Complications of post-chemotherapy retroperitoneal lymph node dissection. J Urol 1995;153(3 Pt 2):976–80.
[24] Heidenreich A, Albers P, Hartmann M, et al. Complications of primary nerve sparing retroperitoneal lymph node dissection for clinical stage I nonseminomatous germ cell tumors of the testis: experience

of the German Testicular Cancer Study Group. J Urol 2003;169(5):1710–4.

[25] Foster RS, Donohue JP. Can retroperitoneal lymphadenectomy be omitted in some patients after chemotherapy? Urol Clin North Am 1998;25(3):479–84.

[26] Steyerberg EW, Keizer HJ, Fossa SD, et al. Prediction of residual retroperitoneal mass histology after chemotherapy for metastatic nonseminomatous germ cell tumor: multivariate analysis of individual patient data from six study groups. J Clin Oncol 1995;13(5):1177–87.

[27] Vergouwe Y, Steyerberg EW, de Wit R, et al. External validity of a prediction rule for residual mass histology in testicular cancer: an evaluation for good prognosis patients. Br J Cancer 2003;88(6):843–7.

[28] Matsuyama H, Yamamoto N, Sakatoku J, et al. Predictive factors for the histologic nature of residual tumor mass after chemotherapy in patients with advanced testicular cancer. Urology 1994;44(3):392–8 [discussion: 398–9].

[29] Onozawa M, Kawai K, Yamamoto T, et al. Clinical parameters that predict histology of postchemotherapy retroperitoneal lymph node mass in testicular cancer. Int J Urol 2004;11(7):535–41.

[30] Herr HW, Sheinfeld J, Puc HS, et al. Surgery for a post-chemotherapy residual mass in seminoma. J Urol 1997;157(3):860–2.

[31] Ravi R, Ong J, Oliver RT, et al. The management of residual masses after chemotherapy in metastatic seminoma. BJU Int 1999;83(6):649–53.

[32] Flechon A, Bompas E, Biron P, et al. Management of post-chemotherapy residual masses in advanced seminoma. J Urol 2002;168(5):1975–9.

[33] Donohue JP, Leviovitch I, Foster RS, et al. Integration of surgery and systemic therapy: results and principles of integration. Semin Urol Oncol 1998; 16(2):65–71.

[34] Richie JP, Garnick MB, Finberg H. Computerized tomography: how accurate for abdominal staging of testis tumors? J Urol 1982;127(4):715–7.

[35] Debono DJ, Heilman DK, Einhorn LH, et al. Decision analysis for avoiding postchemotherapy surgery in patients with disseminated nonseminomatous germ cell tumors. J Clin Oncol 1997;15(4):1455–64.

[36] Rabbani F, Goldenberg SL, Gleave ME, et al. Retroperitoneal lymphadenectomy for post-chemotherapy residual masses: is a modified dissection and resection of residual masses sufficient? Br J Urol 1998;81(2):295–300.

[37] Fossa SD, Qvist H, Stenwig AE, et al. Is postchemotherapy retroperitoneal surgery necessary in patients with nonseminomatous testicular cancer and minimal residual tumor masses? J Clin Oncol 1992; 10(4):569–73.

[38] Stomper PC, Kalish LA, Garnick MB, et al. CT and pathologic predictive features of residual mass histologic findings after chemotherapy for nonseminomatous germ cell tumors: can residual malignancy or teratoma be excluded? Radiology 1991;180(3): 711–4.

[39] Toner GC, Panicek DM, Heelan RT, et al. Adjunctive surgery after chemotherapy for nonseminomatous germ cell tumors: recommendations for patient selection. J Clin Oncol 1990;8(10):1683–94.

[40] Oldenburg J, Alfsen GC, Lien HH, et al. Postchemotherapy retroperitoneal surgery remains necessary in patients with nonseminomatous testicular cancer and minimal residual tumor masses. J Clin Oncol 2003;21(17):3310–7.

[41] Steyerberg EW, Marshall PB, Keizer HJ, et al. Resection of small, residual retroperitoneal masses after chemotherapy for nonseminomatous testicular cancer: a decision analysis. Cancer 1999;85(6): 1331–41.

[42] Fossa SD, Ous S, Lien HH, et al. Post-chemotherapy lymph node histology in radiologically normal patients with metastatic nonseminomatous testicular cancer. J Urol 1989;141(3):557–9.

[43] Carver BS, Bianco FJ Jr, Shayegan B, et al. Predicting teratoma in the retroperitoneum in men undergoing post-chemotherapy retroperitoneal lymph node dissection. J Urol 2006;176(1):100–4.

[44] Donohue JP, Rowland RG, Kopecky K, et al. Correlation of computerized tomographic changes and histological findings in 80 patients having radical retroperitoneal lymph node dissection after chemotherapy for testis cancer. J Urol 1987;137(6): 1176–9.

[45] Albers P, Weissbach L, Krege S, et al. Prediction of necrosis after chemotherapy of advanced germ cell tumors: results of a prospective multicenter trial of the German Testicular Cancer Study Group. J Urol 2004;171(5):1835–8.

[46] Steyerberg EW, Gerl A, Fossa SD, et al. Validity of predictions of residual retroperitoneal mass histology in nonseminomatous testicular cancer. J Clin Oncol 1998;16(1):269–74.

[47] De Wit M, Hartmann M, Brenner W, et al. [18F]-FDG-PET in germ cell tumors following chemotherapy: results of the German multicenter trial. J Clin Oncol. ASCO Annual Meeting Proceedings Part I 2006;24(Suppl 18):4521.

[48] Spermon JR, De Geus-Oei LF, Kiemeney LA, et al. The role of (18)fluoro-2-deoxyglucose positron emission tomography in initial staging and re-staging after chemotherapy for testicular germ cell tumours. BJU Int 2002;89(6):549–56.

[49] Sanchez D, Zudaire JJ, Fernandez JM, et al. 18F-fluoro-2-deoxyglucose-positron emission tomography in the evaluation of nonseminomatous germ cell tumours at relapse. BJU Int 2002;89(9):912–6.

[50] Kollmannsberger C, Oechsle K, Dohmen BM, et al. Prospective comparison of [18F]fluorodeoxyglucose positron emission tomography with conventional assessment by computed tomography scans and serum tumor markers for the evaluation of residual masses

in patients with nonseminomatous germ cell carcinoma. Cancer 2002;94(9):2353–62.

[51] Stephens AW, Gonin R, Hutchins GD, et al. Positron emission tomography evaluation of residual radiographic abnormalities in postchemotherapy germ cell tumor patients. J Clin Oncol 1996;14(5): 1637–41.

[52] De Santis M, Becherer A, Bokemeyer C, et al. 2-18fluoro-deoxy-D-glucose positron emission tomography is a reliable predictor for viable tumor in postchemotherapy seminoma: an update of the prospective multicentric SEMPET trial. J Clin Oncol 2004;22(6):1034–9.

[53] Johns Putra L, Lawrentschuk N, Ballok Z, et al. 18F-fluorodeoxyglucose positron emission tomography in evaluation of germ cell tumor after chemotherapy. Urology 2004;64(6):1202–7.

[54] Ganjoo KN, Chan RJ, Sharma M, et al. Positron emission tomography scans in the evaluation of postchemotherapy residual masses in patients with seminoma. J Clin Oncol 1999;17(11):3457–60.

[55] Beck SD, Foster RS, Bihrle R, et al. Outcome analysis for patients with elevated serum tumor markers at postchemotherapy retroperitoneal lymph node dissection. J Clin Oncol 2005;23(25):6149–56.

[56] Albers P, Ganz A, Hannig E, et al. Salvage surgery of chemorefractory germ cell tumors with elevated tumor markers. J Urol 2000;164(2):381–4.

[57] International Germ Cell Cancer Collaborative Group. International Germ Cell Consensus Classification: a prognostic factor-based staging system for metastatic germ cell cancers. J Clin Oncol 1997; 15(2):594–603.

[58] Beck SD, Patel MI, Sheinfeld J. Tumor marker levels in post-chemotherapy cystic masses: clinical implications for patients with germ cell tumors. J Urol 2004; 171(1):168–71.

[59] Wood DP Jr, Herr HW, Motzer RJ, et al. Surgical resection of solitary metastases after chemotherapy in patients with nonseminomatous germ cell tumors and elevated serum tumor markers. Cancer 1992; 70(9):2354–7.

[60] Eastham JA, Wilson TG, Russell C, et al. Surgical resection in patients with nonseminomatous germ cell tumor who fail to normalize serum tumor markers after chemotherapy. Urology 1994;43(1):74–80.

[61] Coogan CL, Foster RS, Rowland RG, et al. Postchemotherapy retroperitoneal lymph node dissection is effective therapy in selected patients with elevated tumor markers after primary chemotherapy alone. Urology 1997;50(6):957–62.

[62] Waples MJ, Messing EM. Redo retroperitoneal lymphadenectomy for germ cell tumor. Urology 1993; 42(1):31–4.

[63] Donohue JP. Retroperitoneal lymphadenectomy: the anterior approach including bilateral suprarenal-hilar dissection. Urol Clin North Am 1977; 4(3):509–21.

[64] Donohue JP, Zachary JM, Maynard BR. Distribution of nodal metastases in nonseminomatous testis cancer. J Urol 1982;128(2):315–20.

[65] Donohue JP, Thornhill JA, Foster RS, et al. Retroperitoneal lymphadenectomy for clinical stage A testis cancer (1965 to 1989): modifications of technique and impact on ejaculation. J Urol 1993;149(2): 237–43.

[66] Lange PH, Chang WY, Fraley EE. Fertility issues in the therapy of nonseminomatous testicular tumors. Urol Clin North Am 1987;14(4):731–47.

[67] Aprikian AG, Herr HW, Bajorin DF, et al. Resection of postchemotherapy residual masses and limited retroperitoneal lymphadenectomy in patients with metastatic testicular nonseminomatous germ cell tumors. Cancer 1994;74(4):1329–34.

[68] Sheinfeld J. Postchemotherapy retroperitoneal lymph node dissection and resection of residual masses for germ cell tumors of the testis. In: Vogelzang NJ, Scardino PT, Shipley WU, et al, editors. Comprehensive textbook of genitourinary oncology. 3rd edition. Philadelphia: Lippincott Williams and Wilkins; 2006. p. 616–23.

[69] Weissbach L, Boedefeld EA. Localization of solitary and multiple metastases in stage II nonseminomatous testis tumor as basis for a modified staging lymph node dissection in stage I. J Urol 1987; 138(1):77–82.

[70] Foster RS. Modified retroperitoneal lymphadenectomy. BJU Int 2004;94(6):941–55.

[71] Nelson JB, Chen RN, Bishoff JT, et al. Laparoscopic retroperitoneal lymph node dissection for clinical stage I nonseminomatous germ cell testicular tumors. Urology 1999;54(6):1064–7.

[72] Janetschek G, Hobisch A, Peschel R, et al. Laparoscopic retroperitoneal lymph node dissection. Urology 2000;55(1):136–40.

[73] Carver BS, Shayegan B, Motzer RJ, et al. The incidence and implications of disease outside a modified template in men undergoing post-chemotherapy retroperitoneal lymph node dissection (PC-RPLND) for metastatic non-seminomatous germ cell tumors (NSGCT). J Urol 2006;175 (Suppl 4):192.

[74] Coogan CL, Hejase MJ, Wahle GR, et al. Nerve sparing post-chemotherapy retroperitoneal lymph node dissection for advanced testicular cancer. J Urol 1996;156(5):1656–8.

[75] Nonomura N, Nishimura K, Takaha N, et al. Nerve-sparing retroperitoneal lymph node dissection for advanced testicular cancer after chemotherapy. Int J Urol 2002;9(10):539–44.

[76] Fizazi K, Tjulandin S, Salvioni R, et al. Viable malignant cells after primary chemotherapy for disseminated nonseminomatous germ cell tumors: prognostic factors and role of postsurgery chemotherapy–results from an international study group. J Clin Oncol 2001;19(10):2647–57.

[77] Karanikolas N, Serio A, Vickers A, et al. Viable germ cell tumor (GCT) identified at post-chemotherapy retroperitoneal lymph node dissection (PC-RPLND): the significance of risk assignment and adjuvant chemotherapy. J Urol 2006;175(Suppl 4):191.
[78] NCCN Prostate Cancer Panel. NCCN guidelines on testicular cancer. Available at: *http://www.nccn.org/professionals/physician_gls/PDF/testicular.pdf*. Accessed June 13, 2006.
[79] Mosharafa AA, Foster RS, Koch MO, et al. Complications of post-chemotherapy retroperitoneal lymph node dissection for testis cancer. J Urol 2004;171(5):1839–41.
[80] Gels ME, Nijboer AP, Hoekstra HJ, et al. Complications of the post-chemotherapy resection of retroperitoneal residual tumour mass in patients with non-seminomatous testicular germ cell tumours. Br J Urol 1997;79(2):263–8.
[81] McKiernan JM, Motzer RJ, Bajorin DF, et al. Reoperative retroperitoneal surgery for nonseminomatous germ cell tumor: clinical presentation, patterns of recurrence, and outcome. Urology 2003;62(4):732–6.
[82] Heidenreich A, Ohlmann C, Hegele A, et al. Repeat retroperitoneal lymphadenectomy in advanced testicular cancer. Eur Urol 2005;47(1):64–71.
[83] Tait D, Peckham MJ, Hendry WF, et al. Post-chemotherapy surgery in advanced non-seminomatous germ-cell testicular tumours: the significance of histology with particular reference to differentiated (mature) teratoma. Br J Cancer 1984;50(5):601–9.
[84] Gelderman WA, Schraffordt Koops H, Sleijfer DT, et al. Results of adjuvant surgery in patients with stage III and IV nonseminomatous testicular tumors after cisplatin-vinblastine-bleomycin chemotherapy. J Surg Oncol 1988;38(4):227–32.
[85] Mandelbaum I, Yaw PB, Einhorn LH, et al. The importance of one-stage median sternotomy and retroperitoneal node dissection in disseminated testicular cancer. Ann Thorac Surg 1983;36(5):524–8.
[86] Tiffany P, Morse MJ, Bosl G, et al. Sequential excision of residual thoracic and retroperitoneal masses after chemotherapy for stage III germ cell tumors. Cancer 1986;57(5):978–83.
[87] Gerl A, Clemm C, Schmeller N, et al. Sequential resection of residual abdominal and thoracic masses after chemotherapy for metastatic non-seminomatous germ cell tumours. Br J Cancer 1994;70(5):960–5.
[88] See WA, Laurenzo JF, Dreicer R, et al. Incidence and management of testicular carcinoma metastatic to the neck. J Urol 1996;155(2):590–2.
[89] Hartmann JT, Candelaria M, Kuczyk MA, et al. Comparison of histological results from the resection of residual masses at different sites after chemotherapy for metastatic non-seminomatous germ cell tumours. Eur J Cancer 1997;33(6):843–7.
[90] Gels ME, Hoekstra HJ, Sleijfer DT, et al. Thoracotomy for postchemotherapy resection of pulmonary residual tumor mass in patients with nonseminomatous testicular germ cell tumors: aggressive surgical resection is justified. Chest 1997;112(4):967–73.
[91] Steyerberg EW, Keizer HJ, Messemer JE, et al. Residual pulmonary masses after chemotherapy for metastatic nonseminomatous germ cell tumor. Prediction of histology. ReHiT study group. Cancer 1997;79(2):345–55.
[92] Weisberger EC, McBride LC. Modified neck dissection for metastatic nonseminomatous testicular carcinoma. Laryngoscope 1999;109(8):1241–4.
[93] Hahn TL, Jacobson L, Einhorn LH, et al. Hepatic resection of metastatic testicular carcinoma: a further update. Ann Surg Oncol 1999;6(7):640–4.
[94] McGuire MS, Rabbani F, Mohseni H, et al. The role of thoracotomy in managing postchemotherapy residual thoracic masses in patients with nonseminomatous germ cell tumours. BJU Int 2003;91(6):469–73.
[95] Eskicorapci SY, Ekici S, Atsu MN, et al. Resection of pulmonary metastases following chemotherapy for high stage testicular tumors. Int J Urol 2004;11(8):634–9.

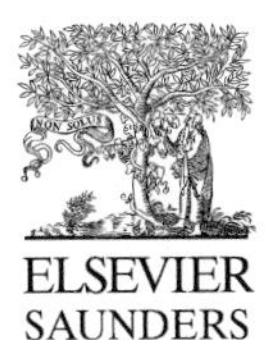
ELSEVIER
SAUNDERS

Urol Clin N Am 34 (2007) 219–225

UROLOGIC
CLINICS
of North America

Post Chemotherapy RPLND in Patients with Elevated Markers: Current Concepts and Clinical Outcome

Stephen D.W. Beck, MD[a,*], Richard S. Foster, MD[a], Richard Bihrle, MD[a], Lawrence H. Einhorn, MD[a,b], John P. Donohue, MD[a]

[a]*Department of Urology, Indiana University School of Medicine, 535 North Barnhill Drive, Suite 420, Indiana Cancer Pavilion, Indianapolis, IN 46202, USA*

[b]*Department of Medicine, Section of Hematology and Oncology, Indiana University School of Medicine, 535 North Barnhill Drive, Suite 420, Indiana Cancer Pavilion, Indianapolis, IN 46202, USA*

With the advent of cisplatin-based chemotherapy, nonseminomatous germ cell tumor (NSGCT) became a highly curable malignancy. A unique aspect of NSGCT is the complementary role of post-chemotherapy surgery in achieving cure of these patients.

Approximately 70% of patients who present with metastatic testis cancer and receive standard cisplatin-based chemotherapy as initial treatment for their disease experience a complete response with normalization of serum tumor markers and resolution of radiographic disease. Patients not achieving a complete response are candidates for subsequent management. Partial remission is usually defined as either persistent serum tumor marker elevation or persistent radiographic disease. Persistent radiographic disease is composed histologically of one of four entities: necrosis-fibrosis, teratoma, germ cell carcinoma, or non–germ cell carcinoma (malignant transformation of teratoma). Removal of teratoma is therapeutic, as this histologic subtype is chemoresistant. The surgical removal of either germ-cell cancer or non–germ cell cancer confers both a staging benefit (some patients will receive postoperative chemotherapy) as well as a therapeutic benefit, as select patients will be cured with surgery alone.

* Corresponding author.
E-mail address: sdwbeck@iupui.edu (S.D.W. Beck).

Persistent serum tumor marker elevation after chemotherapy has historically been considered a relative contraindication to surgery because of supposed systemic disease and low chance of cure with local therapy alone. These patients have typically been treated with subsequent salvage chemotherapy. Over the past 15 years, however, several centers have experienced surgical cures in this population. In this article we will review the pathologic and clinical outcomes and determine the therapeutic value of retroperitoneal lymph node dissection in patients with elevated serum tumor markers at time of post-chemotherapy surgery.

Retroperitoneal pathology

Expected pathology at post chemotherapy retroperitoneal lymph node dissection (PCRPLND) in patients with marker normalization after first-line chemotherapy reveals fibrosis/necrosis in 40% to 50%. Approximately 35% to 40% of patients display mature or immature teratomatous elements, with active germ-cell cancer identified in fewer than 10% of patients [1]. After second-line chemotherapy, the probability of active germ-cell cancer at PCRPLND increases to 50% [2].

In the population with elevated serum tumor markers at time of surgery, the reported incidence of active germ-cell cancer ranges from 40% to 81% (Table 1). In a recent review at Indiana University analyzing 114 patients who had undergone

0094-0143/07/$ - see front matter
doi:10.1016/j.ucl.2007.02.006

Table 1
Clinical and pathologic features of patients undergoing post chemotherapy with elevated serum tumor markers

	Wood et al, 1992 [5]	Coogan et al, 1997 [9]	Eastham et al, 1994 [8]	Murphy et al, 1993 [10]	Albers et al, 2000 [4]	Ravi et al, 1998 [11]	Beck et al, 2005 [3]
No. patients	15	15	16	48	30	30	114
Retroperitoneal pathology							
Cancer	12	6	13	—	18	14	61
Teratoma	1	7	2	—	3	8	39
Fibrosis	2	2	1	—	7	8	14
Tumor marker							
AFP	10	12	8	31	9	20	59
HCG	2	3	5	16	10	7	51
AFP/HCG	3	0	3	1	11	3	4

Abbreviations: AFP, alpha-fetoprotein; HCG, human chorionic gonadotropin; —, unknown.

surgery with elevated serum tumor markers, retroperitoneal pathology revealed germ-cell cancer in 53.5% [3]. For the 50 patients receiving first-line chemotherapy alone before surgery, the incidence of active germ-cell cancer was 28%, compared with 75.8% for the 64 patients receiving second-line chemotherapy (P = .0001). Despite elevated serum tumor markers, and presumed active disease, surgical pathology revealed teratoma in 34.2% and fibrosis in 12.3%. In this series, clinical parameters predictive of teratoma/fibrosis included declining serum tumor markers, low serum human chorionic gonadotropin (βHCG) (<100), and first-line chemotherapy only. Other series have also reported an incidence of teratoma or fibrosis ranging from 20% to 40% [4,5], despite elevated serum tumor markers at time of PCRPLND. A possible explanation for nonviable germ-cell elements and not finding active germ-cell cancer at RPLND in light of elevated serum tumor markers is unrecognized germ-cell elements in the pathologic specimen. Alternatively, the elevated presurgical tumor makers may not be related to active germ-cell cancer, with false-positive HCG related to marijuana use, or cross-reactivity with lactate dehydrogenase (LDH), and false-positive alpha-fetoprotein (AFP) elevation because of hepatic dysfunction. Likewise, the subset with declining serum tumor markers at PCRPLND may have normalized given time, with retroperitoneal pathology more resembling that of a standard PCRPLND. van der Gaast [6], and Beck and colleagues [7] have hypothesized a slow-leak phenomenon from post-chemotherapy cystic teratoma as an explanation for presurgical serum AFP elevation. Although the explanation remains unclear, teratoma or fibrosis is identified in the surgical specimen in up to half the cases at surgery, and as we will see later in this article, carries an improved overall prognosis. In the Indiana series, cerebral metastases were identified early postoperatively in three patients felt to harbor only fibrosis. All three patients died of progressive cancer underscoring the importance of an extensive metastatic evaluation.

Survival

Published studies evaluating the therapeutic benefit of post-chemotherapy surgery in patients with elevated serum tumor markers have reported survival rates ranging from 33% to 75% [4,5,8–11]. Ravi and colleagues [11] reported a disease-free survival in 17 (57%) of 30 marker-positive patients at a median follow-up of 57 months (range: 2 to 150). Most of these studies have reported more favorable outcomes in patients with an elevated serum AFP (as opposed to βHCG), and stable serum tumor markers at time of surgery [5,9,10].

In the Indiana experience, the 5-year overall survival for the 114 patients (50 patients receiving first-line, and 64 receiving second-line chemotherapy, respectively, before surgery) was 53.9% (Fig. 1A). Sixty-one patients (53.5%) are alive and the median follow-up time for survivors was 72 months (range: 24 to 168). All patients alive had a minimum follow-up of 2 years. Fifty-three patients died of disease with a median time to death of 8.0 months (range: 1 to 84). Survival distribution based on serum marker elevation and retroperitoneal pathology is seen in Fig. 1B, C, respectively. The 5-year overall survival based on pathology was 31.4%, 77.5%, and 85.7% for germ-cell cancer, teratoma, and fibrosis, respectively (P = .0001). The 5-year overall survival for the primary chemotherapy group was 81.1%.

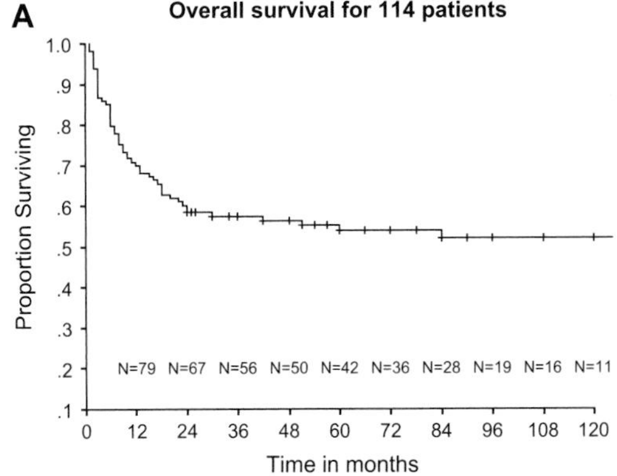

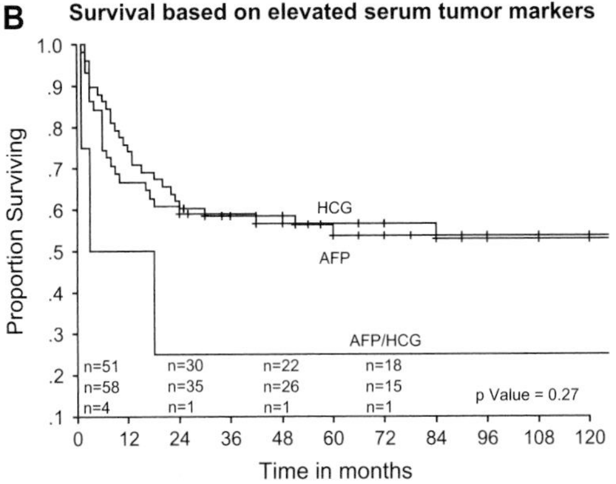

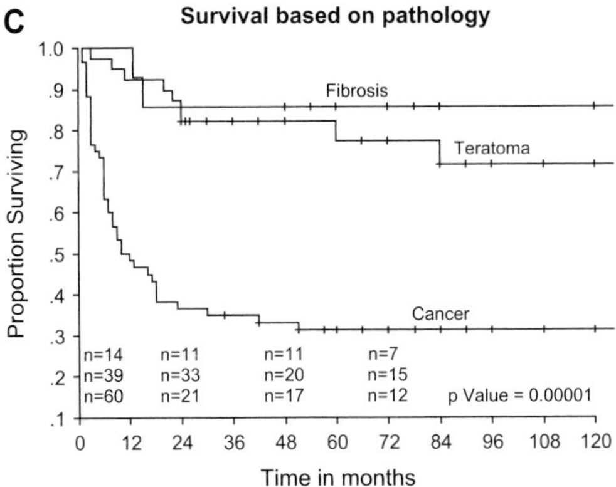

Fig. 1. (*A*) Overall survival for the 114 patients in the study cohort. The majority of patients who relapsed and died did so by 24 months. (*B*) Overall survival for the 114 patients based on serum tumor marker elevation. There was no difference in survival for the 51 patients with an elevated HCG and the 58 patients with an elevated AFP. Only four patients had elevation of both serum tumor markers. (*C*) Overall survival categorized by retroperitoneal pathology. The 5-year overall survival was 31.4%, 77.5%, and 85.7% for germ-cell cancer, teratoma, and fibrosis, respectively ($P = .0001$).

The median survival time for the 64 patients in the salvage group was 15 months (95% confidence interval, 9.0 to 21 months) with a 5-year overall survival of 33.3% ($P = .0001$).

Univariate survival analysis—Indiana experience

In the cohort of 114 patients, 18 variables were subjected to univariate analysis for prognostic significance (Table 2). The following factors were associated with an adverse prognosis: presurgery serum βHCG and AFP levels as both continuous and categorical variables, serum tumor marker status (rising versus declining) before surgery, history of marker normalization, first-line versus salvage chemotherapy, redo RPLND, retroperitoneal pathology, and unresectable disease. Number of sites of disease and adjuvant chemotherapy did not influence survival on univariate analysis.

Multivariable survival analysis—Indiana experience

Eight factors significant on univariate analysis were entered into the multivariate regression analysis using the Cox proportional hazards model. Serum AFP higher than 1000 (five patients), βHCG higher than 1000 (four patients), and unresectable disease (three patients) were excluded from multivariable analysis because of small numbers. Four variables were determined to have independent prognostic significance for survival in the Cox model: βHCG status (rising versus declining or plateau), serum AFP level (continuous variable), redo RPLND, and germ-cell cancer in the surgical specimen (Table 3).

In subset analysis, retroperitoneal pathology, with a 5-year overall survival of 36.9%, 96.5%, and 100% for germ-cell cancer, teratoma, and fibrosis, respectively ($P = .00001$), was the single predictor of outcome on multivariable analysis for the 50 patients in the induction group. Significant variables predictive of outcome for the 64 patients in the salvage group are listed in Table 3. Pathology was not predictive of outcome in this group with no statistical difference in 5-year survival (29.6%, 40.4%, and 50%) for germ-cell cancer, teratoma, and fibrosis, respectively ($P = .20$).

Prognostic variables

The collective literature has demonstrated a therapeutic benefit of post-chemotherapy

Table 2
Results of univariate analysis

	No. of patients	No. of events	5-Year survival, %	Survival, (mo) Median	95% CI	P value
Continuous variables						
Initial HCG	43	12	—	—	—	.110
Initial AFP	53	23	—	—	—	.700
Presurgery HCG	55	26	—	—	—	.002
Presurgery AFP	59	26	—	—	—	.018
Categorical variables						
Presurgery HCG						
<100	42	16	64.0	—	—	.003
>100	13	10	23.0	7	2.0–12.0	—
<1000	51	22	58.6	—	—	.01
>1000	4	4	0.0	3	0.0–20.0	—
Presurgery AFP						
>100	30	10	65.0	—	—	.044
>100	32	19	40.0	22	0.0–46.0	—
<1000	57	24	56.6	—	—	.0019
>1000	5	5	0.0	11	9.0–13.0	—
Presurgery HCG status						.0001
Declining	15	1	93.3	—	—	—
Plateau	18	8	60.0	84	—	—
Rising	22	17	22.7	6	0.0–12.0	—
Presurgery AFP status						.0103
Declining	7	1	85.7	—	—	—
Plateau	11	2	81.8	—	—	—
Rising	44	26	38.7	23	0.0–55.0	—
Serum tumor marker						.272
AFP	58	26	53.7	—	—	—
HCG	51	23	56.6	—	—	—
AFP/HCG	4	3	25.0	3	0.0–20.0	—
Sites of disease						.999
1	74	34	54.8	—	—	—
2	31	14	53.0	—	—	—
3	8	4	50.0	22	—	—
Redo RPLND						<.0001
No	90	33	63.9	—	—	—
Yes	23	19	16.3	9	7.0–11.0	—

Abbreviations: AFP, alpha-fetoprotein; HCG, human chorionic gonadotropin; RPLND, retroperitoneal lymph node dissection; —, unknown.

surgery in patients with elevated serum tumor markers. The 5-year overall survival in select patients undergoing surgery was 55%. Despite elevated serum tumor markers, only 50% of patients harbored germ-cell cancer, of whom one third had a long-term survival with no observed benefit from adjuvant chemotherapy. Risk factors negatively associated with survival included a rising preoperative serum βHCG, an elevated serum AFP (continuous variable), redo RPLND, and germ-cell cancer in the surgical specimen.

Germ-cell cancer in the Indiana series was present in 61 (53.5%) of 114 patients with elevated serum tumor markers undergoing post-chemotherapy surgery. Active germ-cell cancer in the retroperitoneum increased risk of death by 2.5-fold; however, surgery provided a cure for a third of these patients at 5 years with no observed benefit from adjuvant chemotherapy. Even in the presence of poor prognostic clinical and pathologic features, including elevated serum tumor markers and germ-cell cancer in the surgical specimen, RPLND remains a treatment option in this population because of its therapeutic benefit.

In the management of residual retroperitoneal disease after chemotherapy, incomplete initial surgical resection necessitating "redo" surgery portends a poor prognosis. Donohue and colleagues

Table 3
Results of multivariable analysis

	Relative risk (95% CI)	*P* value
Entire cohort		
AFP (continuous)	1.0 (1.0–1.0)	.048
HCG (continuous)	1.0 (1.0–1.0)	.546
AFP status[a]	0.49 (0.89–2.7)	.413
HCG status[a]	5.06 (1.36–18.8)	.015
Preoperative HCG>100	1.077 (0.43–2.67)	.872
Redo RPLND	2.86 (1.49–5.47)	.001
Cancer versus teratoma/fibrosis	2.65 (1.25–5.58)	.011
Induction versus salvage	0.722 (0.31–1.66)	.445
Chemotherapy	—	—
History of marker normalization	1.74 (0.68–4.46)	.247
Induction group		
AFP (continuous)	1.0 (0.998–1.003)	.852
History of marker normalization	1.62 (0.294–8.96)	.579
Adjuvant chemotherapy	0.42 (0.93–1.88)	.258
Cancer versus teratoma/fibrosis	23.1 (3.38–157.9)	.001
Salvage group		
HCG (continuous)	1.0 (1.0–1.0)	.436
HCG versus AFP	2.88 (1.2–6.76)	.015
AFP status[a]	2.04 (0.537–7.74)	.295
HCG status[a]	5.49 (1.46–20.5)	.011
Redo RPLND	3.63 (1.77–7.43)	.001
Cancer versus teratoma/fibrosis	1.84 (0.824–4.12)	.137

Abbreviations: AFP, alpha-fetoprotein; HCG, human chorionic gonadotropin; RPLND, retroperitoneal lymph node dissection; —, unknown.

[a] Marker status reflects statistics for rising markers versus plateau/declining.

[12] reported a 63% (118/188) survival for patients undergoing "redo" PCRPLND versus 86% (529/613) for initial PCRPLND. Likewise, in a contemporary series, Memorial Sloan-Kettering reported a 67% 5-year disease-specific survival for 57 patients undergoing redo surgery [13]. In the Indiana series of patients with elevated serum tumor markers before surgery, 23 patients underwent a "redo" PCRPLND with a 5-year overall survival of 16% compared with 64% for the 90 patients undergoing initial post-chemotherapy surgery (P = .0001). Redo RPLND, probably the only prognostic variable not absolutely dictated by the biological aggressiveness of the disease, largely reflects prior inadequate retroperitoneal technique, underscoring the importance of complete surgical resection at initial RPLND.

Role of adjuvant chemotherapy

Postoperative chemotherapy appears to improve disease-free recurrence in patients with germ-cell cancer after first-line chemotherapy but not when given after second-line chemotherapy [2]. This lack of benefit in the salvage setting is thought to be secondary to the development of tumor chemoresistance. Persistently elevated serum tumor markers after systemic therapy implies a degree of chemoresistance and in the current series adjuvant chemotherapy did not improve patient survival. In the Albers series of 30 patients with elevated serum tumor markers undergoing surgery, only 6 of the 18 patients with viable cancer in the residual tumor specimen received postoperative chemotherapy, of whom 4 have remained free of disease, 1 died of disease, and 1 has progressive disease [4]. The Royal London Hospital, in their series of 30 patients, cautioned that in "... managing these patients do not continue indefinitely with chemotherapy in the face of persistently elevated markers and remember that surgery has a cure rate in its own right" [11]. In the Indiana cohort, the 5-year overall survival for patients with germ-cell cancer receiving (18 patients) and not receiving (42 patients) adjuvant chemotherapy was 44.4% and 25.7%, respectively (P = .067). Administration of adjuvant chemotherapy to patients in the first-line subset must be individualized. Patients with declining markers (resembling patients undergoing standard PCRPLND) are not platinum refractory and we would recommend two courses of adjuvant etoposide and cisplatin. Patients with rising serum tumor markers during or after chemotherapy should be considered platinum refractory and we would not recommend postoperative chemotherapy.

Patient selection

An initial tenet in the management of testicular cancer was the exclusion of surgery for patients with elevated serum tumor markers, with chemotherapy the preferred treatment. This dogma has held true in the management of clinical stage Is disease (elevated serum tumors markers with no radiographic evidence of metastatic disease) [14,15] as well as for the vast majority of patients with marker elevation after chemotherapy. However, there are sufficient data demonstrating a clear therapeutic benefit of surgery in this population proving that even when chemorefractory, and despite elevated serum tumor markers, not all disease is systemic and, moreover, can be cured with aggressive surgery. This being stated, it is with strict selection, identifying disease likely chemorefractory and likely not systemic, that enables surgery to be potentially curative in this uncommon clinical setting. As general guidelines, selection to proceed with surgery include (1) declining or plateau serum tumor markers after chemotherapy, (2) slowly rising markers after an initial complete response to either first- or second-line chemotherapy, (3) radiographic resectable residual disease in one or two sites, and (4) rising markers with resectable disease after exhausting all chemotherapeutic agents.

A more difficult population is the patient with *rising* serum tumor markers during or within 4 weeks of receiving platinum-based chemotherapy. These patients are platinum refractory and should be considered candidates for either high-dose chemotherapy with stem-cell transplantation or surgery. The philosophy at Indiana would be to proceed with surgery (coined "desperation surgery," as this population with rising markers are chemorefractory and will harbor active disease) if the residual disease is surgically resectable in one or two anatomic sites. The rationale for surgery in this clinical setting is threefold. One, the patient may be cured with surgery alone avoiding the morbidity of high-dose chemotherapy. Second, if progression does occur after surgery, high-dose chemotherapy may still be administered in hopes for cure. However, third, if high-dose chemotherapy is administered initially and the patient progresses and is now unresectable, the opportunity of cure with surgery is lost. The outcome of these patients with *rising* serum tumor markers undergoing *desperation* surgery is currently being evaluated at our institution.

Summary

Approximately 50% of patients undergoing post-chemotherapy surgery with elevated serum tumor markers are alive at 5 years. Half of these patients are found to harbor residual viable nonteratomatous germ-cell tumor with a third alive at 5 years with no observed benefit from adjuvant chemotherapy. These studies demonstrate that a subset of patients with elevated serum tumor markers after chemotherapy are curable with surgery. The decision to proceed with surgery in lieu of second- or third-line chemotherapy includes identifying both patients felt unlikely to obtain a complete response with systemic therapy (and thus require surgery), and patients with resectable tumors that are potentially curable with surgery. Identifying prognostic variables predictive of outcome at surgery including a rising preoperative βHCG, elevated AFP (continuous variable), redo RPLND, and germ-cell cancer in the surgical specimen along with clinical and surgical experience should aid in determining the appropriate integration of surgery and chemotherapy in this population.

References

[1] Steyerberg EW, Keizer HJ, Fossa SD, et al. Prediction of residual retroperitoneal mass histology after chemotherapy for metastatic nonseminomatous germ cell tumor: multivariate analysis of individual patient data from six study groups. J Clin Oncol 1995; 13(5):1177–87.

[2] Fox EP, Weathers TD, Williams SD, et al. Outcome analysis for patients with persistent nonteratomatous germ cell tumor in postchemotherapy retroperitoneal lymph node dissections. J Clin Oncol 1993; 11(7):1294–9.

[3] Beck SD, Foster RS, Bihrle R, et al. Outcome analysis for patients with elevated serum tumor markers at postchemotherapy retroperitoneal lymph node dissection. J Clin Oncol 2005;23(25): 6149–56.

[4] Albers P, Ganz A, Hannig E, et al. Salvage surgery of chemorefractory germ cell tumors with elevated tumor markers. J Urol 2000;164(2):381–4.

[5] Wood DP Jr, Herr HW, Motzer RJ, et al. Surgical resection of solitary metastases after chemotherapy in patients with nonseminomatous germ cell tumors and elevated serum tumor markers. Cancer 1992; 70(9):2354–7.

[6] van der Gaast A, Hoekstra JW, Croles JJ, et al. Elevated serum tumor markers in patients with testicular cancer after induction chemotherapy due to a reservoir of markers in cystic differentiated mature teratoma. J Urol 1991;145(4):829–31.

[7] Beck SD, Patel MI, Sheinfeld J. Tumor marker levels in post-chemotherapy cystic masses: clinical implications for patients with germ cell tumors. J Urol 2004; 171(1):168–71.

[8] Eastham JA, Wilson TG, Russell C, et al. Surgical resection in patients with nonseminomatous germ cell tumor who fail to normalize serum tumor markers after chemotherapy. Urology 1994;43(1):74–80.

[9] Coogan CL, Foster RS, Rowland RG, et al. Postchemotherapy retroperitoneal lymph node dissection is effective therapy in selected patients with elevated tumor markers after primary chemotherapy alone. Urology 1997;50(6):957–62.

[10] Murphy BR, Breeden ES, Donohue JP, et al. Surgical salvage of chemorefractory germ cell tumors. J Clin Oncol 1993;11(2):324–9.

[11] Ravi R, Ong J, Oliver RT, et al. Surgery as salvage therapy in chemotherapy-resistant nonseminomatous germ cell tumours. Br J Urol 1998;81(6):884–8.

[12] Donohue JP, Leviovitch I, Foster RS, et al. Integration of surgery and systemic therapy: results and principles of integration. Semin Urol Oncol 1998;16(2):65–71.

[13] McKiernan JM, Motzer RJ, Bajorin DF, et al. Reoperative retroperitoneal surgery for nonseminomatous germ cell tumor: clinical presentation, patterns of recurrence, and outcome. Urology 2003;62(4):732–6.

[14] Davis BE, Herr HW, Fair WR, et al. The management of patients with nonseminomatous germ cell tumors of the testis with serologic disease only after orchiectomy. J Urol 1994;152(1):111–3 [discussion: 114].

[15] Saxman SB, Nichols CR, Foster RS, et al. The management of patients with clinical stage I nonseminomatous testicular tumors and persistently elevated serologic markers. J Urol 1996;155(2):587–9.

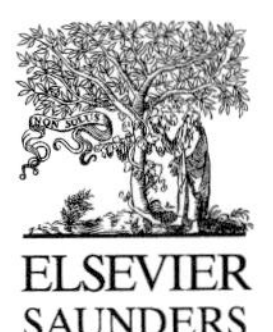

ELSEVIER
SAUNDERS

Urol Clin N Am 34 (2007) 227–233

UROLOGIC CLINICS of North America

Reoperative Retroperitoneal Surgery

Joel Sheinfeld, MD[a,b,*], Pramod Sogani, MD, FACS[a,b]

[a]*Department of Urology, Sidney Kimmel Center for Prostate and Urologic Cancers, Memorial Sloan-Kettering Cancer Center, 353 East 68th Street, New York, NY 10021, USA*

[b]*Department of Urology, Weill College of Medicine, 525 East 68th Street, New York, NY 10021, USA*

The management of patients with testicular cancer has evolved significantly over the past 25 years, largely as a result of the ability of cisplatin-based chemotherapy to cure advanced disease [1]. The appropriate integration of systemic chemotherapy and surgery has resulted in overall survival rates greater than 90% for patients with testicular cancer [2].

Retroperitoneal lymph node dissection (RPLND) remains a critical component in the management of germ-cell tumor (GCT) in both the primary and post-chemotherapy setting; and when properly performed, is a therapeutic procedure and not limited to diagnosis and staging [3,4]. Unfortunately, some patients will relapse in the retroperitoneum after RPLND and require reoperative retroperitoneal surgery. Emerging data on patients suffering late relapse and/or requiring reoperative retroperitoneal surgery clearly indicate that the liberal use of effective cisplatin-based chemotherapy will not compensate for inadequate initial surgery [3,5,6]. Therefore, surgical margins and templates should not be compromised in an attempt to preserve ejaculation. Complete surgical resection of metastatic retroperitoneal disease has been shown to be a significant and independent variable in relapse-free survival for patients with both low-stage and advanced nonseminomatous germ-cell tumor (NSGCT) [3,7].

This article will describe the clinical presentation, disease sites, histologic findings, and postoperative morbidity for patients undergoing reoperative retroperitoneal surgery. In addition, the clinical outcome and possible etiologies for retroperitoneal recurrences are discussed.

Testicular tumors and patterns of metastasis

One feature of testis GCTs that has significantly affected its successful management is the predictable and systematic pattern of metastatic spread from the primary site to the retroperitoneal lymph nodes and subsequently to the lung and posterior mediastinum [8,9]. Lymphatic spread is common to all histologic subtypes of GCT, although choriocarcinoma often metastasizes hematogenously [9]. Anatomic studies in the early 1900s identified the primary lymphatic drainage of the testis to the area of its embryologic origin, the retroperitoneal lymph nodes adjacent to the aorta and inferior vena cava [8]. The primary "landing zone" for the right-sided testicular tumors includes the interaortocaval region, followed by the precaval and preaortic nodes, while that for left-sided tumors is the para-aortic and preaortic nodes [8,10–12]. Furthermore, multiple mapping studies have clearly shown that multifocality and contralateral spread increase with pathologic stage, particularly with right-sided tumors, and that more caudal deposits of metastatic disease to distal iliac, pelvic, and inguinal nodes usually reflects retrograde spread secondary to bulky retroperitoneal disease [9–12].

Retroperitoneal lymph node dissection

There are several reasons to treat the retroperitoneal lymph node in patients with testicular

* Corresponding author. Department of Urology, Sidney Kimmel Center for Prostate and Urologic Cancers, Memorial Sloan-Kettering Cancer Center, 353 East 68th Street, New York, NY 10021.

E-mail address: sheinfej@mskcc.org (J. Sheinfeld).

doi:10.1016/j.ucl.2007.02.008

urologic.theclinics.com

cancer. First, based on the results of RPLND and surveillance series, the retroperitoneum is the initial and often only site of metastatic spread in up to 90% of patents with GCT [9,13]. Second, accurate clinical staging of the retroperitoneum continues to have an approximately 30% error rate despite improved radiographic imaging [9]. Third, untreated retroperitoneal lymph node metastases are usually fatal [8,13]. In autopsy studies of patients who died of GCT, metastases of brain, bone, and liver were late events and usually associated with bulky retroperitoneal disease [8,14,15]. Furthermore, the retroperitoneum is the most common site for late relapse of both teratoma and viable GCT [6,16,17].

RPLND has been well established in the management of NSGCT since 1948; however, its role and the surgical templates and techniques have undergone considerable change over the past 30 years [8]. Initially, RPLND included all the nodal tissue between both ureters down to the bifurcation of the common iliac arteries and as well as both suprahilar regions. In the pre-cisplatin era very extensive dissection of all lymph nodes was necessary given the absence of effective alternative therapy [8]; however, extensive suprahilar dissection can result in increased renovascular and pancreatic complications as well as increased incidence of chylous ascites [8]. In an effort to reduce surgical morbidity, the original suprahilar dissections were replaced by the bilateral infrahilar RPLND.

Historically, bilateral infrahilar RPLND was associated with the loss of antegrade ejaculation because of damage to the paravertebral sympathetic ganglia, postganglionic sympathetic fibers, and/or the hypogastric plexus [8]. The incidence of retrograde ejaculation is related to the extent of the retroperitoneal dissection [8,18,19].

In an effort to preserve antegrade ejaculation, a number of side-specific modified templates have been proposed, variably limiting contralateral dissection, particularly below the level of the inferior mesenteric artery (IMA) [8,20,21]. The highest rates of antegrade ejaculation are reported with "nerve-sparing" techniques in which the sympathetic fibers, hypogastric plexus, and postganglionic sympathetic fibers are prospectively identified, dissected, and preserved [8,18,22].

Retroperitoneal relapse after RPLND

Although tumor recurrence in the retroperitoneum after RPLND is rare, unresected retroperitoneal disease appears to be an underestimated and, consequently, underreported phenomenon. There are several reasons that may explain this apparent discrepancy. First, the use of postoperative cisplatin-based chemotherapy may eliminate occult micrometastatic disease. Second, routine postoperative CT scanning is not routinely performed for follow-up after RPLND, with many centers relying on chest radiographs and serum tumor markers. Third, specifying sites of recurrence, particularly in the retroperitoneum, is often omitted in multiple reports. Finally, a better appreciation and understanding of late relapse suggests that prolonged follow-up will progressively unmask retroperitoneal failures in patients who underwent initial suboptimal RPLND [8,23–25].

With very rare exception, retroperitoneal recurrences after RPLND should always be considered surgical failures, whether they result from a technical error(s) or an inappropriately reduced template [24–26]. Donohue and colleagues [7] stated that "...in many of these cases there was a relative lack of RPLND experience and/or resolve at the time of the initial procedure." Given the demographics of testicular cancer, the "relative lack of RPLND experience" is not surprising. Each year there are approximately 8500 new cases of testicular cancer diagnosed in the United States; and approximately 1200 RPLNDs are performed in over 100 urology residency programs (Residency Review Committee [RRC] 2000–2004). Indiana University and Memorial Sloan-Kettering Cancer Center (MSKCC) each perform over 100 RPLNDs per year and, according to statistics from the RRC of the American Board of Urology [27] for the years 2000 to 2004, urology residents averaged approximately five RPLNDs during their 4-year program (Table 1). These data are pertinent as there is emerging and compelling evidence from the urologic and general surgery literature that increased surgical volume

Table 1
Residency Review Committee. RPLND statistics for urology programs (2000–2004)

Year	Programs, n	Residents, n	RPLND, n
2000	106	229	1129
2001	106	232	1193
2002	104	223	1077
2003	109	234	1253
2004	108	229	1294

correlates with improved clinical outcome for many complex procedures [28–30].

Modified templates and retroperitoneal mapping studies

In 1988 Jewett and Torbey [31] stated that "all modified dissections introduce a risk of incomplete resection of involved nodes." In general, ipsilateral lymph nodes are resected between the level of the renal vessels and the bifurcation of the common iliac artery, contralateral dissection is limited or omitted, and interartocaval nodes are variably resected for left-sided primary tumors [8]. All modified RPLND templates limit dissection in anatomic regions felt to be at reduced risk for metastatic disease based on anatomic mapping studies of retroperitoneal metastases by Ray and colleagues, Donohue and colleagues, and Weissbach and Boedefeld [10–12]. Unfortunately, the mapping studies have significant limitations that may have also contributed to underestimating the extent of retroperitoneal metastasis. First, the mapping studies lack adequate postoperative follow-up; therefore, the rate of extratemplate recurrence is unknown [10–12]. Without clinical follow-up, sample error by the surgeon and/or pathologist cannot be assessed. There was no follow-up reported in the studies by Ray and colleagues [10] or Donohue and colleagues [11]. Weissbach and Boedefeld [12] reported a median follow-up of only 22 months for node-negative patients and noted three retroperitoneal relapses. Second, the Weissbach study was a multicenter study involving 46 centers and 50 surgeons introducing significant surgical variability [12]. Third, as stated previously, it is not possible to accurately assess additional potential sites of metastasis in patients who received postoperative chemotherapy. All patients with pathologic stage II B disease in the Weissbach study participated in a randomized adjuvant chemotherapy trial and received either two or four cycles of PVB (cisplatin, vinblastine, bleomycin) [12]. Fourth, although uncommon, the potential impact that renal and renovascular anatomic variants may have on testicular lymphovascular drainage is not described. Furthermore, the variable insertion of the right gonadal vein(s) at various levels of the inferior vena cava (IVC) and/or right renal vein as well as additional branches to the pelvis and Gerota's fascia may influence potential sites of metastatic disease. Chang and colleagues [32] demonstrated that 5% of patients with retroperitoneal disease harbor disease in the spermatic cord specimen, either within the vessel or in the adjacent tissue, and that incomplete resection may result in paracolic recurrence.

Recently, Eggener and colleagues [20] evaluated 500 patients with CS I-IIA NSGCT who underwent primary RPLND at MSKCC and analyzed the incidence of extratemplate disease for five modified RPLND templates (Weissbach, MSKCC, Indiana, JHU, Innsbruck) in the 191 patients with positive nodes. Depending on the template, overall extratemplate disease ranged from 3% to 23%, including 1% to 11% for patients with low-volume retroperitoneal disease. The histologic distribution of extratemplate disease was not significantly different from in-template disease [20]. For right-sided modified templates, the most common sites of extratemplate disease were the para-aortic nodes (Weissbach, Indiana, Innsbruck, and JHU templates) and preaortic nodes (JHU) [20]. In 2002, Leibovich and colleagues [33] reported that 28 (5%) of 607 patients with right-sided NSGCT who underwent RPLND at Indiana University had positive nodes only in the preaortic or para-aortic region.

For left-sided modified templates that excluded the interaortocaval region, disease would have been unresected in 23 (88%) of 26 patients [20].

A similar analysis by Carver and colleagues [34] of 532 patients with advanced NSGCT who underwent post-chemotherapy RPLND (PC-RPLND) at MSKCC showed a significant number of patients with extratemplate disease. Of 269 patients with viable GCT or teratoma in the retroperitoneal specimen, 7% to 32% had evidence of extra template disease, depending on the limits of the modified template. Again, there was no difference in the histologic distribution of extratemplate disease compared with in-template disease [34].

The most common site(s) of recurrent or residual mass prompting reoperation following either 1° RPLND or PC- RPLND for both right- and left-sided tumors are the left para-aortic area and the left hilar region. In the MSKCC series [3], 34 (53%) of 64 retroperitoneal masses resected at reoperation involved recurrences in the left para-aortic and/or hilar region. Similarly, three (50%) of six retroperitoneal recurrences reported by Cespedes and Peretsman [23] occurred in the left perihilar area. There are two reasons for this. First, as previously noted, this region is excluded in many modified templates for right-sided primary tumors [3,20,34]. Second, there are increased technical demands required to obtain adequate exposure to be able to meticulously dissect the left renal vessels and completely resect the lymph nodes in this area. The technical aspects of adequate exposure, pancreatic mobilization, vascular control, and adequate dissection are beyond the scope of this article and are described elsewhere [3,8].

Clinical implications of incomplete surgical resection

Several investigators have clearly and consistently shown the prognostic significance of complete resection of retroperitoneal disease [3,7]. Stenning and colleagues [35] reported that the risk of disease progression for patients *without* complete resection of all residual masses was approximately four times the risk for those with complete resection [35,36].

Data from Indiana University and more recently, MSKCC, clearly show that patients requiring reoperative retroperitoneal surgery are significantly compromised regardless of other risk factors [3,7]. Donohue and colleagues [7] reported that the relapse rates for primary versus redo post-chemotherapy surgery were 20.6% and 51.6%, respectively. Furthermore, the survival rates decrease from 84% in the primary PC-RPLND group to 55% in the redo group. McKiernan and colleagues [3] reported a 56% disease-specific survival for patients requiring reoperation compared with 90% for those undergoing initial PC-RPLND (Fig. 1) [3].

Survival is also compromised in patients requiring reoperative retroperitoneal surgery following initial primary RPLND. In the MSKCC series, 5-year survival dropped from 99.3% to 86.0% for 22 patients requiring redo-RPLND [3]. Of note 20 (90%) of the 22 patients had received cisplatin-based chemotherapy between the first and second operation, including three or four cycles of induction cisplatin-based chemotherapy because of incomplete resection. This underscores the fact that effective cisplatin-based chemotherapy will not compensate for inadequate surgery.

The findings of multiple series underscore the need for meticulous and complete resection of teratomatous elements to avoid local recurrence and possible malignant transformation. McKiernan and colleagues [3] reported that 10 (45%) of 22 patients undergoing primary RPLND and 20 (59%) of 34 patients undergoing PC-RPLND had teratomatous elements present at the initial RPLND before retroperitoneal recurrence. Teratoma is the most common histologic finding in the reoperative setting following both primary RPLND and PC-RPLND, suggesting that incompletely resected teratoma is a lifelong risk factor for redo surgery. Although teratoma is histologically benign, its biologic and clinical potential is unpredictable. Incompletely resected teratoma may grow, obstruct, or invade local structures. Furthermore, they may undergo malignant transformation with development of non-germ cell elements like sarcoma or carcinoma [8].

Unresected teratoma may result in late relapse [8,24,37]. Holzik and colleagues [38] reported two patients who died from progressive malignant transformation of teratoma after suffering late relapse in the retroperitoneum following prior resection of mature teratoma. Loehrer and associates [37] noted that 10 (19%) of 51 patients with teratoma developed late recurrence. Most recurrences developed locally implying incomplete resection and a significant proportion had undergone malignant transformation [8]. McKiernan and colleagues [3] reported only a 20% survival rate in patients whose reoperative retroperitoneal specimen was teratoma with malignant transformation (TMT).

In the reoperative setting, the most significant factors that affect survival are serum tumor marker status at reoperation, histologic findings at surgery, and completeness of resection [3,39,40]. McKiernan and colleagues [3] reported a 52% 2-year survival in 10 patients who underwent reoperative surgery with elevated markers compared with 80% with normal markers. The disease-specific survival rate for patients with resected teratoma or fibrosis was 80% that dropped to 44% and 20%, respectively, if viable GCT or TMT was found [3].

Morbidity of reoperative surgery

Reoperative retroperitoneal surgery can be a technically demanding procedure because of extensive adhesions and significant desmoplastic reaction secondary to prior surgery and chemotherapy, and extravasated blood and/or lymphatic fluid. In 1993, Waples and Messing [41] described nine patients undergoing extensive reoperative retroperitoneal surgery and reported a mean anesthetic time of 9.5 hours and mean blood loss of 6.3 L. Perioperative complications occurred in five (56%) patients and included common bile duct injury requiring pancreatic jejunostomy,

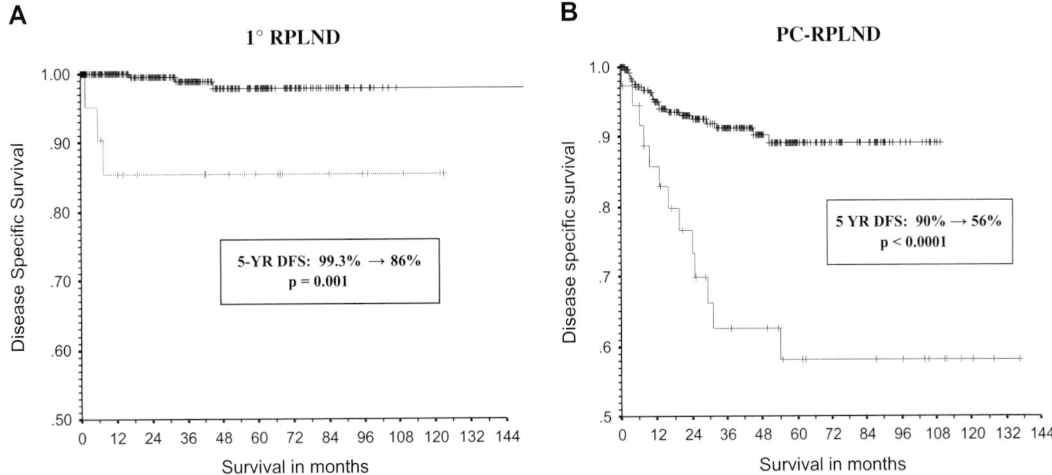

Fig. 1. Adverse impact of redo-RPLND. Disease-specific survival for patients undergoing reoperative retroperitoneal surgery following primary RPLND (*A*) and PC-RPLND (*B*). (*Data from* McKiernan JM, Motzer RJ, Bajorin DF, et al. Reoperative RPLND for germ-cell tumor: clinical presentation, patterns of recurrence, and outcome. Urology 2003;62:732.)

chylous ascites requiring peritoneovenous shunting, and aortic injury resulting in lower-extremity amputation. Sexton and colleagues [42] recently reported the M.D. Anderson experience of 21 patients who underwent repeat RPLND and noted a 29% and 48% intraoperative and postoperative complication rate, respectively. Dissecting in an aortic subadventitial plane was reported in two cases, one requiring aortic grafting [42]. Postoperatively, the most common complications were prolonged ileus and/or partial small-bowel obstruction, and chylous ascites. There was one postoperative death attributable to a pulmonary embolus [42].

In 2003, McKiernan [3] reported the reoperative retroperitoneal surgery experience from MSKCC and noted an overall 27% complication rate, not significantly different from the Indiana experience reported by Bainel (21%) for PC-RPLND without reoperation [3,43]. There was one death attributable to pulmonary embolus. The most common complications in this series of 61 reoperations were lymphocele [4], ileus [3], wound infection [2], small bowel obstruction (SBO) [2], ureteral injury [2] and renal infarction [1,3].

The data suggest that reoperative retroperitoneal surgery can be performed with acceptable morbidity in dedicated tertiary centers with experienced surgeons [3,7,8,42]. Careful preoperative planning, excellent exposure, and strict adherence to basic surgical principles are critical to minimize perioperative morbidity [8]. Achieving a complete resection is critical to avoid a repeat local recurrence and optimize the clinical outcome; sacrificing adjacent organs (kidney, bowel, spleen) or graft replacement of a great vessel may be necessary [8,44]. It is important to rule out occult systemic disease to minimize risk of extraretroperitoneal relapse.

Summary

Although RPLND is both a diagnostic and therapeutic procedure, it must always be performed with therapeutic intent. An uncontrolled retroperitoneum can result in late relapse, reoperative surgery, and compromised clinical outcome.

Incomplete resection of metastatic retroperitoneal disease has been shown to be a significant and independent adverse prognostic variable for patients with NSGCT. A substantial proportion of patients undergoing primary RPLND and PC-RPLND will have unresected extratemplate disease if modified templates are used. Therefore, surgical margins and templates should not be compromised in an attempt to preserve ejaculation. With prospective nerve-sparing techniques preserving antegrade ejaculation in the majority of patients, the argument and need for modified templates is less compelling.

It has become apparent that the anatomic mapping studies, which provided the basis for modified templates, have significant limitations. The left para-aortic region is the most frequent site for surgical failure after RPLND. Teratomatous elements are commonly found in the retroperitoneum of patients undergoing reoperative surgery. Effective cisplatin-based chemotherapy will not reliably compensate for inadequate initial surgery. Reoperative surgery can be performed with acceptable morbidity in tertiary centers with experienced surgeons. The proper integration of reoperative surgery and chemotherapy can salvage almost 70% of patients with retroperitoneal relapse after initial suboptimal RPLND.

Acknowledgment

This work is supported by the Craig Tifford Foundation and the Fred S. Strauss Fund.

The authors gratefully acknowledge the expert assistance of Asha D. Mathew.

References

[1] Sheinfeld J. Treatment of patients with testis cancer: introduction. Urol Oncol 2005;23:222.

[2] Sheinfeld J. The role of adjuvant post-chemotherapy surgery for nonseminomatous germ cell tumors: current concepts and controversies. Semin Urol Oncol 2002;20:262–71.

[3] McKiernan JM, Motzer RJ, Bajorin DF, et al. Reoperative RPLND for germ cell tumor: clinical presentation, patterns of recurrence, and outcome. Urology 2003;62:732–6.

[4] Carver BS, Sheinfeld J. Therapeutic efficacy of laparoscopic RPLND: unproved and untested. Am J Urol Rev 2004;2:427–31.

[5] Baniel J, Foster RS, Einhorn LH, et al. Late relapse of clinical stage I testicular cancer. J Urol 1995;154:1370–2.

[6] Baniel J, Foster RS, Gonin R, et al. Late relapse of testicular cancer. J Clin Oncol 1995;13:1170–6.

[7] Donohue JP, Leviovitch I, Foster RS, et al. Integration of surgery and systemic therapy: results and principles of integration. Semin Urol Oncol 1998;16:65–71.

[8] Sheinfeld J, McKiernan J, Bosl GJ. Surgery of testicular tumors. In: Walsh PC, Retik AB, Vaughan ED Jr, et al, editors. Campbell's urology. Philadelphia: WB Saunders; 2000. p. 2920–44.

[9] Stephenson AJ, Sheinfeld J. The role of retroperitoneal lymph node dissection in the management of testicular cancer. Urol Oncol 2004;22:225–35.

[10] Ray B, Hajdu SI, Whitmore WF Jr. Proceedings: Distribution of retroperitoneal lymph node metastases in testicular germinal tumors. Cancer 1974;33:340–8.

[11] Donohue JP, Zachary JM, Maynard BR. Distribution of nodal metastases in nonseminomatous testis cancer. J Urol 1982;128:315–20.

[12] Weissbach L, Boedefeld EA. Localization of solitary and multiple metastases in stage II nonseminomatous testis tumor as basis for a modified staging lymph node dissection in stage I. J Urol 1987;138:77–82.

[13] Whitmore WF Jr. Surgical treatment of adult germinal testis tumors. Semin Oncol 1979;6:55–68.

[14] Johnson DE, Appelt G, Samuels ML, et al. Metastases from testicular carcinoma. Study of 78 autopsied cases. Urology 1976;8:234–9.

[15] Bredael JJ, Vugrin D, Whitmore WF Jr. Autopsy findings in 154 patients with germ cell tumors of the testis. Cancer 1982;50:548–51.

[16] George DW, Foster RS, Hromas RA, et al. Update on late relapse of germ cell tumors: a clinical and molecular analysis. J Clin Oncol 2003;21:113–22.

[17] Sharp DS, Carver BS, Eggener SE, et al. Clinical outcome of patients managed for late relapse of germ cell tumor. Proc ASCO 2006;24:4550.

[18] Jewett MA, Kong YS, Goldberg SD, et al. Retroperitoneal lymphadenectomy for testis tumor with nerve sparing for ejaculation. J Urol 1988;139:1220–4.

[19] Lange PH, Narayan P, Fraley EE. Fertility issues following therapy for testicular cancer. Semin Urol 1984;2:264–74.

[20] Eggener SE, Carver BS, Parekh DJ, et al. Incidence and predictors of disease outside a modified retroperitoneal lymph node dissection template in clinical stage (CS) I-IIA nonseminomatous germ cell testicular cancer. J Urol 2007;177:937–43.

[21] Sheinfeld J, Herr HW. Role of surgery in management of germ cell tumor. Semin Oncol 1998;25:203–9.

[22] Donohue JP, Foster RS, Rowland RG, et al. Nerve-sparing retroperitoneal lymphadenectomy with preservation of ejaculation. J Urol 1990;144:287–91.

[23] Cespedes RD, Peretsman SJ. Retroperitoneal recurrences after retroperitoneal lymph node dissection for low-stage nonseminomatous germ cell tumors. Urology 1999;54:548–52.

[24] Sheinfeld J. Risks of the uncontrolled retroperitoneum [editorial]. Ann Surg Oncol 2003;10:100–1.

[25] Carver BS, Sheinfeld J. Germ cell tumors of the testis. Ann Surg Oncol 2005;12:871–80.

[26] Sheinfeld J. Laparoscopic retroperitoneal lymph node dissection: description of the nerve-sparing technique [editorial]. Urology 2002;60:343.

[27] Statistics. Residency Review Committee (RRC). American Board of Urology 2000–2004.

[28] Ho V, Heslin MJ, Yun H, et al. Trends in hospital and surgeon volume and operative mortality for cancer surgery. Ann Oncol 2006;13:851–8.

[29] Begg CB, Cramer LD, Hoskins WJ, et al. Impact of hospital volume on operative mortality for major cancer surgery. JAMA 1998;280:1747–51.

[30] Konety BR, Dhawan V, Allareddy V, et al. Impact of hospital and surgeon volume on in-hospital mortality for radical cystectomy: data from the Heatlh Care Utilization Project. J Urol 2005;173:2085–9.

[31] Jewett MAS, Torbey C. Nerve sparing techniques in retroperitoneal lymphadenectomy in patients with low stage testicular cancer. Semin Urol 1988; 233–7.

[32] Chang S, Mohseni H, Rabbani F, et al. Paracolic recurrence: the importance of wide excision of spermatic cord at retroperitoneal lymph node dissection (RPLND). J Urol 2002;167:94–6.

[33] Leibovich BS, Foster RS, Mosharafa AA, et al. Unusual sites of metastasis in low stage testis cancer. J Urol 2002;167:683A.

[34] Carver BS, Shayegan B, Motzer RJ, et al. The incidence and implications of disease outside a modified template in men undergoing post-chemotherapy retroperitoneal lymph node dissection (PC-RPLND) for metastatic non-seminomatous germ cell tumor (NSGCT). J Urol 2006;175:593A.

[35] Stenning SP, Parkinson MC, Fisher C, et al. Post-chemotherapy residual masses in germ cell tumor patients. Cancer 1998;83:1409–19.

[36] Sheinfeld J. Commentary on retroperitoneal surgery following induction chemotherapy for advanced NSGCT. Am J Urol Rev 2003;1:267–70.

[37] Loehrer PJ Sr., Hui S, Clark S, et al. Teratoma following cisplatin-based combination chemotherapy for nonseminomatous germ cell tumors: a clinicopathological correlation. J Urol 1986;135:1183–9.

[38] Holzik MF, Hoekstra HJ, Mulder NH, et al. Non-germ cell malignancy in residual or recurrent mass after chemotherapy for nonseminomatous testicular germ cell tumor. Ann Surg Oncol 2003;10:131–5.

[39] Fox EP, Weathers TD, Williams SD, et al. Outcome analysis for patients with persistent nonteratomatous germ cell tumor in photochemotherapy retroperitoneal lymph node dissections. J Clin Oncol 1993;11:1294–9.

[40] Murphy BR, Breeden ES, Donohue JP, et al. Surgical salvage of chemorefractory germ cell tumors. J Clin Oncol 1993;11:324–9.

[41] Waples MJ, Messing EM. Redo retroperitoneal lymphadenectomy for germ cell tumor. Urology 1993; 42:1–4.

[42] Sexton WJ, Wood CG, Kim R, et al. Repeat retroperitoneal lymph node dissection for metastatic testis cancer. J Urol 2003;169:1353–6.

[43] Baniel J, Foster RS, Rowland RG, et al. Complications of post-chemotherapy retroperitoneal lymph node dissection. J Urol 1995;153:976–80.

[44] Nash PA, Leibovitch I, Foster RS, et al. En bloc nephrectomy in patients undergoing post-chemotherapy retroperitoneal lymph node dissection for nonseminomatous testis cancer: indications, implications and outcomes. J Urol 1998;159:707–10.

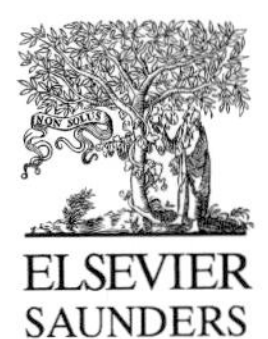

ELSEVIER
SAUNDERS

Urol Clin N Am 34 (2007) 235–243

UROLOGIC
CLINICS
of North America

Management of Non-Retroperitoneal Residual Germ Cell Tumor Masses

Mark H. Katz, MD, James M. McKiernan, MD*

Department of Urology, Columbia University College of Physicians and Surgeons, New York Presbyterian Hospital, Columbia University Medical Center, 161 Fort Washington Avenue, 11th Floor, New York, NY 10032, USA

In the year 2007, approximately 8000 new cases of and 400 deaths attributable to testicular cancer are expected in the United States [1]. The incidence of testicular cancer, the most common cancer in men between the ages of 20 and 35, continues to increase in the United States and Europe [2,3]. Testicular cancer has become a paradigm for the successful multidisciplinary approach to solid tumors. The overall cure rate for testicular cancer is now greater than 90% compared with cure rates of 60% to 65% in the 1960s [4]. Although the management of testicular cancer has yielded dramatic results, the outcomes are highly dependent on appropriate management. Surgery remains an integral component of management, but the implementation of reliable serum tumor markers, improvements in imaging technology, and the refinement in chemotherapeutic strategies have changed its role in the treatment of testicular cancer.

The standard of care for patients who have advanced (stage III/IV) germ cell tumors (GCTs) is cisplatin-based chemotherapy. The integration of surgery after systemic therapy has become an important component of treatment, and has resulted in survival rates of 70% to 80% for advanced GCT [4,5]. Surgical exploration and resection of residual retroperitoneal masses after chemotherapy is generally recommended for patients who have normalized serum tumor markers. The patient's prognosis is related to previous serum tumor marker level, prior treatment burden, and histology of the resected specimen (necrosis, teratoma, or viable GCT). Although variables, such as a residual mass less than 1.5 cm, a greater than 90% reduction in size of the mass after chemotherapy, and the absence of teratoma in the primary tumor, have been used to obviate surgery, there are no standard guidelines for observation versus adjunctive resection [6–8]. Because surgery provides no additional benefit for residual masses composed of necrosis, several investigators have attempted to reliably predict histology in postchemotherapy specimens. Unfortunately, the results of these studies have been conflicting. It seems that no group of criteria can accurately predict necrosis and thus avoid the need for postchemotherapy retroperitoneal lymph node dissection (RPLND).

This article focuses on the management of residual masses outside of the retroperitoneum. Non-retroperitoneal postchemotherapy residual masses are frequently encountered in patients who have advanced GCTs and must be managed by clinicians from various specialties, including urology, general and thoracic surgery, and otolaryngology. Common sites for residual lesions include the thorax (mediastinum and lung), neck, and nonpulmonary visceral organs, such as the liver. Topics addressed in this article include the ability to predict the histology of extra-retroperitoneal residual masses, indications for surgery, survival outcomes, perioperative complications, and management after surgery.

Causes of non-retroperitoneal residual masses

Testicular cancer most frequently metastasizes by way of the lymphatics to the retroperitoneal

* Corresponding author.
E-mail address: jmm23@columbia.edu (J.M. McKiernan).

doi:10.1016/j.ucl.2007.02.004

lymph nodes. Dissemination to more distant sites is not uncommon, however. Up to 35% of patients who have advanced testicular cancer demonstrate residual masses at more than one site after initial chemotherapy [9]. Although hematogenous metastases, particularly with choriocarcinoma, to the lung, liver, bone, or brain may occur, the most common mechanism for spread outside of the retroperitoneum is through contiguous lymphatics to the mediastinum. Although cisplatin-based chemotherapy often suffices for the management of patients who have metastases outside of the retroperitoneum, consolidation surgical resection is frequently necessary. A large, multicenter, retrospective review examined the sites of residual masses after induction chemotherapy for advanced GCT [10]. Some 27%, 15%, 4%, 2%, and 0.5% of patients demonstrated residual disease in the mediastinum, lungs, neck, liver, and brain, respectively. Another study reported that approximately 10% to 20% of cases who had supradiaphragmatic metastases require at least one thoracic surgical procedure for the excision of persistent radiographic abnormalities after chemotherapy [11]. Resection of other sites (eg, liver, bone, and brain) is less common. Hahn and colleagues [12] reported that only 57 of the 2219 patients (2.5%) who underwent postchemotherapy RPLND at the University of Indiana also had hepatic resection of residual disease.

Predicting histology in non-retroperitoneal residual masses

The ability to predict the histology of postchemotherapy residual masses, both within and outside the retroperitoneum, is important because the prognosis and management differ for tumors composed of viable GCT, teratoma, and necrosis. For masses within the retroperitoneum, logistic regression analysis has attempted to identify parameters that are predictive of necrosis. This identification is critical because additional surgery, although therapeutic for teratoma and viable GCT, is not beneficial for those who have residual necrosis. Current investigations indicate that within the retroperitoneum necrosis composes approximately 40% of residual masses, teratoma another 40%, and viable GCT the remaining 20% [13]. Reported variables that predict necrosis are small (< 1.5 cm) residual lesions, a greater than 90% reduction in the mass after chemotherapy, and the absence of teratomatous elements in the primary tumor [6,14–16]. These findings have been inconsistent in the literature. Because of the inability to accurately predict postchemotherapy histology in the retroperitoneum, the most conservative approach is to resect all residual radiographic lesions. The histology of the postchemotherapy RPLND specimen subsequently dictates further treatment if necessary.

For residual masses outside of the retroperitoneum, research efforts have focused on the histologic concordance between residual masses in the retroperitoneum and other distant sites (eg, thoracic, hepatic, and cervical). If necrosis in the retroperitoneum could accurately predict necrosis at other sites, patients could be safely spared the morbidity of additional surgery.

Residual thoracic disease (pulmonary and mediastinal)

The most recent Memorial Sloan-Kettering Cancer Center (MSKCC) experience of 86 patients who underwent synchronous (within 2 months of each other) and 44 patients who underwent asynchronous (thoracotomy > 2 months after RPLND) thoracotomy and RPLND procedures for residual disease revealed an overall histologic discordance rate of 28% and 57%, respectively [17]. A worse histology was found in the chest approximately one third of the time. Hartmann and colleagues [18] examined 27 patients who required at least two surgical interventions for multiple sites of residual disease after first-line cisplatin-based chemotherapy. Eight of 27 (30%) patients demonstrated dissimilar histologic findings at the multiple sites. In the subset of patients who underwent retroperitoneal and thoracic resections, less favorable histology was found in 2 patients in the retroperitoneum and in 1 patient in the thorax. In a study from Norway, investigators found discordant pathology in 7 of 15 (47%) patients who had metastatic testicular cancer who underwent at least two postchemotherapy resections for residual tumor [19]. Brenner and colleagues [20] reported on their experience of simultaneous resection for retroperitoneal, thoracic, and cervical residual masses after chemotherapy in 24 patients. Six patients (25%) demonstrated discordant pathology in the chest and retroperitoneum, 1 with viable tumor only in the chest and 2 with viable tumor only in the retroperitoneum. Another retrospective review of 31 patients undergoing thoracotomy for residual pulmonary lesions revealed dissimilarity between the retroperitoneal and pulmonary histology in

50% of the patients [21]. This study included 3 patients (15%) who had viable tumor found in the pulmonary specimen but not in the RPLND. Toner and colleagues [22] found that the size of postchemotherapy pulmonary metastases did not predict final histology, and that patients who have bilateral pulmonary lesions may have a different histology in each lung. Six of 14 patients who had pulmonary nodules smaller than 1 cm had either teratoma [5] or viable GCT [1]. Three of 8 patients who underwent bilateral thoracotomy had different histologies in each lung. Mandelbaum and colleagues [23] and Tiffany and colleagues [24] found dissimilar patterns of histology in thoracic and retroperitoneal specimens in 29% and 35% of patients, respectively. The above studies consistently demonstrate a significant discordance rate, on average of approximately one third of cases, between postchemotherapy RPLND and thoracic histology. The inability of the RPLND specimen to accurately predict histology outside of the retroperitoneum has led most investigators to conclude that all sites of disease should be resected.

In 1998, Tognini and colleagues [25] updated the Indiana University experience first presented by Mandelbaum and colleagues [23] in 1983. A total of 143 patients underwent postchemotherapy resection of retroperitoneal and thoracic masses under the same anesthetic. There was thoracic and retroperitoneal histologic concordance in 78% of those who had retroperitoneal necrosis, in 70% who had teratoma, and in 69% who had viable cancer. Analyzing only those deemed uncomplicated by Indiana University criteria (standard induction chemotherapy, normalization of serum tumor markers, and no previous attempts at surgical resection) demonstrated that 18 of 21 (86%) patients who had necrosis in the retroperitoneum revealed the same pathology in the chest. This finding led the authors to conclude that in uncomplicated cases a finding of necrosis in the retroperitoneum allows for observation of residual thoracic tumors. In 1997, an international, multi-institutional study of 215 patients who had testicular cancer used logistic regression analysis to help predict residual pulmonary histology after chemotherapy [26]. The histology at RPLND was the strongest predictor of pulmonary histology. Necrosis was found at thoracotomy in 89% of patients who had necrosis in the RPLND specimen. When RPLND histology was necrosis and the primary tumor was teratoma negative, the probability of necrosis at thoracotomy increased to 93%. The authors concluded that the necessity of thoracotomy is doubtful in some patients in whom the pulmonary histology is likely to be necrosis (ie, necrosis at RPLND and teratoma-negative primary tumor). Given the strong predictive value of the RPLND histology, the authors also recommended that RPLND be performed before thoracotomy is considered. The above studies from Tognini and colleagues [25] and Steyerberg and colleagues [26] suggest that necrosis at RPLND in a subset of patients may be predictive enough to preclude thoracotomy. Moreover, using a logistic regression model with multiple variables may better predict which patients benefit from close follow-up rather than resection. It seems evident that despite the above compelling data, however, no regression model or set of variables can perfectly predict thoracic histology. We still advocate the resection of all residual disease in the thorax to ensure that no viable tumor or teratoma remains in situ.

Residual disease at other sites

There is a paucity of data comparing residual RPLND histology with histology at non-retroperitoneal sites other than the thorax. In a report of 16 patients who had residual neck masses, histologic discordance was seen in 7 (44%) patients [27]. Rivoire and colleagues [28] reviewed 37 patients who underwent liver resection after chemotherapy for GCT. Twenty-seven of the patients had additional synchronous abdominal resections, 20 of which were RPLND. Eleven of the 27 (41%) patients demonstrated histologic discordance of the two sites. Six of these 11 individuals had the more adverse histology in the liver. These discordance rates further support the rationale for resecting all sites of residual disease if technically feasible. Table 1 summarizes the histologic discordance between postchemotherapy RPLND and non-retroperitoneal residual masses.

A small proportion of men presenting with advanced, life-threatening testicular cancer may be treated with platinum-based chemotherapy before radical orchiectomy. After the appropriate course of primary systemic chemotherapy, these patients subsequently undergo delayed orchiectomy. Because this is a rare clinical scenario, there is a paucity of data on the effect of chemotherapy on the primary tumor. There are, however, a few studies examining the histology of orchiectomy specimens after chemotherapy and the histologic concordance of the testicular primary with other

Table 1
Histologic discordance between retroperitoneal and non-retroperitoneal postchemotherapy residual masses

Source, year	No. patients	% Discordance
Mandelbaum et al, 1983 [23]	24	29
Donohue et al, 1987 [6]	24	29
Tiffany et al, 1986 [24]	23	35
Qvist et al, 1991 [19]	15	47
Brenner et al, 1996 [20]	24	25
Hartmann et al, 1997 [18]	27	30
Gels et al, 1997 [21]	20	50
Mohseni et al, 2002 [27]	16	44
McGuire et al, 2003 [17]	105	38

postchemotherapy sites of disease. One of the largest studies on this topic from Indiana University examined 160 patients who underwent postchemotherapy orchiectomy and RPLND [29]. They found teratoma in 31% and viable GCT in 25% of the orchiectomy specimens. Of the patients who had viable GCT in the testis after chemotherapy, 42.5% demonstrated a complete response (necrosis/scar) in the RPLND specimen. Moreover, there was less than 50% histologic concordance between the testicular and RPLND specimens. These results confirm that, like residual disease at other sites, postchemotherapy orchiectomy is indicated regardless of the response to chemotherapy at metastatic sites.

The management of brain metastases has traditionally been recognized as a separate clinical entity. The blood–brain barrier and cerebral edema are unique features of intracranial GCT, and the major concern has been the ability to obtain cytotoxic levels of chemotherapeutic drugs in the brain. Prognosis is based on the features of brain involvement. Mahalati and colleagues [30] and Spears and colleagues [31] have divided patients into three groups: (1) brain metastases at presentation, (2) isolated relapses in the brain, and (3) brain metastases with progressive disease. Oftentimes, residual intracranial disease is managed with a multimodality approach, including surgery, radiotherapy, and additional chemotherapy. Mahalati and colleagues [30] reviewed their experience of 11 patients who had nonseminomatous GCT brain metastases. Patients were divided into the three groups described above. Four of 5 patients in group 1 were still alive (mean follow-up 13 months, range 3–47 months). Three of 5 patients in group 1 received chemotherapy, craniotomy, and radiotherapy. Radiation therapy was given to those who had viable GCT in the specimen. The authors concluded that surgery was indicated for single residual brain lesions amenable to resection in patients in groups 1 and 2. Surgery was not performed for patients who had multiple brain metastases and progressive disease.

Indications for postchemotherapy surgery

Generally accepted indications for postchemotherapy resection include patients who have residual radiographic disease and normalized serum tumor markers (α-fetoprotein and human chorionic gonadotropin). The added benefit of resection must be weighed against the morbidity of additional surgery. Removal of residual viable cancer offers therapeutic benefit and can be curative in a subset of patients. The excision of residual teratoma is also beneficial because teratoma possesses the potential to undergo malignant transformation, and to continue to grow, obstruct, and invade adjacent structures (growing teratoma syndrome). Because teratomas are chemoresistant, surgical extirpation is the only cure. Unfortunately clinicians cannot reliably predict the histology of residual masses within and outside of the retroperitoneum. The studies presented above demonstrate a reasonable correlation between retroperitoneal and non-retroperitoneal histology, suggesting that perhaps necrosis discovered in the retroperitoneum obviates additional surgery [25]. Furthermore, certain subgroups of patients, such as those considered uncomplicated by Indiana University criteria, seem to demonstrate a stronger correlation between retroperitoneal and thoracic histology. Investigators have also used logistic regression models incorporating multiple variables to help predict the postchemotherapy histology of lesions outside the retroperitoneum [26]. On multivariate analysis, factors such as RPLND histology and pathology of the primary tumor proved to be strong predictors of thoracic histology. Remarkably, the size of the residual pulmonary nodules was not predictive of histology. This finding contrasted with an earlier study demonstrating that the size of postchemotherapy retroperitoneal masses was a strong predictor of histology [32]. McGuire and colleagues [33] applied the logistic regression model described by Steyerberg and colleagues [26] to 70 patients who had no teratoma in the primary tumor and necrosis at RPLND and found teratoma or viable GCT in the thorax in 24% of patients.

Our interpretation of the above data is that no single variable or regression model can predict histology outside of the retroperitoneum with enough accuracy to safely preclude resection. Several studies have demonstrated that a significant proportion of patients who have necrosis in the retroperitoneum demonstrate teratoma or viable GCT at other sites [21,25]. Postchemotherapy resection of non-retroperitoneal residual masses provides important prognostic information and is curative in most patients who have teratoma and in a subset of those who have viable GCT. In an effort to maintain optimum survival, all sites of residual disease should be resected regardless of size. In patients who have multiple or bilateral residual pulmonary nodules, excision of all disease is still recommended if technically feasible.

Management of synchronous retroperitoneal and non-retroperitoneal disease

It is not uncommon to have postchemotherapy residual disease at multiple sites within and outside the retroperitoneum. Presurgical planning is individualized and may require coordination with multiple surgical specialties based on tumor location, including urology, general and thoracic surgery, and otolaryngology. To minimize the number of surgical procedures, resection of residual disease at multiple sites under one anesthetic seems appropriate if there is no significant increase in complications. Some earlier reports described multiple sequential surgeries to excise all residual masses [9,24]. These retrospective series demonstrated few major perioperative complications. In 1983, Mandelbaum and colleagues [23] described the first one-stage procedure for simultaneous thoracic and retroperitoneal residual disease in 24 patients. Eighteen patients underwent median sternotomy and 6 had thoracotomy for residual thoracic disease, followed by RPLND under the same anesthetic. There were no perioperative deaths or major complications. When compared with the entire cohort of 72 patients who underwent resection of residual thoracic disease, the subset undergoing combined excision only had a slightly prolonged ileus without other additional morbidity. Long-term survival was similar in the overall and combined groups (74% and 83%, respectively).

In 1996, investigators from MSKCC reviewed their experience with 24 patients who underwent simultaneous retroperitoneal and thoracic resection of postchemotherapy residual masses [20]. In addition, 3 of these patients also underwent formal neck dissection to remove an anterior cervical mass. Three patients were excluded from the single-stage operative approach because of poor pulmonary function. All patients had midline abdominal incisions for the RPLND, and the incision was extended to a thoracoabdominal approach in 2 patients. The other 22 patients received separate thoracic incisions. More than half of the patients received high-risk or salvage chemotherapy, 5 had undergone previous RPLND, and 2 demonstrated elevated α-fetoprotein levels before surgery. Fourteen patients underwent modified rather than complete RPLND because the frozen section demonstrated only necrosis. The overall 5-year survival was 79%. This study demonstrated that simultaneous resection of abdominal, thoracic, and cervical residual masses was a feasible and safe alternative to multiple staged procedures. A retrospective study from Indiana University reviewed 143 patients who underwent resection of residual retroperitoneal and chest disease under the same anesthetic [25]. Fifty of the 143 cases (35%) were classified as having a complicated postoperative course. When compared with the overall group who underwent postchemotherapy RPLND at Indiana University during the same time period, major and minor complications were significantly higher in the subset of 143 patients who underwent the combined approach. No single major or minor complication was more likely in the patients who underwent the combined procedure. The investigators concluded that a combined removal of retroperitoneal and thoracic disease was reasonable based on morbidity. The possibility of added complications was offset by the elimination of additional surgical procedures.

Patients who have residual hepatic lesions frequently undergo synchronous resections. Hahn and colleagues [12] reviewed the Indiana University experience with resection of residual hepatic disease in 57 patients. Concomitant procedures were performed in 53 of 60 (87%) liver resections, including 37 RPLNDs. Complications occurred in 18 procedures (30%), 15 (83%) of which entailed synchronous resections at multiple sites. Chylous ascites is a well-known complication associated with synchronous liver resection [13].

The above studies demonstrate that a combined approach under the same anesthetic for retroperitoneal and non-retroperitoneal lesions is acceptable based on morbidity in this relatively young and healthy patient population. Appropriate patient selection is imperative, and preoperative evaluation must reveal adequate pulmonary function. The combined procedure must be technically feasible with acceptable blood loss and reasonable time constraints. Because of the nature of the combined procedure, a multidisciplinary approach must be coordinated with surgeons from various specialties.

Survival outcomes

The outcome for patients undergoing postchemotherapy surgery for non-retroperitoneal masses depends on the histology of the resected specimen. Investigators from MSKCC reported that 48 of 50 (96%) patients who had fibrosis at thoracotomy and 18 of 22 (82%) who had completely resected teratoma were disease-free at a median follow-up of 24 months [17]. Only 3 of 12 (25%) patients who had resected viable cancer demonstrated no evidence of disease, however. Multivariate analysis revealed that viable GCT in the thoracic and RPLND specimens were independent predictors against disease-free survival. An earlier study from MSKCC revealed a 79% 5-year overall survival rate for 24 patients who underwent simultaneous excision of retroperitoneal, thoracic, and neck (3 patients) residual masses after chemotherapy [20]. Two patients in the cohort had elevated levels of α-fetoprotein before surgery. Only 3 patients (13%) had viable tumor in the specimen. Kesler and colleagues [34] reviewed 268 patients who had testicular GCT who required at least one surgical procedure to remove residual mediastinal disease after chemotherapy. Thirty-five percent of patients received second-line chemotherapy before removal of residual thoracic disease. The overall 5- and 10-year survivals were 86% and 74%, respectively. Five- and 10-year disease-free survivals were 80% and 63%, respectively. Multivariate analysis revealed that a more adverse histology (ie, viable GCT versus teratoma versus necrosis) was an independent predictor of worse long-term survival. Another study from the Netherlands analyzed 31 patients who underwent resection of residual pulmonary masses after chemotherapy [21]. With a median follow-up of 80 months, the 5-year and 10-year survival rates were 87% and 82%, respectively. Only 4 patients demonstrated viable tumor on final pathology, none of whom had viable tumor at RPLND. Three of 4 (75%) patients who had viable tumor were alive without evidence of disease. Mohseni and colleagues [27] reported on 16 patients who had a residual neck lesion who underwent resection of 61 residual masses in multiple sites. Ten patients had teratoma, 3 demonstrated viable GCT, and 3 revealed necrosis. All of the patients who had teratoma and 1 of 3 who had viable GCT had no evidence of disease after complete resection.

Based on these data, the overall survival for patients undergoing resection of non-retroperitoneal postchemotherapy masses seems to be approximately 80% at 5- and 10-year follow up. Overall survival data must be interpreted with caution because all of the studies represent a heterogeneous patient population, with many patients undergoing salvage chemotherapy regimens and some having elevated serum tumor markers at the time of surgery. Moreover, each study has different proportions of patients who have viable GCT, teratoma, and necrosis in the specimens. As demonstrated by McGuire and colleagues [17], patients who have necrosis or teratoma in the residual tumor have a markedly improved outcome compared with those having viable GCT. Subsets of patients who have viable GCT do demonstrate a durable response after excision of residual lesions. This finding highlights the importance of a complete resection whenever technically feasible.

Patients who have nonpulmonary visceral metastases are believed to have a poor prognosis. At Indiana University, 57 patients underwent 60 hepatic resections for residual disease over a 34-year period [12]. Eighty-nine percent of patients who had necrosis were alive with no evidence of disease at a median follow-up of 47 months in contrast with 29% of patients who had viable GCT and normal preoperative serum tumor markers. The authors concluded that hepatic resection is safe and efficacious except in the subset of patients who have elevated preoperative serum tumor markers. Other smaller studies investigating residual hepatic disease have recommended resection based on the size of the lesions or close follow-up and delayed excision for enlarging masses [28,35].

The most recent data from MSKCC reviewed the outcomes of 130 patients who underwent postchemotherapy resection of extra-retroperitoneal masses either concurrently or within 6 weeks of postchemotherapy RPLND [36]. This study analyzed patients who had disease at all sites outside of the retroperitoneum, including the lungs, mediastinum, neck, and liver. They found that the 5-year progression-free survival and disease-free survival for this group were 74% and 85%, respectively. These outcomes were significantly worse when compared with a cohort of 402 patients who only demonstrated residual disease in the retroperitoneum. On multivariate analysis, extra-retroperitoneal pathology (teratoma and viable tumor) was a significant predictor of disease progression. These data suggest that residual extra-retroperitoneal disease confers an adverse prognosis, and, again, highlight the importance of aggressive surgical resection of all residual masses.

Complications

Fortunately, patients undergoing surgery for advanced testicular cancer are relatively young and healthy men. Large-volume residual disease, postchemotherapy desmoplastic reaction, and prior exposure to bleomycin increase the technical difficulty and perioperative demands of the surgery. Perioperative mortality was approximately 1% in a large series of patients undergoing mediastinal resection [34]. Nonfatal complications have been reported in approximately 0% to 30% of patients [9,12,20,21,34]. Complications specific to postchemotherapy non-retroperitoneal surgery arise from pulmonary, lymphatic, infectious, and vascular causes.

Pulmonary complications include atelectasis, which is treated by vigorous pulmonary physiotherapy; pneumonia, which is managed with appropriate antibiotics; pneumothorax, which is managed with oxygen and observation or chest tube drainage; and adult respiratory distress syndrome (ARDS). ARDS is a complication that may be fatal or require prolonged mechanical ventilation in an intensive care unit. Prior exposure to bleomycin is a risk factor for ARDS. Clinicians must judiciously monitor perioperative fluid administration and avoid exposure to unnecessarily high concentrations of inspired oxygen in bleomycin-treated patients.

Chylothorax occurs secondary to injury of the thoracic duct or its tributaries and has been reported in approximately 2% to 4% of cases [20,34]. Familiarity with lymphatic anatomy in the chest and meticulous lymphostasis can minimize this complication. Clinical presentation includes shortness of breath and desaturation, similar to patients who have a significant pneumothorax. Chest radiograph or CT demonstrates a pleural effusion, and thoracentesis is diagnostic. Chylous fluid has a characteristic milky or turbid appearance with a fat content of 4 to 40 g/L and a total protein content of greater than 30 g/L. Thoracentesis may provide symptomatic relief, but many patients require chest tube drainage. Chylous ascites occurs in approximately 2% to 3% of patients undergoing RPLND but is more prevalent in patients undergoing simultaneous hepatic resection [13,28]. Dietary management of chylous leakage includes a low-fat diet with medium-chain triglycerides or total parenteral nutrition.

Intra-abdominal abscess formation has been reported in patients undergoing hepatic resection and must be managed with intravenous antibiotics and drainage [12,28]. Major vascular injuries are uncommon in experienced centers. One large study of 268 patients who underwent resection of residual mediastinal disease reported bleeding necessitating reoperation in 1.4% of cases [34].

Management after resection of residual masses

The histology of the resected residual masses guides further treatment. Patients who have necrosis require no more immediate treatment and should be followed with careful surveillance. Completely resected teratoma also does not warrant further systemic therapy. Patients who have residual viable cancer, however, may be treated with additional cisplatin-based chemotherapy. Fox and colleagues [37] reviewed 580 postchemotherapy RPLNDs at a single institution and found 133 patients who had viable nonteratomatous GCT. Seventy percent (19 of 27) of those who received primary chemotherapy followed by two additional courses of postoperative chemotherapy after complete resection remained disease-free, whereas 100% (7 of 7) who did not undergo additional chemotherapy relapsed. Thirty-six percent (9 of 25) of patients who had a complete resection after salvage chemotherapy and subsequently received postoperative chemotherapy remained disease-free compared with 43% (12 of 28) of those who received no additional chemotherapy. Only 9% (4 of 43) of patients who had an incomplete resection were disease-free at the time of publication. The authors concluded that two additional courses of cisplatin-based chemotherapy after complete resection of viable GCT was safe and reduced the risk for relapse in patients who initially underwent primary chemotherapy. Additional standard chemotherapy was not beneficial in those who received preoperative salvage chemotherapy. An international, multicenter, retrospective review assessed the value of postchemotherapy surgery in patients who had viable GCT who initially received cisplatin-based chemotherapy [10]. An analysis of 238 patients, 53.5% of whom demonstrated residual masses outside the retroperitoneum, revealed that complete resection, 10% or fewer viable malignant cells, and good International Germ Cell Consensus Classification (IGCCC) were independent predictors of improved progression-free and overall survival. Recipients of postoperative chemotherapy demonstrated a significantly improved progression-free survival compared with nonrecipients. There was no significant difference in overall survival between the postoperative chemotherapy recipients and nonrecipients, however. On multivariate analysis, postoperative chemotherapy was associated with an improved progression-free survival ($P < .001$) but no improvement in overall survival ($P = .26$). Patients were assigned to one of three risk groups based on the above-mentioned prognostic indicators (complete resection, <10% viable malignant cells, and good IGCCC): those who had no risk factors (favorable group), those who had one risk factor (intermediate group), and those who had two or three risk factors (poor-risk group). Recipients of postoperative chemotherapy in the intermediate-risk group revealed an improved progression-free and overall survival compared with nonrecipients. Patients in the favorable-risk group faired well with or without additional chemotherapy and those in the poor-risk group did poorly regardless of additional systemic therapy. The above results highlight the importance of a complete resection of viable GCT and suggest that patients who have favorable characteristics (complete resection, ≤10% viable malignant cells, and good IGCCC) may not require postoperative chemotherapy.

Summary

Over the past 2 to 3 decades, the role of postchemotherapy surgery for advanced GCT has undergone a remarkable transformation. With the introduction of cisplatin-based chemotherapy and refinements in imaging technology, postchemotherapy surgery has become an integral component of the multimodality approach to treating advanced GCT. This combined approach has resulted in cure rates of approximately 80% in patients who have advanced GCT. We believe that postchemotherapy surgery is indicated for patients who have residual radiographic disease and normalized serum tumor markers. The benefit of postchemotherapy surgery both within and outside of the retroperitoneum depends on the histology of the resected specimen. Unfortunately, no set of variables can accurately predict necrosis and thus obviate the need for surgery. Multiple studies have demonstrated that histology in the RPLND specimen does not correlate well enough with other sites of residual disease, such as the mediastinum and lungs, to preclude their resection. Emerging evidence suggests that at least intermediate-risk patients benefit by receiving additional chemotherapy. The complex integration of multiple surgical specialists, aggressive evaluation, and proactive resection of persistent non-retroperitoneal masses is imperative in the effective management of male GCT.

References

[1] Jemal A, Siegel R, Ward E, et al. Cancer statistics, 2007. CA Cancer J Clin 2007;57:43–66.

[2] Bergstrom R, Adami HO, Mohner M, et al. Increase in testicular cancer incidence in six European countries: a birth cohort phenomenon. J Natl Cancer Inst 1996;88:727–33.

[3] McKiernan JM, Goluboff ET, Liberson GL, et al. Rising risk of testicular cancer by birth cohort in the United States from 1973 to 1995. J Urol 1999; 162:361–3.

[4] Einhorn LH. Testicular cancer as a model for a curable neoplasm: The Richard and Hinda Rosenthal Foundation Award Lecture. Cancer Res 1981;41: 3275–80.

[5] Bosl G, Bajorin D, Sheinfeld J, et al. Cancer of the testis. In: DeVita V, Hellman S, Rosenberg S, editors. Cancer: principles and practice of oncology. Philadelphia: JB Lippincott; 2000. p. 1491–518.

[6] Donohue JP, Rowland RG, Kopecky K, et al. Correlation of computerized tomographic changes and histological findings in 80 patients having radical retroperitoneal lymph node dissection after chemotherapy for testis cancer. J Urol 1987;137:1176–9.

[7] Bajorin DF, Herr H, Motzer RJ, et al. Current perspectives on the role of adjunctive surgery in combined modality treatment for patients with germ cell tumors. Semin Oncol 1992;19:148–58.

[8] Sheinfeld J, Bajorin D, Solomon M. Management of postchemotherapy residual masses in advanced germ cell tumors. AUA Update Series 1997;17:18–24.

[9] Gerl A, Clemm C, Schmeller N, et al. Sequential resection of residual abdominal and thoracic masses after chemotherapy for metastatic non-seminomatous germ cell tumors. Br J Cancer 1994;70:960–5.

[10] Fizazi K, Tjulandin S, Salvioni R, et al. Viable malignant cells after primary chemotherapy for disseminated nonseminomatous germ cell tumors: prognostic factors and role of postsurgery chemotherapy—results from an international study group. J Clin Oncol 2001;19:2647–57.

[11] Kesler KA, Donohue JP. Combined urologic and thoracic approaches for advanced or disseminated testis cancer. Atlas Urol Clin North Am 1999;7: 79–94.
[12] Hahn TL, Jacobson L, Einhorn LH. Hepatic resection of metastatic testicular carcinoma: a further update. Ann Surg Oncol 1999;6:640–4.
[13] Sheinfeld J, McKiernan JM, Bosl GJ, et al. Surgery of testicular tumors. In: Walsh PC, Retik AB, Vaughan ED, editors. Campbell's urology. 8th edition. Philadelphia: Saunders; 2002. p. 2920–44.
[14] Carter GE, Lieskovsky G, Skinner DG, et al. Reassessment of the role of adjunctive surgical therapy in the treatment of advanced germ cell tumors. J Urol 1987;138:1397–401.
[15] Stomper PC, Jochelson MS, Garnick MB, et al. Residual abdominal masses after chemotherapy for nonseminomatous testicular cancer: correlation of CT and histology. AJR Am J Roentgenol 1985; 145:743–6.
[16] Gelderman WA, Schraffordt Koops H, Sleijfer DT, et al. Results of adjuvant surgery in patients with stage III and IV nonseminomatous testicular tumors after cisplatin-vinblastine-bleomycin chemotherapy. J Surg Oncol 1988;38:227–32.
[17] McGuire MS, Rabbani F, Mohseni H, et al. The role of thoracotomy in managing postchemotherapy residual thoracic masses in patients with nonseminomatous germ cell tumors. BJU Int 2003;91:469–73.
[18] Hartmann JT, Candelaria M, Kuczyk MA, et al. Comparison of histological results from resection of residual masses at different sites after chemotherapy for metastatic non-seminomatous germ cell tumors. Eur J Cancer 1997;33:843–7.
[19] Qvist HL, Fossa SD, Ous S, et al. Post-chemotherapy tumor residuals in patients with advanced nonseminomatous testicular cancer. Is it necessary to resect all residual masses? J Urol 1991;145:300–3.
[20] Brenner PC, Herr HW, Morse MJ, et al. Simultaneous retroperitoneal, thoracic, and cervical resection of postchemotherapy residual masses in patients with metastatic nonseminomatous germ cell tumors of the testis. J Clin Oncol 1996;14:1765–9.
[21] Gels ME, Hoekstra HJ, Sleijfer DT, et al. Thoracotomy for postchemotherapy resection of pulmonary residual tumor mass in patients with nonseminomatous testicular germ cell tumors. Aggressive surgical resection is justified. Chest 1997;112:967–73.
[22] Toner GC, Panicek DM, Heelan RT, et al. Adjunctive surgery after chemotherapy for nonseminomatous germ cell tumors: recommendations for patient selection. J Clin Oncol 1990;8:1683–94.
[23] Mandelbaum I, Yaw PB, Einhorn LH, et al. The importance of one-stage median sternotomy and retroperitoneal node dissection in disseminated testicular cancer. Ann Thorac Surg 1983;36:524–8.
[24] Tiffany P, Morse MJ, Bosl G, et al. Sequential excision of residual thoracic and retroperitoneal masses after chemotherapy for stage III germ cell tumors. Cancer 1986;57:978–83.
[25] Tognini PG, Foster RS, McGraw P, et al. Combined post-chemotherapy retroperitoneal lymph node dissection and resection of chest tumor under the same anesthetic is appropriate based on morbidity and tumor pathology. J Urol 1998;159:1833–5.
[26] Steyerberg EW, Keizer JH, Messemer JE, et al. Residual pulmonary masses after chemotherapy for metastatic nonseminomatous germ cell tumor. Prediction of histology. Cancer 1997;79:345–55.
[27] Mohseni HF, Rabbani F, Leon A, et al. Management and clinical outcome of patients with germ cell tumor and a postchemotherapy residual neck mass. J Urol 2002;167:693A.
[28] Rivoire M, Elias D, De Cian F, et al. Multimodality treatment of patients with liver metastases from germ cell tumors: the role of surgery. Cancer 2001; 92:578–87.
[29] Liebovitch I, Little JS Jr, Foster RS, et al. Delayed orchiectomy after chemotherapy for metastatic nonseminomatous germ cell tumors. J Urol 1996;155: 952–4.
[30] Mahalati K, Bilen CY, Ozen H, et al. The management of brain metastases in nonseminomatous germ cell tumors. BJU Int 1999;83:457–61.
[31] Spears WT, Morphis JG 2nd, Lester SG, et al. Brain metastases and testicular tumors: long-term survival. Int J Radiat Oncol Biol Phys 1992;22: 17–22.
[32] Steyerberg EW, Keizer HJ, Fossa SD, et al. Prediction of residual retroperitoneal mass histology after chemotherapy for metastatic nonseminomatous germ cell tumor: multivariate analysis of individual patient data from six study groups. J Clin Oncol 1995;13:1177–87.
[33] McGuire M, Rabbani F, Mohseni H, et al. The role of thoracotomy in the management of postchemotherapy residual thoracic masses. J Urol 1999;161: 703A.
[34] Kesler KA, Brooks J, Rieger KM, et al. Mediastinal metastases from testicular nonseminomatous germ cell tumors: patterns of dissemination and predictors of long-term survival with surgery. J Thorac Cardiovasc Surg 2003;125:913–23.
[35] Copson E, McKendrick J, Hennessey N, et al. Liver metastases in germ cell cancer: defining a role for surgery after chemotherapy. BJU Int 2004;94: 552–8.
[36] Shayegan B, Carver BS, Motzer RJ, et al. Impact of residual extra-retroperitoneal masses in patients with advanced non-seminomatous germ cell testicular cancer. AUA abstract # 449, 2006.
[37] Fox EP, Weathers TD, Williams SD, et al. Outcome analysis for patients with persistent nonteratomatous germ cell tumor in postchemotherapy retroperitoneal lymph node dissections. J Clin Oncol 1993; 11:1294–9.

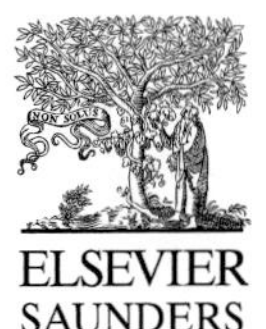
ELSEVIER
SAUNDERS

Urol Clin N Am 34 (2007) 245–251

UROLOGIC
CLINICS
of North America

Adult and Pediatric Testicular Teratoma

Brett S. Carver, MD, Hikmat Al-Ahmadie, MD, Joel Sheinfeld, MD*

Department of Urology and Pathology, Memorial Sloan-Kettering Cancer Center, 1275 York Avenue, New York, NY 10021, USA

Testicular cancer is the most common malignancy in men 20 to 35 years of age and accounts for approximately 1% of all male malignancies. The American Cancer Society [1] estimates that in 2006 there will be 8250 new cases of testicular cancer in the United States and approximately 370 men will die of the disease. The successful multidisciplinary approach for the management of testicular cancer has resulted in survival rates of greater than 90% overall [2]. Germ-cell tumors (GCT) of the testis can be divided into two major subgroups based on histology: seminoma and nonseminoma. Nonseminomatous histologies including embryonal cell carcinoma, yolk sac tumor, choriocarcinoma, and teratoma account for approximately 50% of all GCT. In approximately 60% of cases, more than one histologic pattern is identified, with the most frequent combination being embryonal carcinoma, yolk sac tumor, and teratoma. In its pure form, teratomas compromise approximately 3% of testicular GCT in adults and 38% of tumors in infants and children [3,4]. Teratoma has diverse biologic potential unrelated to the degree of maturity of the histologic components. In this review we will discuss the histologic variants, clinical management, and implications of teratoma.

Pathology of teratoma

Teratoma is a neoplasm of germ-cell origin that is composed of several types of tissue representing different germinal layers (endoderm, mesoderm, ectoderm), forming somatic-type tissue in various stages of maturation and differentiation. Based on findings of genetic studies, it is now recommended to consider teratoma as a single entity regardless of the degree of maturation and differentiation of the tissue comprising it [5]. Infantile teratomas are diploid and follow a benign course. Genetic studies (karyotyping and comparative genomic hybridization) tumors have failed to demonstrate chromosomal changes in these tumors. In contrast, teratomas in adult testes are hypotriploid and have genetic changes similar to those seen in other components of GCTs.

On gross examination, teratomas are usually nodular and firm with a variably cystic and solid cut surface. The cysts may be filled with keratinous material or clear serous or mucoid fluid. The solid areas may contain translucent, gray-white nodules representing cartilage. Hair or melanin-containing tissue may also be rarely seen. Areas of immature tissue are mostly solid and may have an encephaloid, hemorrhagic, or necrotic appearance.

Fig. 1 demonstrates the microscopic appearance of the various histologic subtypes of teratoma. Microscopically, mature elements contain well-differentiated tissues resembling normal postnatal tissue and typically including structures derived from the three germ layers. Tissue of ectodermal origin maybe represented by nests of squamous epithelium with or without cyst formation and keratinization. Neural tissue may be encountered as foci of neuroglia. Structures of endodermal origin are represented by glandular epithelium of enteric or respiratory type. Other glandular tissue such as pancreatic, mucus-producing, prostate, and thyroid may be found. Mesodermal elements are represented by cartilage,

* Corresponding author. Department of Urology, Sidney Kimmel Center for Prostate and Urologic Cancers, 353 East 68th Street, New York, NY 10021.

E-mail address: sheinfej@mskcc.org (J. Sheinfeld).

0094-0143/07/$ - see front matter
doi:10.1016/j.ucl.2007.02.013

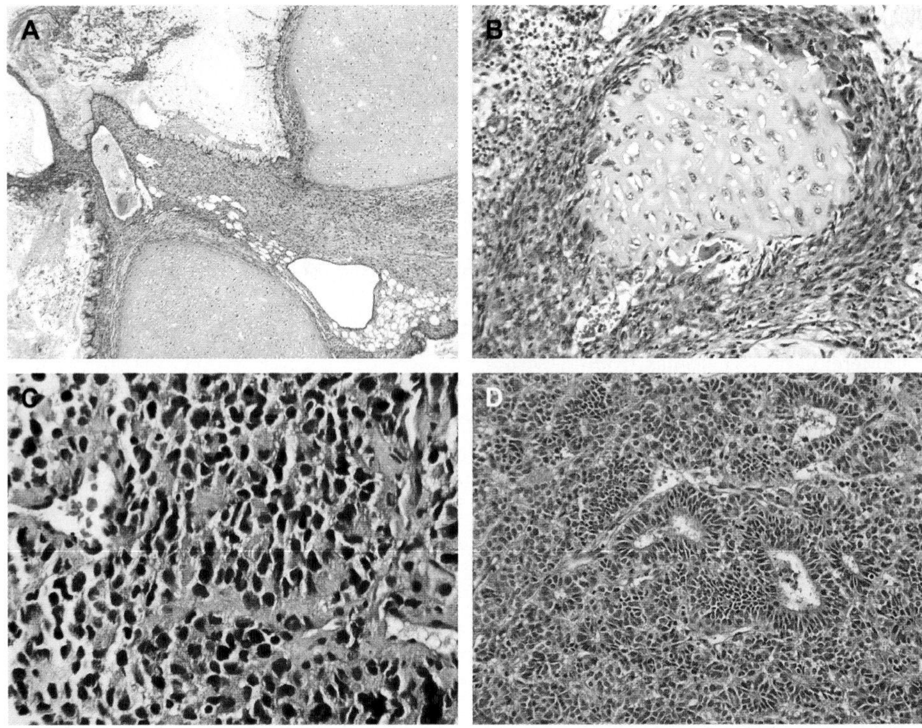

Fig. 1. Teratoma with various types of mature tissue elements including enteric-type epithelium, cartilage, smooth muscle, and adipose tissue (*A*). Teratoma with immature tissue elements resembling fetal-type cartilage and undifferentiated mesenchyme (*B*). Teratoma with somatic-type malignancies: rhabdomyosarcoma (*C*) and primitive neuroectodermal tumor (*D*).

bone, adipose tissue, fibrous tissue, and, most commonly, muscle. Attempts at organ formation are frequently identified with smooth muscle encircling glands of respiratory or enteric morphology.

Immature, fetal-type tissue may also consist of ectodermal, endodermal, and/or mesodermal elements. It usually occurs as islands of immature neuroepithelium resembling that of the developing embryonic neural tube. Immature tissue may also have an organoid arrangement with blastematous and primitive tubular structures resembling that of the developing kidney or lung. Embryonic skeletal muscle, cartilage, and nonspecific cellular stroma may also be encountered. There is no point, however, in grading the degree of immaturity in such tumors in adults because they derive from invasive malignant GCTs and they may have metastases even if they appear totally mature.

Teratoma with somatic-type malignancies refers to the development of independently evolving, malignant neoplasms of the type typically encountered in other organs and tissues, eg, sarcomas and carcinomas. Usually derived from one of the teratomatous elements, these tumors are characterized by an invasive or expansile proliferation of malignant cells that overgrow the surrounding GCT. The most common somatic-type malignancy seen in GCT is sarcoma of various types, particularly those of striated muscle differentiation (ie, rhabdomyosarcoma). Primitive neuroectodermal tumors have also been increasingly identified in association with GCT. Adenocarcinomas, squamous carcinomas, and neuroendocrine carcinomas may also be associated with GCT.

Low-stage pure testicular teratoma

Prepubertal

The reported incidence of testicular tumors in children ranges from 0.5 to 2.0 cases per 100,000 boys [6]. Testicular teratoma is the second most common prepubertal testis tumor following yolk sac tumor and occurs with a relative frequency ranging from 13% to 60% [7–9]. On sonographic evaluation, teratomas may demonstrate the appearance of cystic areas with intervening septa and solid areas. In contrast to the cystic appearance of teratomas, other testis tumors in children are typically solid, with the exception of the rare cystic granulosa cell tumor or simple testicular cysts. The presence of calcifications in the tumor is another helpful sonographic finding associated with teratomas; however, the diagnosis must be verified by pathologic examination.

Serum alpha-fetoprotein (AFP) levels are also useful in differentiating teratomas from yolk sac tumors. Teratomas do not stain positively for AFP by immunohistochemistry, and elevated serum AFP levels are not reported in patients with these tumors. In contrast, greater than 90% of yolk sac tumors stain immunohistochemically for AFP, the majority of which also are associated with elevated serum AFP levels [10,11]. Therefore, serum AFP levels should always be obtained during the initial evaluation of a testicular tumor in the prepubertal child.

The natural history of prepubertal testicular teratomas differs significantly from testis teratomas in the adult. Metastasis from testicular teratomas in prepubertal children has not been reported, while similar tumors occurring after puberty are known to metastasize [6,12]. Based on this, the treatment of choice for prepubertal testicular teratomas is orchiectomy; however, recent studies with long-term follow-up have demonstrated the safety and efficacy of testis-sparing surgery [13].

Postpubertal

While teratomatous elements are found in 55% to 80% of primary nonseminomatous germ-cell tumors (NSGCTs) in adults, only 2% to 6% of cases are composed of pure teratoma [14,15]. The ultrasonographic and pathologic appearance of pure teratomas is similar in the prepubertal and postpubertal testis. As previously discussed, serum tumor markers are usually not elevated in patients with a pure testicular teratoma. Although pure testicular teratomas have a benign clinical course in prepubertal children, in adults metastases have been reported in 29% to 76% of cases at initial presentation (Table 1) [12,16,17]. Furthermore, retroperitoneal metastases have been identified in approximately 20% of patients with clinical stage I pure testicular teratoma treated with primary retroperitoneal lymph node dissection (RPLND) [16,18].

Table 1
The incidence of metastatic disease at initial presentation in men with pure testicular teratoma

Reference	Total no. of patients with pure teratoma	Patients with metastases, n (%)
Rabbani et al [12]	29	22 (76)
Leibovitch et al [16]	41	23 (56)
Simmonds et al [17]	14	4 (29)

The standard treatment for all germ-cell testicular tumors in adults is a radical orchiectomy performed through an inguinal approach. However, controversy exists concerning the management of the retroperitoneum in patients with clinical stage I pure teratoma. The treatment options for these patients include primary RPLND or surveillance. The incidence of retroperitoneal metastases in patients with clinical stage I disease is approximately 30% and increases to 75% for patients with clinical stage IIA disease [12,16,18]. For patients undergoing a primary RPLND for pure testicular teratoma, the histologic finding in the retroperitoneal lymph nodes of teratoma or viable GCT is present in approximately 30% and 20% of patients, respectively [12]. The significance of viable GCT in the retroperitoneum of patients with pure testicular teratoma implies that either a small-volume viable NSGCT was not detected on pathologic analysis of the orchiectomy specimen, or these retroperitoneal metastases occurred before the viable GCT elements in the testis underwent necrosis or regression ("burnt-out lesion"). The survival rate for patients with low-volume disease following primary RPLND approaches 100% [12,16,18].

Studies have demonstrated that even in properly selected patients with pure testicular teratoma, approximately 20% of patients will relapse during surveillance [17,19]. The retroperitoneum is the most common site of relapse, followed by the lungs or elevated serum tumor marker (STM) alone. Survival rates after therapy for surveillance range from 95% to 100% and are comparable to that of primary RPLND [17,19]. For patients with clinical stage I NSGCT on surveillance, a number of factors predictive of retroperitoneal or systemic failure have been identified, such as a primary tumor stage of T2 (cIb) or greater, lymphovascular invasion, and/or the histologic finding of embryonal cell carcinoma predominance [20,21]. Several of these factors may also be helpful in selecting patients with pure testicular tumors for surveillance protocols. Patient compliance is the most important selection criteria for entry into a surveillance program because strict adherence to frequent follow-up evaluations is critical. Because patients with pure testicular teratoma do not have elevated serum tumor markers at presentation and because of the increased incidence of harboring teratoma in the retroperitoneum and the potential for late relapse, strict vigilance is required for surveillance protocols.

Advanced-stage pure testicular teratoma

Approximately two thirds of patients with NSGCTs, including those with pure testicular teratomas, will present with advanced metastatic disease. This group of patients with pure testicular teratomas typically have had regression of other viable nonseminomatous germ-cell elements in the testis. Heidenreich and colleagues [18] reported that 80% of patients with advanced pure testicular teratomas had evidence of scars or calcifications in the testicular parenchyma suggestive of a "burnt-out" tumor. Therefore, serum tumor markers are frequently elevated, and viable GCTs such as embryonal cell carcinoma or yolk sac tumor are frequently present in the metastatic sites. These patients are managed initially with chemotherapy according to the International Germ Cell Cancer Collaborative Group (IGCCCG) risk criteria, followed by postchemotherapy RPLND (PC-RPLND). The postchemotherapy histologic findings in the retroperitoneal specimen reveal fibrosis, teratoma, and viable GCT, in 44%, 50%, and 6% of patients, respectively [12]. Following the multidisciplinary management of advanced metastatic testicular teratoma, the disease-free survival rate is excellent with approximately 90% of patients remaining continuously free of disease [12,16].

The impact of teratoma in mixed nonseminomatous germ-cell tumors

Although pure testicular tumors in adults are rare, teratoma is present frequently in combination with other histologic subtypes. In approximately 60% of cases, more than one histologic pattern is identified, with the most frequent combination being embryonal carcinoma, yolk sac tumor, and teratoma. The impact of teratomatous elements in the orchiectomy specimen of men with NSGCT has been evaluated by several investigators. Teratomatous elements are present in the retroperitoneum in 20% of men undergoing primary RPLND and 40% of men undergoing PC-RPLND for metastatic NSGCT [12,16,22]. Teratoma in the orchiectomy specimen has been shown to predict for teratoma in the retroperitoneum in men with both low- and high-volume retroperitoneal disease [22–24]; however, the absence of teratoma in the primary tumor does not exclude the finding of teratoma in the retroperitoneum. The Indiana group reported that 82% of men with teratoma in the orchiectomy specimen undergoing PC-RPLND will have teratoma in the retroperitoneum compared with approximately 48% of men without teratoma in the orchiectomy specimen [23]. Previously, Beck and colleagues [24] reported that teratoma in the orchiectomy specimen and the volume of the retroperitoneal metastasis were significant predictors for teratoma in the retroperitoneum. We have reported in our series of men undergoing PC-RPLND that teratoma was found in the retroperitoneum in 67% of men with teratoma in the orchiectomy specimen and in 28% of men without teratoma in the orchiectomy specimen (Table 2) [22]. Although the presence of teratoma in the

Table 2
The incidence of teratoma in the retroperitoneum for men undergoing PC-RPLND at Memorial Sloan-Kettering Cancer Center [22]

	Total no. patients	Teratomatous elements in the retroperitoneum (%)
Teratoma in the orchiectomy		
Yes	224	150 (67)
No	308	85 (28)
RP nodal size postchemotherapy		
Normal (≤ 1 cm)	154	35 (23)
1–2 cm	83	29 (35)
2–5 cm	173	96 (56)
> 5 cm	98	67 (68)
Percent reduction RP nodal size		
≥ 90%	46	9 (20)
90%–50%	221	65 (29)
50%–0%	173	104 (60)
Enlarging RP nodal mass	49	46 (94)

Abbreviations: PC-RPLND, postchemotherapy retroperitoneal lymph node dissection; RP, retroperitoneal.

orchiectomy specimen is predictive for teratoma in the retroperitoneum, 20% to 30% of patients with a normal postchemotherapy retroperitoneum on CT imaging and no teratoma in the primary tumor harbored teratoma in the retroperitoneum [22,25]. Therefore, we continue to recommend PC-RPLND in all patients.

Additionally, the presence of teratomatous elements in the orchiectomy specimen has previously been reported to predict for an incomplete clinical response to induction chemotherapy in patients with advanced NSGCT [26,27]. Rabbani and colleagues [26] reported that in patients treated with cisplatin-based chemotherapy for stage II–III testicular NSGCT, those with teratoma in the primary tumor had a significantly lower radiologic response (23%) compare with patients with no teratoma in the primary tumor (54%).

Retroperitoneal teratoma in men with advanced testicular NSGCT

Teratomatous elements are present in the retroperitoneum in approximately 40% of men undergoing PC-RPLND for metastatic NSGCT [22]. Despite the mature histologic appearance of some teratomas, there are significant advantages to complete resection. First, teratoma may grow, obstruct, or invade adjacent structures and become unresectable. Second, there is the risk of transformation to somatic-type malignancies, such as sarcoma or carcinoma. Last, teratoma may result in late relapses.

The finding of residual teratoma in the retroperitoneum following chemotherapy has been assumed to be a favorable prognostic factor; however, several series have reported a high frequency of recurrences (Table 3) [28–31]. Loehrer and colleagues [28] reported on 51 patients who had surgical resections of teratoma after cisplatin-based chemotherapy. Twenty (39%) patients relapsed with either histologically proven teratoma (10 patients) or viable GCT (10 patients). Sonneveld and colleagues [29] reported on 51 patients with retroperitoneal teratoma following chemotherapy for NSGCT. In their series, nine patients suffered a relapse, with growing teratoma in 56%, teratoma with somatic-type malignancy in 33%, and viable GCT in 11%. We recently reported on the clinical outcome of 210 men undergoing PC-RPLND for teratoma [31]. Overall, relapse occurred in 30 patients and the 10-year probability of freedom from recurrence was 80%. Of the patients who suffered a relapse, 50% relapsed with teratomatous elements and 50% relapsed with viable GCT. For patients relapsing following resection of teratoma, 17% relapsed with somatic-type malignancy.

Loehrer and colleagues [28] reported that on univariate analysis, initial tumor burden, somatic-type malignancy in the resected specimen, and the site of residual disease (mediastinum) predicted for disease relapse after postchemotherapy resection of residual teratoma. Additionally, it has been shown that recurrence of teratoma is related to the completeness of the surgical resection [29]. We demonstrated that increasing postchemotherapy retroperitoneal nodal size and intermediate or poor IGCCCG risk classification were independent predictors of disease recurrence following complete resection of teratoma [31]. In our series, following complete resection of residual teratoma, the 10-year probability of freedom from recurrence and disease-specific survival is 80% and 92% respectively, highlighting the successful integration of chemotherapy and postchemotherapy surgery [31].

Taken together, these data demonstrate that complete surgical resection of teratoma is the treatment of choice for this chemoresitant tumor. Furthermore, approximately 20% to 30% of patients with normal postchemotherapy retroperitoneal CT imaging will harbor teratoma in the retroperitoneum following treatment with chemotherapy for metastatic NSGCT, demonstrating that the retroperitoneum remains difficult to stage clinically [22,25]. We have demonstrated an excellent clinical outcome for men undergoing PC-RPLND for residual masses less than 2 cm (5-year probability of freedom from recurrence 94%), justifying an aggressive surgical approach for all patients with NSGCT who achieve marker-negative status after chemotherapy, and

Table 3
The clinical outcome of men following PC-RPLND resection of teratoma

Reference	No. of patients	Patients with recurrence, n (%)
Loehrer et al [28]	51	20 (39)
Sonneveld et al [29]	51	9 (18)
Fossa et al [30]	37	5 (14)
Carver et al [31]	210	30 (14)

Abbreviation: PC-RPLND, postchemotherapy retroperitoneal lymph node dissection.

underscoring the need for complete surgical resection as the treatment of choice for patients with residual teratoma [31].

Teratoma with somatic-type malignancy

Teratoma with somatic-type malignancy (malignant transformation) is characterized by the presence of malignant tissues of the type encountered in other organs and tissues, such as sarcoma of various types, particularly rhabdomyosarcoma and chondrosarcoma, as well as squamous carcinoma, adenocarcinoma, neuroblastoma, and primitive neuroectodermal tumors. The incidence of malignant transformation is approximately 3% to 6% in men undergoing PC-RPLND following induction or salvage chemotherapy and increases to 12% to 18% in men undergoing reoperative PC-RPLND and in those suffering later relapse [32–34]. Whereas there appears to be no difference in clinical outcome for men with mature and immature teratoma, the histologic finding of teratoma with somatic-type malignancy has been associated with a poor prognosis [32,35,36]. Comiter and colleagues [35] reported on 21 patients undergoing therapy for teratoma with somatic-type malignancy, and with a median follow-up of 50 months 17 of patients relapsed. Motzer and colleagues [32] reported on 46 patients with somatic-type malignancy managed with chemotherapy and/or surgical resection. With a median follow-up of 34 months, 25 remained disease free. Because teratoma with malignant transformation is generally resistant to standard chemotherapy, complete surgical resection, particularly of a solitary site, remains the treatment of choice. Donadio and colleagues [36] reported on 10 patients with somatic-type malignancy who received chemotherapy tailored to the histology of the malignant cell type. In this series, seven patients achieved a partial response to chemotherapy and three achieved durable long-term survival. Therefore, chemotherapy regimens should be administered based on the histology of the somatic-type malignancy, although prognosis is still guarded, and complete surgical resection remains of paramount importance.

Summary

Teratoma, while histologically benign, has diverse biologic potential. The capacity of teratoma to demonstrate local aggressive growth, distant spread, and transformation to a somatic malignancy highlights the unpredictability of this GCT. Given the chemoresitant nature of teratoma, complete surgical resection and control of the retroperitoneum is the treatment of choice.

References

[1] American Cancer Society. Cancer facts and figures 2006. Available at: www.cancer.org. Accessed August 1, 2006.

[2] Sheinfeld J, Herr HW. Role of surgery in management of germ cell tumor. Semin Oncol 1998;25:203–9.

[3] Walsh C, Rushton HG. Diagnosis and management of teratomas and epidermoid cysts. Urol Clin North Am 2000;27:509–18.

[4] Mostofi FK, Sesterhenn IA, Davis CJ. Anatomy and pathology of testis cancer. In: Vogelzang NJ, Scardino PT, Shipley WU, et al, editors. Comprehensive textbook of genitourinary oncology. 2nd edition. Philadelphia: Lippincott Williams and Wilkins; 2000. p. 909–26.

[5] Woodward PJ, Heidenreich A, Looijenga LHJ. Germ cell tumours. In: Eble JN, Sauter G, Epstein JL, et al, editors. Pathology and genetics of tumours of the urinary system and male genital organs. Lyon (France): IARCPress; 2004. p. 221–49.

[6] Brosman SA. Tumors: male genital tract. In: Kelalis PP, King LR, Belman AB, editors. Clinical pediatric urology. 3rd edition. Philadelphia: WB Saunders; 1985. p. 1202–19.

[7] Brosman S. Testicular tumors in prepubertal children. Urology 1979;13:581–8.

[8] Brown NJ. Teratoma and yolk sac tumors. J Clin Pathol 1976;29:1021–5.

[9] Houser R, Izant RJ, Perskey L. Testicular tumors in children. Am J Surg 1965;110:876–92.

[10] Fernandes ET, Etaubanas E, Rao BN, et al. Two decades of experience with testicular tumors in children at St Jude Children's Research Hospital. J Pediatr Surg 1989;24:677–81.

[11] Grady R, Ross J, Kay R. Epidemiological features of testicular teratoma in a prepubertal population. J Urol 1997;158:1191–2.

[12] Rabbani F, Farivar-Mohseni H, Leon A, et al. Clinical outcome after retroperitoneal lymphadenectomy of patients with pure testicular teratoma. Urology 2003;62:1092–6.

[13] Rushton HG, Belman AB, Sesterhenn I, et al. Testicular sparing surgery for prepubertal teratoma of the testis: a clinical and pathologic study. J Urol 1990; 144:726–30.

[14] Sesterhenn IA, Weiss RB, Mostofi FK, et al. Prognosis and other clinical correlates of pathologic review in stage I and II testicular carcinoma: a report from the testicular cancer intergroup study. J Clin Oncol 1992;10:69–78.

[15] Stevens MJ, Norman AR, Fischer C, et al. Prognosis of testicular teratoma differentiated. Br J Urol 1994;73:701–6.

[16] Leibovitch I, Foster RS, Ulbright TM, et al. Adult primary pure teratoma of the testis: the Indiana experience. Cancer 1995;75:2244–50.

[17] Simmonds PD, Lee AHS, Theaker JM, et al. Primary pure teratoma of the testis. J Urol 1996;155:939–42.

[18] Heidenreich A, Moul JW, McLeod DG, et al. The role of retroperitoneal lymphadenectomy in mature teratoma of the testis. J Urol 1997;157:160–3.

[19] Read G, Stenning SP, Cullen MH, et al. Medical Research Council prospective study of surveillance for stage I testicular teratoma. J Clin Oncol 1992;10:1762–8.

[20] Pohar K, Rabbani F, Bosl G, et al. Results of retroperitoneal lymph node dissection for clinical stage I and II pure embryonal carcinoma of the testis. J Urol 2003;170:1155–8.

[21] Sogani PC, Perrotti M, Herr HW, et al. Clinical stage I testis cancer: long-term outcome of patients on surveillance. J Urol 1998;159:855–8.

[22] Carver BS, Bianco FJ, Shayegan B, et al. Predicting teratoma in the retroperitoneum for men undergoing post-chemotherapy retroperitoneal lymph node dissection. J Urol 2006;176:100–3.

[23] Debono DJ, Heilman DK, Einhorn LH, et al. Decision analysis for avoiding postchemotherapy surgery in patients with disseminated nonseminomatous germ cell tumors. J Clin Oncol 1997;15:1455–64.

[24] Beck SD, Foster RS, Bihrle R, et al. Teratoma in the orchiectomy specimen and volume of metastasis are predictors of retroperitoneal teratoma in post-chemotherapy nonseminomatous testis cancer. J Urol 2002;168:1402–4.

[25] Fossa SD, Ous S, Lien HH, et al. Post-chemotherapy lymph node histology in radiologically normal patients with metastatic nonseminomatous testicular cancer. J Urol 1989;141:557–9.

[26] Rabbani F, Gleave ME, Coppin CM, et al. Teratoma in primary testis tumor reduces complete response rates in the retroperitoneum after primary chemotherapy: case for primary retroperitoneal lymph node dissection in stage IIB germ cell tumors with teratomatous elements. Cancer 1996;78:480–6.

[27] Steyerberg EW, Keizer HJ, Fossa SD, et al. Prediction of residual retroperitoneal mass histology after chemotherapy for metastatic nonseminomatous germ cell tumor: multivariate analysis of individual patient data from six study groups. J Clin Oncol 1995;13:1177–87.

[28] Loehrer PJ, Hui S, Clark S, et al. Teratoma following cisplatin-based combination chemotherapy for nonseminomatous germ cell tumors: a clinicopathological correlation. J Urol 1986;135:1183–9.

[29] Sonneveld DJ, Sleifer DT, Koops HS, et al. Mature teratoma identified after post-chemotherapy surgery in patients with disseminated nonseminomatous testicular germ cell tumors. Cancer 1998;82:1343–51.

[30] Fossa SD, Aass N, Ous S, et al. Histology of tumor residuals following chemotherapy in patients with advanced nonseminomatous testicular cancer. J Urol 1989;142:1239–42.

[31] Carver BS, Shayegan B, Serio A, et al. Long-term clinical outcome following post-chemotherapy retroperitoneal lymph node dissection in men with residual teratoma. J Clin Oncol 2007;25:1033–7.

[32] Motzer RJ, Amsterdam A, Prieto V, et al. Teratoma with malignant transformation: diverse malignant histologies arising in men with germ cell tumors. J Urol 1998;159:133–8.

[33] Baniel J, Foster RS, Gonin R, et al. Late relapse of testicular cancer. J Clin Oncol 1995;13:1170–6.

[34] McKiernan JM, Motzer RJ, Bajorin DF, et al. Reoperative retroperitoneal surgery for nonseminomatous germ cell tumor: clinical presentation, patterns of recurrence, and outcome. Urology 2003;62:732–6.

[35] Comiter CV, Kibel AS, Richie JP, et al. Prognostic features of teratomas with malignant transformation: a clinicopathological study of 21 cases. J Urol 1998;159:859–63.

[36] Donadio AC, Motzer RJ, Bajorin DF, et al. Chemotherapy for teratoma with malignant transformation. J Clin Oncol 2003;21:4285–91.

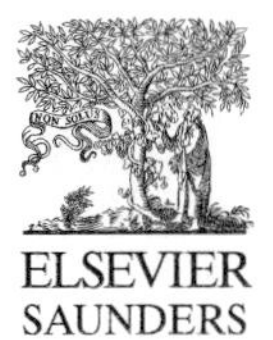
ELSEVIER
SAUNDERS

Urol Clin N Am 34 (2007) 253–258

UROLOGIC CLINICS of North America

Late Relapse of Testis Cancer

Yaron Ehrlich, MD[a], Jack Baniel, MD[a,b,*]

[a]*Department of Urology, Rabin Medical Center–Beilinson Campus, Petah Tikva 49100, Israel*
[b]*Sackler Medical School, Tel Aviv University, P.O. Box 39040, Tel Aviv 69978, Israel*

The introduction of cisplatin-based chemotherapy for the treatment of testicular germ-cell tumors (GCTs) in the late 1970s transformed testicular cancer into a model of a curable neoplasm [1]. Its combination with surgery in men with advanced disease has led to a cure rate of approximately 80% [2]. Relapse occurs in about 10% of patients, mostly in the first 2 years after treatment [3,4].

Reports of late relapse, beyond 2 years, date back to the early 1970s [5]; however, the first to describe late relapse of GCT as a unique clinical entity were Einhorn and colleagues [6] from Indiana University. In the past decade, further data from Indiana University and other leading cancer centers have consistently shown that late-relapse GCT behaves differently from primary or early-relapse GCT in terms of tumor biology and response. The aim of the present review was to outline the clinical characteristics, tumor biology, and therapeutic outcome of late relapse.

Definition

Late relapse of GCT is defined as follows:

- Initial diagnosis of seminomatous or nonseminomatous testicular GCT.
- Recurrence of GCT established by biopsy, marker elevation, or growth at a previously stable GCT site.
- Interval of more than 2 years since successful treatment of the initial GCT.

To establish the diagnosis, the presence of a second primary testicular neoplasm or extragonadal GCT and secondary causes of marker elevation should be excluded. Physical examination and ultrasound of the remaining testicle are of major importance. A false-positive elevation of beta-human chorionic gonadotropin (HCG) can occur from cross-reaction of substances such as marijuana or luteinizing hormone (LH). LH is elevated in hypogonadism, and may be reduced in these cases by administration of testosterone. A false-positive elevation of alpha-fetoprotein (AFP) can occur in association with liver disease or drug abuse (alcohol or cocaine).

Incidence

The first report from Indiana University [6] included 81 patients who were diagnosed with late-relapse GCT from 1979 to 1992. Although the true incidence of late relapse could not be calculated because many of the patients were referrals who were initially treated outside the university center, the incidence could be deducted by limiting the study population to men with stage II/III testicular cancer who entered first-line chemotherapy protocols at Indiana University. This analysis yielded 17 men with late relapse out of a total of 590 men treated for primary GCT during the study period (2.9%). Accordingly, data from Memorial Sloan-Kettering Cancer Center (MSKCC) showed a 3% rate of GCT relapse at 2 years after receipt of first-line chemotherapy for viable GCT, for an incidence of 3.1 per 1000 years of follow-up [7]. Similar rates ranging from 2.3% to 4.3% have been reported from European centers [8–10].

Late relapse of stage I GCT has also been described. Studies of surveillance programs [11–16] comprising a total of 1419 patients with stage

* Corresponding author. Department of Urology, Rabin Medical Center, Beilinson Campus, Petah Tikva 49100, Israel.

E-mail address: edithr@clalit.org.il (J. Baniel).

0094-0143/07/$ - see front matter
doi:10.1016/j.ucl.2007.02.012

I GCT patients managed by orchiectomy and active surveillance recorded an overall late relapse rate of 1.9%. Similar rates were observed among seminomatous and nonseminomatous GCT.

Patient characteristics

In most of the patients in the MSKCC [7] and Indiana University [6,17] series, the pathological diagnosis of the initial tumor was nonseminomatous GCT (Table 1). However, these data should be interpreted with caution because of the bias inherent in series from major specialized centers, which include many patients with advanced disease who either failed first-line chemotherapy or had unresectable tumors at diagnosis and were referred for further treatment. The findings of Dieckmann and colleagues [18] in an unselected group of patients with late relapse may represent the actual incidence more accurately. These authors reported that of 122 patients from 24 institutions in Germany with a diagnosis of late-relapse GCT, 50 (41%) had had a primary pure testicular seminoma. Gerl and colleagues [9] found a similar risk for late relapse in patients with nonseminomatous and seminomatous GCT.

The time to relapse according to several large studies ranges widely, from 2 to 32 years, with a median of 7 to 10 years [6,7,17]. Although many years may pass before a person becomes symptomatic, the time to relapse beyond the third year is unpredictable, often leading patients and physicians to stop follow-up after this point. Accordingly, studies report that 60% to 72% of late relapses are detected by the presence of symptoms, and only 28% to 40% by elevated markers or abnormal radiographic studies [7,17]. In the series presented by Dieckmann and colleagues [18], patients were diagnosed earlier, at a median interval of 4 years to late relapse, and more cases (61%) were detected during routine follow-up. The proportion of patients presenting with symptoms appeared to be directly associated with the length of follow-up.

The most common site of late relapse is the retroperitoneum (47% to 83% of patients), followed by the lungs and mediastinum. Accordingly, the most common symptoms are back and abdominal pain. Several studies found that in 48% to 65% of patients who later developed late recurrences, the initial tumor was limited to the retroperitoneum [6,7,17]. Less common sites of relapse are the cervical nodes, liver, bone, and brain [5–7,9,10,17–19]. In 57% of patients, the disease is limited to one anatomical site [17].

Most patients with late relapse of nonseminomatous GCT have elevated levels of tumor markers. AFP is the predominant marker in this subgroup (76% to 52% of patients), followed by HCG (28% to 10% of patients) [5–7,9,17,18]. In some cases (10% of patients with nonseminomatous GCT), HCG is the only elevated marker at late relapse [18]. The increase in AFP may precede the radiologic detection of late relapse by 2 to 44

Table 1
Patient characteristics at late relapse

Characteristic	Baniel et al 1995 [6]	George et al 2003 [17]	Gerl et al 1997 [9]	Ronnen et al 2005 [7]
No. of patients	81	83	25	29
Time to relapse, y, n (%)				
2–5	34 (42)	23 (28)	11 (44)	6 (21)
>5	47 (58)	60 (72)	14 (56)	23 (79)
Pure seminoma	2 (2)	3 (4)	1 (4)	0
Nonseminoma	79 (98)	80 (96)	24 (96)	29 (100)
Elevated markers	54/76 (71)	55/82 (67)	17/24 (71)	NA
Recurrence pathology, N (%)				
Cancer	66 (81)	66/80 (83)	22 (88)	NA
Teratoma	15 (19)	14/80 (17)	3 (12)	NA
Tumor site, n (%)				
Retroperitoneum	43 (53)	39 (47)	12 (48)	24 (83)
Lungs	19 (23)	21 (25)	2 (8)	11 (38)
Mediastinum	10 (12)	8 (10)	8 (32)	8 (28)

Abbreviation: NA, not applicable.

months [5,9,17], reflecting the slow-growing nature of some of the tumors. The predominance of AFP as a marker of late relapse in nonseminomatous GCT might be explained by the finding at Indiana University that yolk-sac tumor was the most common germ-cell subtype in the patients with recurrences [17].

Late-relapsing seminomatous GCT has somewhat different characteristics. Dieckmann and colleagues [18] found that 80% of the late-recurring seminomas in their series developed in patients with a first stage I tumor. The estimated risk of recurrence was 0.6% for patients after adjuvant radiotherapy for stage I seminomatous GCT [20,21], and 1.9% for patients on surveillance programs [12,13,16]. Late relapse after radiation therapy for stage I seminomatous GCT tends to occur outside the radiation field [20,21]. LDH is the predominant marker at late relapse in this subgroup (52%), followed by HCG (33%) and AFP (9%) [18].

Risk factors for late relapse

Late relapse has been well documented after first-line and salvage chemotherapy [6,7], and it has been described after primary retroperitoneal lymph node dissection (RPLND) for low-stage nonseminomatous GCT [6,22], after postchemotherapy RPLND [7,23], and after adjuvant radiotherapy for stage I seminomatous GCT [20,21]. Late relapse may even appear during surveillance for stage I testicular GCT [13]. Thus, although previous treatment modalities may change the clinical behavior of the tumor, the propensity of GCT to relapse late is inherent in its biology.

MSKCC experience with first-line chemotherapy for good-risk GCT by International Germ Cell Consensus Classification criteria showed a lower rate of late relapse [24] compared with previously reported data from unselected patients treated with first-line chemotherapy in the same institute [7]. Although Gerl and colleagues [9] also reported a lower rate of late relapse in "good-risk" nonseminomatous GCT (Medical Research Council criteria), others did not find the initial stage of disease to be an independent predictor of late relapse [6,8,19].

Dieckmann and colleagues [18] found that early first relapse after treatment of nonseminomatous GCT is a risk factor for a second, late relapse, reported in 19% of their series. Gerl and colleagues [9] calculated a cumulative relapse risk of 9.4% at 5 years for individuals with early relapse.

The more than 300 patients with late relapse reported in the literature did not have common characteristics, making the identification of patients at risk very difficult.

Teratoma and inadequate control of the retroperitoneum

Teratoma seems to play an important role in late relapse. In the Indiana University experience, 60% of patients with late recurrence had teratoma, either alone or in combination with other cell types [25]. Non–germ-cell malignant tumors, mostly sarcomas and adenocarcinoma, were detected in 23% of patients with late recurrence. The malignant transformation of teratoma was believed to be responsible for this finding [26]. Others have suggested that mature teratoma may retain its ability to dedifferentiate into viable GCT over many years [27], thereby accounting for the entire spectrum of histologies at late relapse.

The excision of all masses after chemotherapy, within and outside the boundaries of the retroperitoneum, is integral to the cure of nonseminomatous GCT [28]. Studies have shown that approximately 40% of all resected postchemotherapy residual masses were teratomas [29]. Patients who initially had large bulky retroperitoneal tumors with teratomatous elements were at increased risk of relapse [27].

At the time of postchemotherapy RPLND, teratomatous masses may grow large and adhere to vital organs, making complete resection difficult. By the same token, microscopic teratoma inside normal-appearing lymph nodes may escape removal if a policy of tumorectomy-only is applied. Wood and colleagues [30], in a study of 113 patients undergoing bilateral template postchemotherapy RPLND for nonseminomatous GCT, identified tumor outside the boundaries of the modified template in 14 patients (12%), 9 of whom had micrometastases outside a palpable mass. In a study by Oldenburg and colleagues [31], 26% of patients with residual mass of up to 2 cm at the time of postchemotherapy RPLND had a teratoma in the retroperitoneum.

Adequate control of the retroperitoneum might reduce the risk of relapse at a site that is difficult and costly to monitor. Sonneveld and colleagues [23] showed that incomplete resection of teratoma led to late-relapsing teratoma and non–germ-cell tumors. The proper extent of postchemotherapy surgical resection and methods for patient selection for the procedure remain controversial [32]. The current policy of leading referral centers in North America is to perform bilateral template postchemotherapy RPLND. In Indiana University, no late retroperitoneal relapses were noted after this procedure [6].

Treatment of late-relapsing tumor

Surgery

Surgery is the preferred treatment modality for resectable tumors at late relapse [7,9,17,33]. This is true for patients with marker-negative tumor masses who are at risk of teratoma and non-GCT, and patients with marker-positive resectable tumor at a single site. If the tumor is completely resected and tumor markers normalize postoperatively, the patient will probably not benefit from adjuvant chemotherapy [9].

In the early Indiana University series, 20% of patients were managed with surgery alone, and 69% of them remained disease-free [6]. Eight years later, the Indiana University group updated their study on late relapse [17] and found, not surprisingly, that a greater percentage of patients (59%) had been treated with primary surgery, of whom 92% achieved a no evidence of disease (NED) status and 46% were continuously disease-free. Patients rendered disease-free by primary resection of a tumor at only one site fared better than those operated on at more than one site [17].

The most prominent risk factor for treatment failure was the presence of viable cancer at the relapse site [6].

Chemotherapy

As a single modality of therapy, surgery is superior to chemotherapy at producing a durable NED state. Although some late tumors respond to chemotherapy, the disease is rarely cured by this modality alone. This may be explained by the histological characteristics of the late tumors, which are usually viable GCT, teratoma, and teratoma with malignant transformation, which do not respond as readily as primary GCTs to cisplatin-based regimens. With the possible exception of chemotherapy-naïve patients, who are discussed in the next section, the only candidates for chemotherapy are patients with unresectable disease, in whom treatment may make the disease operable or less likely, achieve a durable complete remission. For chemotherapy to be successful, it should be followed by surgery [6,10,17,33]. In the updated study from Indiana University, 32 patients received chemotherapy alone. Only six (19%) achieved complete remission, including five who remained continuously disease-free (of whom three were chemotherapy-naïve). Another 18 patients (56%) were rendered disease-free by postchemotherapy surgery, of whom 12 (38%) remained continuously disease-free [17].

In a selected group of patients referred to the MSKCC for salvage chemotherapy at late relapse, only a regimen of paclitaxel, ifosfamide, and cisplatin followed by surgery was found to be effective; 7 of 29 patients achieved long-term complete remission [7]. Long-term complete remission following chemotherapy alone has also been documented in selected patients [7,17,19].

Chemotherapy in the chemotherapy-naïve patient

Chemotherapy-naïve patients constitute a unique group and include patients with stage I GCT on surveillance or after radiotherapy, and patients with stage II nonseminomatous GCT after primary RPLND. Most of the late-relapse GCTs in chemotherapy-naïve patients [6,12,13,15,17,34], including those exposed to radiotherapy [18,20, 21,35], respond to chemotherapy.

In addition, recurrence can be effectively reduced in stage I seminomas by adjuvant treatment with a single-agent carboplatin regimen. Although data on late relapse in this patient group are still lacking, there is evidence that although not naïve to chemotherapy, they maintain chemosensitivity [34,35].

Treatment of marker-only late relapse

In the study by Gerl and colleagues [9], an increase in AFP occurred in 16 patients with late relapse. In 12 of them, the increase was documented 6 to 44 months (median 27 months) before radiological detection of the tumor. Other reports have confirmed this observation [5,7,17,36]. In one case, late relapse was diagnosed solely on the basis of an elevation in HCG [17]. Positron emission tomography identified the disease site in only a minority of patients. Ultimately, the disease was detected in most patients by computed tomography scan [17]. Given the unfavorable results of chemotherapy at late relapse, it is reasonable to withhold any treatment until the disease site is apparent and amenable to surgical excision.

Recurrent relapse after late relapse

Patients after successful treatment of a late recurrence are at risk of both early and late repeated relapse. In the Indiana University series, 44% of patients with a first relapse had a second one after achieving a NED state [17]. A durable response was achieved in only 30% of patients, mainly by surgery. In almost 20% of cases, the second relapse occurred more than 2 years after complete response of the first late relapse [6]. Elevated AFP levels at first relapse may be associated with a higher risk of second late relapse [6]. The outcome of patients with recurrent relapses is poor.

Molecular analysis of late relapse

The chemotherapy resistance of GCT is an important biological and clinical problem at late relapse. A search for genetic mechanisms suggested that gene amplification may be associated with drug resistance [37]. More recently, KIT and the epidermal growth factor receptor (EGFR) were found to be expressed in a significant proportion of refractory GCTs, either late-relapse tumors or transformed teratoma [38]. Sugimora and colleagues [39], using microarray technology with gene-expression profiling, identified a gene set that can differentiate patients with early- and late-relapse yolk-sac GCT. The most over expressed gene in the late-relapse group was a small nuclear ribonucleoprotein 70-kD polypeptide.

References

[1] Einhorn LH. Testicular cancer as a model for a curable neoplasm: the Richard and Hinda Rosenthal Foundation Award Lecture. Cancer Res 1981;41(9 Pt 1):3275–80.

[2] Bosl GJ, Motzer RJ. Testicular germ-cell cancer. N Engl J Med 1997;337(4):242–53.

[3] Williams SD, Birch R, Einhorn LH, et al. Treatment of disseminated germ-cell tumors with cisplatin, bleomycin, and either vinblastine or etoposide. N Engl J Med 1987;316(23):1435–40.

[4] Bosl GJ, Gluckman R, Geller NL, et al. VAB-6: an effective chemotherapy regimen for patients with germ-cell tumors. J Clin Oncol 1986;4(10):1493–9.

[5] Lipphardt ME, Albers P. Late relapse of testicular cancer. World J Urol 2004;22(1):47–54.

[6] Baniel J, Foster RS, Gonin R, et al. Late relapse of testicular cancer. J Clin Oncol 1995;13(5):1170–6.

[7] Ronnen EA, Kondagunta GV, Bacik J, et al. Incidence of late-relapse germ cell tumor and outcome to salvage chemotherapy. J Clin Oncol 2005; 23(28):6999–7004.

[8] Shahidi M, Norman AR, Dearnaley DP, et al. Late recurrence in 1263 men with testicular germ cell tumors. Multivariate analysis of risk factors and implications for management. Cancer 2002;95(3):520–30.

[9] Gerl A, Clemm C, Schmeller N, et al. Late relapse of germ cell tumors after cisplatin-based chemotherapy. Ann Oncol 1997;8(1):41–7.

[10] Ravi R, Oliver RT, Ong J, et al. A single-centre observational study of surgery and late malignant events after chemotherapy for germ cell cancer. Br J Urol 1997;80(4):647–52.

[11] Gels ME, Hoekstra HJ, Sleijfer DT, et al. Detection of recurrence in patients with clinical stage I nonseminomatous testicular germ cell tumors and consequences for further follow-up: a single-center 10-year experience. J Clin Oncol 1995;13(5):1188–94.

[12] Francis R, Bower M, Brunstrom G, et al. Surveillance for stage I testicular germ cell tumours: results and cost benefit analysis of management options. Eur J Cancer 2000;36(15):1925–32.

[13] Daugaard G, Petersen PM, Rorth M. Surveillance in stage I testicular cancer. APMIS 2003;111(1):76–83.

[14] Nicolai N, Pizzocaro G. A surveillance study of clinical stage I nonseminomatous germ cell tumors of the testis: 10-year follow-up. J Urol 1995;154(3):1045–9.

[15] Boyer MJ, Cox K, Tattersall MH, et al. Active surveillance after orchiectomy for nonseminomatous testicular germ cell tumors: late relapse may occur. Urology 1997;50(4):588–92.

[16] Sogani PC, Perrotti M, Herr HW, et al. Clinical stage I testis cancer: long-term outcome of patients on surveillance. J Urol 1998;159(3):855–8.

[17] George DW, Foster RS, Hromas RA, et al. Update on late relapse of germ cell tumor: a clinical and molecular analysis. J Clin Oncol 2003;21(1):113–22.

[18] Dieckmann KP, Albers P, Classen J, et al. Late relapse of testicular germ cell neoplasms: a descriptive analysis of 122 cases. J Urol 2005;173(3):824–9.

[19] Kuczyk MA, Bokemeyer C, Kollmannsberger C, et al. Late relapse after treatment for nonseminomatous testicular germ cell tumors according to a single center-based experience. World J Urol 2004;22(1):55–9.

[20] Jones WG, Fossa SD, Mead GM, et al. Randomized trial of 30 versus 20 Gy in the adjuvant treatment of stage I testicular seminoma: a report on Medical Research Council Trial TE18, European Organisation for the Research and Treatment of Cancer Trial 30942 (ISRCTN18525328). J Clin Oncol 2005; 23(6):1200–8.

[21] Fossa SD, Horwich A, Russell JM, et al. Optimal planning target volume for stage I testicular seminoma: a Medical Research Council randomized trial. Medical Research Council Testicular Tumor Working Group. J Clin Oncol 1999;17(4):1146–54.

[22] Stephenson AJ, Bosl GJ, Bajorin DF, et al. Retroperitoneal lymph node dissection in patients with low stage testicular cancer with embryonal carcinoma predominance and/or lymphovascular invasion. J Urol 2005;174(2):557–60.

[23] Sonneveld DJ, Sleijfer DT, Koops HS, et al. Mature teratoma identified after postchemotherapy surgery in patients with disseminated nonseminomatous testicular germ cell tumors: a plea for an aggressive surgical approach. Cancer 1998;82(7):1343–51.
[24] Kondagunta GV, Bacik J, Bajorin D, et al. Etoposide and cisplatin chemotherapy for metastatic good-risk germ cell tumors. J Clin Oncol 2005; 23(36):9290–4.
[25] Michael H, Lucia J, Foster RS, et al. The pathology of late recurrence of testicular germ cell tumors. Am J Surg Pathol 2000;24(2):257–73.
[26] Motzer RJ, Amsterdam A, Prieto V, et al. Teratoma with malignant transformation: diverse malignant histologies arising in men with germ cell tumors. J Urol 1998;159(1):133–8.
[27] Loehrer PJ Sr., Hui S, Clark S, et al. Teratoma following cisplatin-based combination chemotherapy for nonseminomatous germ cell tumors: a clinicopathological correlation. J Urol 1986;135(6): 1183–9.
[28] Fizazi K, Tjulandin S, Salvioni R, et al. Viable malignant cells after primary chemotherapy for disseminated nonseminomatous germ cell tumors: prognostic factors and role of postsurgery chemotherapy—results from an international study group. J Clin Oncol 2001;19(10):2647–57.
[29] Steyerberg EW, Keizer HJ, Fossa SD, et al. Prediction of residual retroperitoneal mass histology after chemotherapy for metastatic nonseminomatous germ cell tumor: multivariate analysis of individual patient data from six study groups. J Clin Oncol 1995;13(5):1177–87.
[30] Wood DP Jr, Herr HW, Heller G, et al. Distribution of retroperitoneal metastases after chemotherapy in patients with nonseminomatous germ cell tumors. J Urol 1992;148(6):1812–5.
[31] Oldenburg J, Alfsen GC, Lien HH, et al. Postchemotherapy retroperitoneal surgery remains necessary in patients with nonseminomatous testicular cancer and minimal residual tumor masses. J Clin Oncol 2003;21(17):3310–7.
[32] Foster RS, Beck S, Bihrle R. Secondary surgery in germ cell tumors—when and how extensively should it be performed? World J Urol 2004;22(1):37–40.
[33] Schmoll HJ, Souchon R, Krege S, et al. European consensus on diagnosis and treatment of germ cell cancer: a report of the European Germ Cell Cancer Consensus Group (EGCCCG). Ann Oncol 2004;15(9):1377–99.
[34] Aparicio J, Garcia del Muro X, Maroto P, et al. Multicenter study evaluating a dual policy of postorchiectomy surveillance and selective adjuvant single-agent carboplatin for patients with clinical stage I seminoma. Ann Oncol 2003;14(6):867–72.
[35] Oliver RT, Mason MD, Mead GM, et al. Radiotherapy versus single-dose carboplatin in adjuvant treatment of stage I seminoma: a randomised trial. Lancet 2005;366(9482):293–300.
[36] Muramaki M, Hara I, Miyake H, et al. Clinical study of six cases showing late relapse of germ cell tumors. Int J Urol 2005;12(9):855–8.
[37] Rao PH, Houldsworth J, Palanisamy N, et al. Chromosomal amplification is associated with cisplatin resistance of human male germ cell tumors. Cancer Res 1998;58(19):4260–3.
[38] Madani A, Kemmer K, Sweeney C, et al. Expression of KIT and epidermal growth factor receptor in chemotherapy refractory non-seminomatous germ-cell tumors. Ann Oncol 2003;14(6):873–80.
[39] Sugimura J, Foster RS, Cummings OW, et al. Gene expression profiling of early- and late-relapse nonseminomatous germ cell tumor and primitive neuroectodermal tumor of the testis. Clin Cancer Res 2004; 10(7):2368–78.

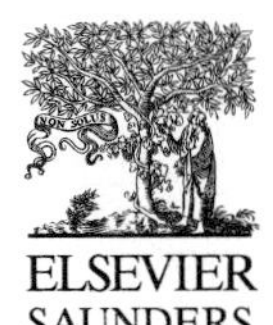

ELSEVIER
SAUNDERS

Urol Clin N Am 34 (2007) 259–268

UROLOGIC
CLINICS
of North America

Short- and Long-Term Complications of Therapy for Testicular Cancer

Melissa R. Kaufman, MD, PhD, Sam S. Chang, MD*

Vanderbilt University, Department of Urologic Surgery, A-1302 Medical Center North, Nashville, TN 37232, USA

Testicular germ-cell carcinoma, although a rare disease accounting for only 1% to 2% of all neoplasms in men, is distinguished by being the most common malignancy afflicting young men under 45 years of age [1,2]. The worldwide incidence of testicular cancer has shown an alarming increase during the past 40 years [3,4], with more than 8000 cases predicted in the United States in 2005 [5]. Fortunately, with this increasing incidence there has been a concomitant decrease in mortality. For low-stage disease, 5-year survival is estimated at greater than 90% [6]. Multimodal treatment strategies have contributed dramatically to this success.

However, the armamentarium used to provide this long-term survival is not without possible significant sequela for this young patient population [7,8]. Herein we review the treatments used for testicular cancer and the complications associated with each modality of therapy (Table 1). The treatment regimen used for any testicular neoplasm depends on histopathology of the specific tumor and is discussed elsewhere. Staging and treatment are based on primary pathology, involvement of regional lymph nodes, and evidence of metastatic disease, as well as levels of serum tumor markers [9]. It is imperative the clinician recognize possible treatment-related morbidity when counseling and monitoring testicular cancer patients.

Surgical complications

The gold standard for treatment of all primary tumors is unilateral radical inguinal orchiectomy with high ligation of the spermatic cord [10]. Inguinal orchiectomy provides not only histopathologic and staging information but also local control of the neoplasm and, potentially, a complete cure for patients with testis-confined disease.

Although morbidity is limited, the most frequent complication from inguinal orchiectomy is bleeding from the spermatic vessels into the scrotum or retroperitoneum. Misinterpretation of retroperitoneal hematomas as metastatic disease may result in unnecessary treatments [11]. Inappropriate scrotal violation, reported in up to 17% of cases, can alter lymphatic drainage and/or contaminate the scrotum with neoplastic cells resulting in a risk of local recurrence between 2.9% and 11% [12–14]. Wide excision of the scrotal scar should be performed in such cases. Additional treatment for seminoma should include extension of the radiation field to include the ipsilateral groin and scrotum, although systemic cytotoxic therapies do not demonstrate a survival advantage.

Orchiectomy can have a damaging psychosocial consequence resulting in impairments in body image and self-perception [15]. Fortunately, most men treated for testicular cancer eventually regain normal body image [16]. Insertion of a testicular prosthesis is a viable option to improve scrotal cosmesis following orchiectomy, although the implant itself is not without possible associated complications such as pain, infection, and lymphadenopathy [17–19]

Retroperitoneal lymph node dissection

Germ-cell tumors can have a propensity for lymphatic metastasis with retroperitoneal metastases

* Corresponding author.
E-mail address: sam.chang@vanderbilt.edu (S.S. Chang).

0094-0143/07/$ - see front matter
doi:10.1016/j.ucl.2007.02.011

Table 1
Treatment complications

	Surgical	Chemotherapy	Radiotherapy
Short term	Bleeding from spermatic vessels Surgical site infection Body image impairment Vascular injury Bowel injury Lymphocele, chylous ascites Ureteral injury Thromboembolic complications Pancreatitis Bowel obstruction	Hematologic toxicity Mucositis Sensory neuropathy Ototoxicity Fatigue Pulmonary toxicity Hemorrhagic cystitis Central nervous system toxicity	Nausea Diarrhea Cutaneous changes Fatigue Anorexia
Long term	Ventral hernia Ejaculatory dysfunction Infertility Bowel obstruction	Leukemia Secondary malignancy Nephrotoxicity Neurotoxicity Ototoxicity Pulmonary toxicity Vascular toxicity Cardiotoxicity Metabolic/hormonal Infertility	Secondary malignancy Cardiotoxicity Infertility

discovered in the lymph nodes of 27% of patients preoperatively deemed to have stage I disease [20–22]. The pattern of lymphatic drainage has been recognized for more than a century and modern analysis has allowed development of strategies for surgical resection of appropriate lymphatic beds via retroperitoneal lymph node dissection (RPLND) [23–27]. Historically, RPLND included a bilateral suprahilar node dissection with associated pancreatic and renovascular complications [28]. RPLND has since evolved to the present standard of modified infrahilar unilateral templates to maximize staging and cancer control while minimizing morbidity [29–31]. However, RPLND is a major surgical procedure and continues to be associated with a variety of potential complications, both short and long term [32,33].

Vascular complications of RPLND

Vascular injury is a rarely reported complication, but can be devastating if unrecognized [32,33]. Vascular injuries are more common in the postchemotherapy RPLND and in those patients with bulky suprahilar disease [7,34]. Injuries to the renal vein are more common on the left because of less spacious anatomy. Careful mobilization of the entire vein and prompt closure of any bleeding are crucial. Complete vascular dissection using the "split and roll" technique can assist in avoiding vascular injury [35]. Renal vein anomalies have been noted in 3.2% of men undergoing RPLND [36]. Preoperative imaging can help in recognizing these vascular anomalies and planning for the appropriate surgical approach.

Bowel complications of RPLND

Direct injury of the bowel during RPLND is rare during primary surgery, and most commonly occurs in the duodenum when resection of large or reactionary masses is attempted [33]. Full-thickness injuries require primary two-layer closure with interposition of omentum to decrease incidence of abscess and fistula. Small bowel fistulas can often be managed conservatively with low-residue diets and intravenous (IV) hyperalimentation. Small bowel obstruction is observed in 0.2% of primary RPLNDs [33], with a higher frequency in the population undergoing bilateral node dissection. Postoperative paralytic ileus is reported in approximately 2% of patients after RPLND and is often responsive to conservative management [32,37].

Lymphatic complications of RPLND

Although rare, lymphoceles that manifest symptoms can occur following transabdominal lymphadenectomy [38]. These are frequently treated with percutaneous surgical drainage with sclerotherapy reserved for persistent drainage

[39], and may occasionally require open drainage and marsupialization.

Transection of major lymphatics, particularly those that drain directly into the cisterna chyli, may result in formation of chylous ascites in around 2% of patients undergoing RPLND [40]. This lymphatic fluid can cause abdominal distention, diaphragmatic irritation, and dyspnea within weeks of surgery. The diagnosis of chylous ascites is confirmed with paracentesis. Treatment strategies include low-fat diets supplemented with medium-chain triglycerides that circumvent small bowel absorption. If these conservative dietary changes are ineffective, IV hyperalimentation is used with or without the somatostatin analogue octreotide [41]. Finally, surgical exploration and ligation or the creation of peritoneovenous shunts may become necessary for recalcitrant cases [33].

Ureteral injury in RPLND

Risk of ureteral injury correlates with post-chemotherapy status, where the incidence is 0.9% [34]. Careful dissection to preserve the adventitial blood supply allows isolation and retraction of the ureter. It is often easiest to locate the ureter at its crossing of the iliac vessels. Immediately recognized injuries should be primarily repaired, but the majority of injuries are often delayed in their presentation and thus close follow-up, particularly in patients with large mass resections, should be helpful in detecting these ureteral complications. In cases with significant retroperitoneal or ureteral involvement, preoperative ureteral stent placement can facilitate dissection and may obviate need for nephrectomy.

General surgical complications of RPLND

Although risk of thromboembolic events is not as pronounced as in pelvic lymph node surgery, prophylaxis for deep vein thrombosis (DVT) should be considered for this major urologic surgery [42]. Routine use of sequential pneumatic compression and early ambulation are commonly used strategies to prevent DVT and associated complications such as pulmonary embolus.

Mobilization and retraction of the duodenum may result in a transient pancreatitis manifested as nausea and emesis in conjunction with elevated serum pancreatic enzymes [43]. Conservative treatment with dietary restriction and/or modification is often sufficient to resolve this temporary pancreatic inflammation.

As in all surgical procedures, wound-healing issues may arise. Superficial infection occurs in approximately 4.8% of patients who have undergone RPLND and is often successfully managed with short-term antibiotic therapy [44]. A recognized late complication is the development of a ventral hernia in 0.8% to 1.6% of patients undergoing RPLND via a midline incision [7,44].

Ejaculatory dysfunction and infertility following RPLND

One of the most troubling long-term morbidities following RPLND is the loss of antegrade ejaculation secondary to intraoperative damage to crucial autonomic nerve fibers. Sympathetic fibers from the thoracolumbar outflow tract decussating around the aortic bifurcation are responsible for seminal emission into the posterior urethra. Ejaculation depends on both autonomic and somatic sacral and lumbar nerves that tighten the bladder neck, relax the external sphincter, and contract the bulbourethral and perineal muscles. Damage to these structures may result in loss of seminal emission or retrograde ejaculation. This loss of antegrade ejaculation is particularly morbid for this young patient population with its associated potential infertility and patients are counseled to consider sperm banking before RPLND. As our understanding of the neuroanatomy associated with ejaculatory dysfunction has evolved, modifications in the techniques used for RPLND have likewise advanced. Current techniques designated as "nerve-sparing" that minimize contralateral dissection and preserve the crucial sympathetic fibers of the hypogastric plexus have resulted in successful return of ejaculation in almost 100% of patients [10,45–47].

Postchemotherapy RPLND

Patients with metastatic germ-cell tumor may undergo cytoreductive chemotherapy before RPLND. Modern imaging has allowed us to identify patients with visible recurrence in the retroperitoneum after primary chemotherapy. RPLND in this patient population may have a higher incidence of complications, up to 35% in some series [32,34,48]. This increased rate reflects a multitude of changes in postchemotherapy patients and likely involves tumor location, size, desmoplastic reaction, and compromised performance status. In addition to the previously mentioned increased incidence of vascular and ureteral injuries in postchemotherapy RPLND patients, neurologic complications also plague this population. Neurologic sequelae range from transient peripheral neuropathies to paraplegia secondary to ischemic spinal cord injury [34,49]. Perioperative management of these RPLND patients must also account for the potential residual toxicities associated with chemotherapy as will be discussed in detail in the following section [50].

Complications of chemotherapy

Before the era of effective chemotherapy, disseminated testicular cancer was uniformly fatal [51]. Fortunately, new therapeutics emerged that have changed the face of testicular cancer [52,53]. The current regimen for chemotherapeutic intervention provides exceptional survival, greater than 80%, even in highly advanced stages of testicular neoplasms [54]. The standard of treatment for patients with disseminated germ-cell tumors is currently a regimen of bleomycin, an antibiotic with antineoplastic activity, etoposide, a DNA topoisomerase inhibitor, and cisplatin, an alkylating agent. This multidrug chemotherapeutic regimen is commonly referred to as BEP. Patients with resistant disease or those who experience relapse will undergo salvage chemotherapy with cisplatin, ifosfamide, and either vinblastine or etoposide. This salvage regimen provides a durable result in approximately 20% to 25% of these previously refractory patients [55]. Even among patients unresponsive to salvage chemotherapy, approximately 25% of patients who undergo high-dose chemotherapy with bone marrow transplantation will have long-term survival. These remarkable and admirable high cure rates are accompanied by long-term sequela for these mostly young survivors of testicular neoplasms [56]. The major categories of identified complications following chemotherapeutic treatment of testicular neoplasms are discussed in the following paragraphs.

Initial chemotherapy

The immediate toxicities associated with administration of BEP chemotherapy are well documented and may include hematologic toxicity (9%), mucositis (25%), sensory neuropathy (20%), ototoxicity (10%), fatigue (39%), and acute pulmonary toxicity (13%) [57]. Salvage chemotherapy regimens that include ifosfamide additionally carry the risk of hemorrhagic cystitis and acute central nervous system toxicity [58,59]. In the mostly young and healthy patient population stricken with testicular cancer, their high performance status allows exceptionally good tolerance to the regimens. Rarely do testicular cancer patients fail to complete their chemotherapeutic cycles secondary to immediate toxicities.

Secondary malignancies

One of the most devastating complications arising from treatment with BEP is the development of therapy-related leukemias, which are frequently refractory to treatment [60,61]. DNA topoisomerase inhibitors, such as etoposide, produce an acute leukemia with an onset 2 to 3 years following treatment. Alkylating agents such as cisplatin may produce leukemia with a prodromal myelodysplastic syndrome that manifests 5 to 7 years following treatment. The risk of leukemia from etoposide treatment is dose related [62]. Risk-benefit analysis has revealed there is one case of therapy-related leukemia per approximately 20 cured patients, with the analysis revealing the benefits of chemotherapeutic intervention outweigh the risks of long-term malignancy [63]. As mentioned above, this risk appears dose related and will thus likely decrease from the recorded 0.5% at 5 years seen with four cycles of BEP when data are available for patients treated with current therapies including lower doses and fewer cycles.

Postchemotherapy testicular cancer survivors are additionally at increased risk for development of secondary primary non–germ-cell malignancies at an incidence of 1.38% [60]. The reported risk is increased over that of the general population for lung cancer, biliary cancer, gastrointestinal cancer, bladder cancer, stomach cancer, and sarcoma [64].

Nephrotoxicity

Nephrotoxicity is a recognized complication of cisplatin-based chemotherapies [7,65]. Clinical presentation may range from metabolic changes such as hypokalemia and hypomagnesemia to acute or chronic renal failure [54]. Approximately one quarter of patients may have a permanent 20% to 30% reduction in glomerular filtration rate; however, most of these patients manifest only moderate clinical symptoms of electrolyte disturbances [66–68].

Neurotoxicity

Cisplatin-based chemotherapy is commonly associated with peripheral neuropathies that are primarily sensory in character [69]. Peripheral digit paresthesia and dysesthesia are common manifestations. Neuronal damage attributable to cisplatin may be present in up to 76% of patients, with clinical symptoms persisting in 20% to 40% [70,71].

A second troubling neurologic consequence of cisplatin-based therapy is ototoxicity, resulting in high-frequency hearing loss and tinnitus [72]. This ototoxicity is dose related and fortunately most patients have subclinical damage or mild symptoms [73].

Pulmonary toxicity

Bleomycin administration has been associated with chronic lung damage that can result in pulmonary fibrosis, and in a small percentage of patients, may eventually result in death. Toxicity is related to total bleomycin dose, exposure to high oxygen concentrations, thoracic radiation, decreased renal function, older age, and history of smoking [74]. Pneumonitis induced by bleomycin typically manifests in the first few months of therapy with symptoms of a nonproductive cough and dyspnea with exertion [75]. Once infectious pneumonitis is excluded, bleomycin is usually discontinued in these patients. Patients receiving bleomycin therapy with suggestions of drug-induced pneumonitis are monitored with pulmonary function tests. A 40% to 60% fall from baseline of the diffusion capacity of carbon monoxide (DLCO), a marker of significant pulmonary compromise, usually terminates bleomycin therapy. Corticosteroids are additionally administered to reduce lung inflammation. In patients who have received bleomycin therapy, it is imperative to perform adequate pulmonary evaluation before future surgical interventions such as RPLND to reduce potential perioperative morbidity [76]. Careful monitoring of fluid management in the bleomycin-treated patient is accomplished by giving a minimal volume to support urine output and hemodynamic stability [50]. In addition, many anesthesiologists promote restriction on the concentration of forced inspired oxygen during surgery; however, studies have demonstrated that inspired oxygen concentration is not an independent risk factor for postoperative pulmonary complications [77].

Vascular toxicity

A strikingly high percentage of patients who undergo chemotherapy with vinblastine and bleomycin for testicular neoplasms manifest episodic vasoconstriction of the digital arteries, commonly referred to as Raynaud's phenomenon [78,79]. These painful spasms manifest on average 10 months following therapy and 20% to 25% of patients may have persistent symptoms for more than 10 years [80]. Neurovascular complications, including cerebrovascular hemorrhage, have been reported following the administration of cisplatin-based therapy for testicular cancer [59,81]. This central nervous system toxicity is postulated to be related to metabolic and vascular abnormalities induced by the chemotherapeutic agent. Clinician awareness of this phenomenon is important in the differential diagnosis of neurologic symptoms in the face of potential brain metastasis.

Cardiotoxicity

Although the mechanism is unknown, patients undergoing cisplatin- and bleomycin-based chemotherapy for testicular cancers are at a greater than twofold increased risk for cardiovascular disease [80,82,83]. Interplay of a variety of metabolic and vascular factors may accelerate atherosclerosis or impact autonomic function [84]. This postchemotherapy cardiac toxicity has been reported to manifest as a devastating myocardial infarction [81,85]. Increases in markers of endothelial injury following cisplatin administration implicate this agent in damage to the endothelium that may contribute to its cardiovascular toxicity [86].

Metabolic and hormonal disturbances

Profound derangements of plasma and intracellular ion concentrations have been demonstrated following treatment with cisplatin-based chemotherapies [87,88]. Alterations in the balance of magnesium and potassium may present as simple fatigue or life-threatening Torsades des pointes. Changes in plasma values may precede a measurable compromise of renal function. Hypomagnesemia may lead to vasospasm of coronary arteries and contribute to the increased incidence of cardiovascular disease in testicular cancer patients treated with platinum-based chemotherapies [89].

Metabolic abnormalities such as increases in serum cholesterol may contribute to long-term cardiovascular pathology in patients treated with chemotherapy, including changes in total testosterone and urinary cortisol [90].

Infertility

Striking men in their prime reproductive years, fertility is a crucial issue to address for the survivor of testicular cancer. Curiously, up to 60% of patients diagnosed with testicular cancer have abnormal semen analysis including lower sperm counts and higher serum follicle-stimulating hormone (FSH) levels [91]. Chemotherapy has well-documented adverse effects on semen quality, particularly with platinum-based regimens [92]. The effects of chemotherapy on fertility have been reported to be less profound than those seen with radiation therapy [93]; however, recent paternity data revealed low-dose chemotherapy and radiation treatments to be equally deleterious to fertility with high-dose chemotherapy resulting in the lowest paternity rates [94]. Hormonal dysfunction, including elevation of FSH following chemotherapy has been correlated with this decreased paternity [95]. The most common manifestations on seminal parameters are impairment of spermatogenesis leading to azoospermia. This phenomenon was found to be dependent on the total dose of cisplatin given [96]. Much of this testicular damage appears to be transient, and may resolve in up to 80% of cases by 5 years [97]. Although decreased sperm counts do not preclude fathering children [98], discussion on sperm cryopreservation and assisted reproductive technologies should be initiated in all patients who must undergo chemotherapy for testicular cancer [99,100].

Miscellaneous complications

A number of case reports of unusual complications following chemotherapy for testicular cancer exist. Osteonecrosis of the femoral head was reported in three testicular cancer patients following BEP chemotherapy and treatment with the commonly prescribed antiemetic ondansetron, a serotonin receptor antagonist, in conjunction with dexamethasone [101]. Bilateral spontaneous pneumothorax was reported after implementation of a salvage chemotherapy regimen [102]. One case of gynecomastia has been reported in a young man in complete remission with normal values of beta-human chorionic gonadotropin (BHCG) following BEP combination chemotherapy [103]. This postchemotherapy gynecomastia resolved spontaneously over an 8-month time period.

Complications of radiation therapy

Following orchiectomy, a treatment for early stage seminoma is retroperitoneal radiation therapy (XRT). Seminoma is exquisitely sensitive to radiation and cure rates for low-stage disease approach 100%. Acute side effects are predominantly gastrointestinal, with mild nausea being reported in approximately half of the patients undergoing XRT [104,105]. Less frequently reported side effects during therapy include diarrhea and cutaneous toxicity. Significant incidences of long-term morbidity in regards to secondary malignancies as well as cardiac disease have been recognized [106,107]. In a substantial cohort of patients treated over a 48-year period at a single institution, standardized mortality ratios for cancer-specific and cardiac-related deaths were 1.61 and 1.91 respectively, indicating significant excess risk in this post-XRT population as compared to controls. Subdiaphragmatic radiotherapy to the para-aortic and ipsilateral iliac has also been found to have a greater deleterious effect on fertility than chemotherapy [93].

Complications of surveillance

For patients with clinical stage I disease with favorable histopathologic features, management options include surveillance following primary orchiectomy [108,109]. Surveillance entails an exceptionally motivated and compliant patient willing to undergo a rigorous regimen of physical exam, serum tumor markers, and radiographic studies [110].

While limiting the morbidity of an invasive surgical procedure or radiation therapy, relapse can and does happen with rates that approach 25% to 35% [111–113]. Up to 30% of patients with the diagnosis of clinical stage I disease are found to have pathologic stage II disease following RPLND, indicating a substantial risk of understaging [20–22]. The majority of patients on surveillance relapse in the first 2 years, although recurrences much later have been reported. Additionally, a substantial proportion of patients on surveillance who relapse will be found with high-volume or systemic disease [114].

Poor adherence with the follow-up regimen is common, elucidating the burden of the clinician to use careful patient selection when offering this option for treatment [115]. In addition to disease recurrence, another complication of surveillance is the significant anxiety and possible negative psychological effect on these young, active patients. Finally, surveillance protocols are unlikely to be cost-effective when compared to primary RPLND or radiation therapy [116].

Summary

With rates of cure greater than 90%, the long-term consequences of treatment for testicular cancer are now being appropriately explored. The stress of the cancer diagnosis and therapy, along with frequent surveillance by imaging, blood analysis, and physician visits can create an environment of disease-focused anxiety. Studies performed on survivors of testicular cancer, however, reveal that most do not suffer from a reduced quality of life [16,117]. Indeed, one study indicated survivors of testicular cancer to be more physically active than the general population [118].

We are privileged to practice during an era of such great success in treatment of these previously devastating germ-cell tumors. The fact that long-term complications are recognized underscores the success of the therapeutic modifications. Continued effort to minimize treatment complications while maintaining and even improving efficacy are paramount.

References

[1] Bosl GJ, Motzer RJ. Testicular germ-cell cancer. N Engl J Med 1997;337:242–53.
[2] Oliver RT. Testis cancer. Curr Opin Oncol 1997;9: 287–94.
[3] Huyghe E, Matsuda T, Thonneau P. Increasing incidence of testicular cancer worldwide: a review. J Urol 2003;170:5–11.
[4] McKiernan JM, Goluboff ET, Liberson GL, et al. Rising risk of testicular cancer by birth cohort in the United States from 1973 to 1995. J Urol 1999; 162:361–3.
[5] Carver BS, Sheinfeld J. Germ cell tumors of the testis. Ann Surg Oncol 2005;12:871–80.
[6] International germ cell consensus classification. A prognostic factor-based staging system for metastatic germ cell cancers. International germ cell cancer collaborative group. J Clin Oncol 1997;15: 594–603.
[7] Abouassaly R, Klein EA, Raghavan D. Complications of surgery and chemotherapy for testicular cancer. Urol Oncol 2005;23:447–55.
[8] Grossfeld GD, Small EJ. Long-term side effects of treatment for testis cancer. Urol Clin North Am 1998;25:503–15.
[9] Richie JP, Steele GS. Neoplasms of the testis. In: Walsh PC, editor. Campbell's urology, Eighth Edition. Philadelphia: Saunders; 2002. p. 2876–919.
[10] Sheinfeld J, McKiernan J, Bosl GJ. Surgery of testicular tumors. In: Walsh PC, editor. Campbell's urology, Eighth Edition. Philadelphia: Saunders; 2002. p. 920–44.
[11] Bochner BH, Lerner SP, Kawachi M, et al. Postradical orchiectomy hemorrhage: should an alteration in staging strategy for testicular cancer be considered? Urology 1995;46:408–11.
[12] Capelouto CC, Clark PE, Ransil BJ, et al. A review of scrotal violation in testicular cancer: is adjuvant local therapy necessary? J Urol 1995;153:981–5.
[13] Leibovitch I, Baniel J, Foster RS, et al. The clinical implications of procedural deviations during orchiectomy for nonseminomatous testis cancer. J Urol 1995;154:935–9.
[14] Giguere JK, Stablein DM, Spaulding JT, et al. The clinical significance of unconventional orchiectomy approaches in testicular cancer: a report from the testicular cancer intergroup study. J Urol 1988; 139:1225–8.
[15] van Basten JP, Jonker-Pool G, van Driel MF, et al. Fantasies and facts of the testes. Br J Urol 1996;78: 756–62.
[16] Fleer J, Hoekstra HJ, Sleijfer DT, et al. Quality of life of survivors of testicular germ cell cancer: a review of the literature. Support Care Cancer 2004; 12:476–86.
[17] Chapple A, McPherson A. The decision to have a prosthesis: a qualitative study of men with testicular cancer. Psychooncology 2004;13:654–64.
[18] Herrinton LJ, Brox T, Greenland S, et al. Regarding: a cohort study of systemic and local complications following implantation of testicular prostheses. Ann Epidemiol 2003;13:73–7.
[19] Turek PJ, Master VA. Safety and effectiveness of a new saline-filled testicular prosthesis. J Urol 2004; 172:1427–30.
[20] Sternberg CN. The management of stage I testis cancer. Urol Clin North Am 1998;25:435–49.
[21] Klepp O, Olsson AM, Henrikson H, et al. Prognostic factors in clinical stage I nonseminomatous germ cell tumors of the testis: multivariate analysis of a prospective multicenter study. Swedish-Norwegian testicular cancer group. J Clin Oncol 1990; 8:509–18.
[22] Lashley DB, Lowe BA. A rational approach to managing stage I nonseminomatous germ cell cancer. Urol Clin North Am 1998;25:405–23.
[23] Whitmore W. Some experience with retroperitoneal lymph node dissection and chemotherapy in the management of testis neoplasms. Br J Urol 1962;34:436–47.

[24] Skinner DG, Leadbetter WF. The surgical management of testis tumors. J Urol 1971;106:84–93.

[25] Donohue JP, Zachary JM, Maynard BR. Distribution of nodal metastases in nonseminomatous testis cancer. J Urol 1982;128:315–20.

[26] Weissbach L, Boedefeld EA. Localization of solitary and multiple metastases in stage II nonseminomatous testis tumor as basis for a modified staging lymph node dissection in stage I. Urol 1987;138:77–82.

[27] Weinstein M. Lymphatic drainage of the testes. Atlas Urol Clin North Am 1999;7:1–7.

[28] Donohue JP, Rowland RG. Complications of retroperitoneal lymph node dissection. J Urol 1981; 125:338–40.

[29] Donohue JP. Nerve-sparing retroperitoneal lymphadenectomy for testis cancer. Evolution of surgical templates for low-stage disease. Eur Urol 1993; 23 (Suppl 2):44–46.

[30] Donohue JP, Thornhill JA, Foster RS, et al. Primary retroperitoneal lymph node dissection in clinical stage A non-seminomatous germ cell testis cancer. Review of the Indiana University experience 1965–1989. Br J Urol 1993;71:326–35.

[31] Foster RS, Donohue JP. Nerve-sparing retroperitoneal lymphadenectomy. Urol Clin North Am 1993;20:117–25.

[32] Baniel J, Sella A. Complications of retroperitoneal lymph node dissection in testicular cancer: primary and post-chemotherapy. Semin Surg Oncol 1999; 17:263–7.

[33] Patel A. Complications of lymphadenectomy. In: Taneja S, Smith R, Ehrlich R, editors. Complications of urologic surgery. Philadelphia: Saunders; 2001. p. 370–86.

[34] Baniel J, Foster RS, Rowland RG, et al. Complications of post-chemotherapy retroperitoneal lymph node dissection. J Urol 1995;153:976–80.

[35] Donohue JP. Retroperitoneal lymphadenectomy: the anterior approach including bilateral suprarenal-hilar dissection. Urol Clin North Am 1977;4: 509–21.

[36] Hoeltl W, Hruby W, Aharinejad S. Renal vein anatomy and its implications for retroperitoneal surgery. J Urol 1990;143:1108–14.

[37] Heidenreich A, Albers P, Hartmann M, et al. Complications of primary nerve sparing retroperitoneal lymph node dissection for clinical stage I nonseminomatous germ cell tumors of the testis: experience of the German testicular cancer study group. J Urol 2003;169:1710–4.

[38] Babaian RJ, Bracken RB, Johnson DE. Complications of transabdominal retroperitoneal lymphadenectomy. Urology 1981;17:126–8.

[39] Karcaaltincaba M, Akhan O. Radiologic imaging and percutaneous treatment of pelvic lymphocele. Eur J Radiol 2005;55:340–54.

[40] Baniel J, Foster RS, Rowland RG, et al. Management of chylous ascites after retroperitoneal lymph node dissection for testicular cancer. J Urol 1993; 150:1422–4.

[41] Shapiro AM, Bain VG, Sigalet DL, et al. Rapid resolution of chylous ascites after liver transplantation using somatostatin analog and total parenteral nutrition. Transplantation 1996;61:1410–1.

[42] Geerts WH, Pineo GF, Heit JA, et al. Prevention of venous thromboembolism: the seventh ACCP conference on antithrombotic and thrombolytic therapy. Chest 2004;126:338S–400S.

[43] Baniel J, Leibovitch I, Foster RS, et al. Hyperamylasemia after post-chemotherapy retroperitoneal lymph node dissection for testis cancer. J Urol 1995;154:1373–5.

[44] Baniel J, Foster RS, Rowland RG, et al. Complications of primary retroperitoneal lymph node dissection. J Urol 1994;152:424–7.

[45] Foster RS, Donohue JP. Retroperitoneal lymph node dissection for the management of clinical stage I nonseminoma. J Urol 2000;163:1788–92.

[46] Donohue JP, Foster RS, Rowland RG, et al. Nerve-sparing retroperitoneal lymphadenectomy with preservation of ejaculation. J Urol 1990;144: 287–91 [discussion 91–2].

[47] Jewett MA, Kong YS, Goldberg SD, et al. Retroperitoneal lymphadenectomy for testis tumor with nerve sparing for ejaculation. J Urol 1988;139: 1220–4.

[48] Chang SS, Smith JA Jr, Girasole C, et al. Beneficial impact of a clinical care pathway in patients with testicular cancer undergoing retroperitoneal lymph node dissection. J Urol 2002;168:87–92.

[49] Leibovitch I, Nash PA, Little JS Jr, et al. Spinal cord ischemia after post-chemotherapy retroperitoneal lymph node dissection for nonseminomatous germ cell cancer. J Urol 1996;155:947–51.

[50] Donat SM. Peri-operative care in patients treated for testicular cancer. Semin Surg Oncol 1999;17: 282–8.

[51] Loehrer PJ Sr, Williams SD, Einhorn LH. Testicular cancer: the quest continues. J Natl Cancer Inst 1988;80:1373–82.

[52] Einhorn LH, Donohue J. Cis-diamminedichloroplatinum, vinblastine, and bleomycin combination chemotherapy in disseminated testicular cancer. Ann Intern Med 1977;87:293–8.

[53] Einhorn LH, Donohue JP. Chemotherapy for disseminated testicular cancer. Urol Clin North Am 1977;4:407–26.

[54] Chaudhary UB, Haldas JR. Long-term complications of chemotherapy for germ cell tumours. Drugs 2003;63:1565–77.

[55] Loehrer PJ Sr, Einhorn LH, Williams SD. VP-16 plus ifosfamide plus cisplatin as salvage therapy in refractory germ cell cancer. J Clin Oncol 1986; 4:528–36.

[56] Gilligan T. Complications of systemic therapy for genitourinary malignancies. AUA Update Series 2005;24.

[57] de Wit R, Roberts JT, Wilkinson PM, et al. Equivalence of three or four cycles of bleomycin, etoposide, and cisplatin chemotherapy and of a 3- or 5-day schedule in good-prognosis germ cell cancer: a randomized study of the European Organization for Research and Treatment of Cancer genitourinary tract cancer cooperative group and the Medical Research council. J Clin Oncol 2001; 19:1629–40.
[58] Ratliff TR, Williams RD. Hemorrhagic cystitis, chemotherapy, and bladder toxicity. J Urol 1998; 159:1044.
[59] Dietrich J, Marienhagen J, Schalke B, et al. Vascular neurotoxicity following chemotherapy with cisplatin, ifosfamide, and etoposide. Ann Pharmacother 2004;38:242–6.
[60] Bokemeyer C, Schmoll HJ. Secondary neoplasms following treatment of malignant germ cell tumors. J Clin Oncol 1993;11:1703–9.
[61] Travis LB, Curtis RE, Storm H, et al. Risk of second malignant neoplasms among long-term survivors of testicular cancer. J Natl Cancer Inst 1997; 89:1429–39.
[62] Pedersen-Bjergaard J, Daugaard G, Hansen SW, et al. Increased risk of myelodysplasia and leukaemia after etoposide, cisplatin, and bleomycin for germ-cell tumours. Lancet 1991;338:359–63.
[63] Kollmannsberger C, Kuzcyk M, Mayer F, et al. Late toxicity following curative treatment of testicular cancer. Semin Surg Oncol 1999;17:275–81.
[64] Wanderas EH, Fossa SD, Tretli S. Risk of subsequent non-germ cell cancer after treatment of germ cell cancer in 2006 Norwegian male patients. Eur J Cancer 1997;33:253–62.
[65] Fossa SD, Aass N, Winderen M, et al. Long-term renal function after treatment for malignant germ-cell tumours. Ann Oncol 2002;13:222–8.
[66] Osanto S, Bukman A, Van Hoek F, et al. Long-term effects of chemotherapy in patients with testicular cancer. J Clin Oncol 1992;10:574–9.
[67] Boyer M, Raghavan D, Harris PJ, et al. Lack of late toxicity in patients treated with cisplatin-containing combination chemotherapy for metastatic testicular cancer. J Clin Oncol 1990;8:21–6.
[68] Hartmann JT, Kollmannsberger C, Kanz L, et al. Platinum organ toxicity and possible prevention in patients with testicular cancer. Int J Cancer 1999;83:866–9.
[69] Thompson SW, Davis LE, Kornfeld M, et al. Cisplatin neuropathy. Clinical, electrophysiologic, morphologic, and toxicologic studies. Cancer 1984;54:1269–75.
[70] Hansen SW, Helweg-Larsen S, Trojaborg W. Long-term neurotoxicity in patients treated with cisplatin, vinblastine, and bleomycin for metastatic germ cell cancer. J Clin Oncol 1989; 7:1457–61.
[71] Roth BJ, Greist A, Kubilis PS, et al. Cisplatin-based combination chemotherapy for disseminated germ cell tumors: long-term follow-up. J Clin Oncol 1988;6:1239–47.
[72] van der Hulst RJ, Dreschler WA, Urbanus NA. High frequency audiometry in prospective clinical research of ototoxicity due to platinum derivatives. Ann Otol Rhinol Laryngol 1988;97:133–7.
[73] Bokemeyer C, Berger CC, Hartmann JT, et al. Analysis of risk factors for cisplatin-induced ototoxicity in patients with testicular cancer. Br J Cancer 1998;77:1355–62.
[74] Ginsberg SJ, Comis RL. The pulmonary toxicity of antineoplastic agents. Semin Oncol 1982;9:34–51.
[75] White DA, Stover DE. Severe bleomycin-induced pneumonitis. Clinical features and response to corticosteroids. Chest 1984;86:723–8.
[76] Goldiner PL, Schweizer O. The hazards of anesthesia and surgery in bleomycin-treated patients. Semin Oncol 1979;6:121–4.
[77] Donat SM, Levy DA. Bleomycin associated pulmonary toxicity: is perioperative oxygen restriction necessary? J Urol 1998;160:1347–52.
[78] Fossa SD, Lehne G, Heimdal K, et al. Clinical and biochemical long-term toxicity after postoperative cisplatin-based chemotherapy in patients with low-stage testicular cancer. Oncology 1995;52: 300–5.
[79] Vogelzang NJ, Bosl GJ, Johnson K, et al. Raynaud's phenomenon: a common toxicity after combination chemotherapy for testicular cancer. Ann Intern Med 1981;95:288–92.
[80] Meinardi MT, Gietema JA, van der Graaf WT, et al. Cardiovascular morbidity in long-term survivors of metastatic testicular cancer. J Clin Oncol 2000;18:1725–32.
[81] Doll DC, Ringenberg QS, Yarbro JW. Vascular toxicity associated with antineoplastic agents. J Clin Oncol 1986;4:1405–17.
[82] Huddart RA, Norman A, Shahidi M, et al. Cardiovascular disease as a long-term complication of treatment for testicular cancer. J Clin Oncol 2003; 21:1513–23.
[83] Fossa SD. Long-term sequelae after cancer therapy—survivorship after treatment for testicular cancer. Acta Oncol 2004;43:134–41.
[84] Nuver J, Smit AJ, Sleijfer DT, et al. Left ventricular and cardiac autonomic function in survivors of testicular cancer. Eur J Clin Invest 2005;35:99–103.
[85] Icli F, Karaoguz H, Dincol D, et al. Severe vascular toxicity associated with cisplatin-based chemotherapy. Cancer 1993;72:587–93.
[86] Licciardello JT, Moake JL, Rudy CK, et al. Elevated plasma von Willebrand factor levels and arterial occlusive complications associated with cisplatin-based chemotherapy. Oncology 1985;42: 296–300.
[87] Ariceta G, Rodriguez-Soriano J, Vallo A, et al. Acute and chronic effects of cisplatin therapy on renal magnesium homeostasis. Med Pediatr Oncol 1997;28:35–40.

[88] Lajer H, Bundgaard H, Secher NH, et al. Severe intracellular magnesium and potassium depletion in patients after treatment with cisplatin. Br J Cancer 2003;89:1633–7.

[89] Lajer H, Daugaard G. Cisplatin and hypomagnesemia. Cancer Treat Rev 1999;25:47–58.

[90] Nuver J, Smit AJ, Wolffenbuttel BH, et al. The metabolic syndrome and disturbances in hormone levels in long-term survivors of disseminated testicular cancer. J Clin Oncol 2005;23:3718–25.

[91] Nijman JM, Schraffordt Koops H, Oldhoff J, et al. Sexual function after surgery and combination chemotherapy in men with disseminated nonseminomatous testicular cancer. J Surg Oncol 1988;38:182–6.

[92] Lampe H, Horwich A, Norman A, et al. Fertility after chemotherapy for testicular germ cell cancers. J Clin Oncol 1997;15:239–45.

[93] Huyghe E, Matsuda T, Daudin M, et al. Fertility after testicular cancer treatments: results of a large multicenter study. Cancer 2004;100:732–7.

[94] Brydoy M, Fossa SD, Klepp O, et al. Paternity following treatment for testicular cancer. J Natl Cancer Inst 2005;97:1580–8.

[95] Huddart RA, Norman A, Moynihan C, et al. Fertility, gonadal and sexual function in survivors of testicular cancer. Br J Cancer 2005;93:200–7.

[96] DeSantis M, Albrecht W, Holtl W, et al. Impact of cytotoxic treatment on long-term fertility in patients with germ-cell cancer. Int J Cancer 1999;83:864–5.

[97] Pont J, Albrecht W, Postner G, et al. Adjuvant chemotherapy for high-risk clinical stage I nonseminomatous testicular germ cell cancer: long-term results of a prospective trial. J Clin Oncol 1996;14:441–8.

[98] Bohlen D, Burkhard FC, Mills R, et al. Fertility and sexual function following orchiectomy and 2 cycles of chemotherapy for stage I high risk nonseminomatous germ cell cancer. J Urol 2001;165:441–4.

[99] Lee SJ, Schover LR, Partridge AH, et al. American Society of Clinical Oncology recommendations on fertility preservation in cancer patients. J Clin Oncol 2006;24:2917–31.

[100] Girasole C, Cookson MS, Smith Jr JA, et al. Sperm banking: use and outcomes in patients treated for testicular cancer. In: Program and abstracts of the American Urologic Association annual meeting. Atlanta (GA), 2006. p. 148 [abstract 456].

[101] van den Berkmortel F, de Wit R, de Rooy J, et al. Osteonecrosis in patients with testicular tumours treated with chemotherapy. Neth J Med 2004;62:23–7.

[102] Loutfi R, Kattan J, Kikano T. Spontaneous pneumothorax following chemotherapy for metastatic germ cell tumor: a case report. J Med Liban 2004;52:115–7.

[103] Uygur MC, Ozen H. Gynecomastia following chemotherapy for testicular cancer. Urol Int 2003;70:253–4.

[104] Classen J, Schmidberger H, Meisner C, et al. Radiotherapy for stages IIa/b testicular seminoma: final report of a prospective multicenter clinical trial. J Clin Oncol 2003;21:1101–6.

[105] Bamberg M, Schmidberger H, Meisner C, et al. Radiotherapy for stages I and IIa/b testicular seminoma. Int J Cancer 1999;83:823–7.

[106] Zagars GK, Ballo MT, Lee AK, et al. Mortality after cure of testicular seminoma. J Clin Oncol 2004;22:640–7.

[107] Chao CK, Lai PP, Michalski JM, et al. Secondary malignancy among seminoma patients treated with adjuvant radiation therapy. Int J Radiat Oncol Biol Phys 1995;33:831–5.

[108] Peckham MJ, Barrett A, Husband JE, et al. Orchidectomy alone in testicular stage I non-seminomatous germ-cell tumours. Lancet 1982;2:678–80.

[109] Thomas J, Aleman M, Dreicer R, et al. Management of stage I nonseminomatous germ-cell tumors. Semin Urol Oncol 2002;20:220–6.

[110] Theodorescu D, Rabbani F, Donat SM. Follow-up of genitourinary malignancies for the office urologist: a practical approach. Part 2: kidney cancer and germ cell cancer of the testis. AUA Update Series 2004;23.

[111] Sturgeon JF, Jewett MA, Alison RE, et al. Surveillance after orchidectomy for patients with clinical stage I nonseminomatous testis tumors. J Clin Oncol 1992;10:564–8.

[112] Chang SS, Sheinfeld J. Clinical stage I nonseminomatous germ cell tumors: treatment options. AUA Update Series 2001;20.

[113] Sogani PC, Perrotti M, Herr HW, et al. Clinical stage I testis cancer: long-term outcome of patients on surveillance. J Urol 1998;159:855–8.

[114] Nicolai N, Pizzocaro G. A surveillance study of clinical stage I nonseminomatous germ cell tumors of the testis: 10-year followup. J Urol 1995;154:1045–9.

[115] Fossa SD, Jacobsen AB, Aass N, et al. How safe is surveillance in patients with histologically low-risk non-seminomatous testicular cancer in a geographically extended country with limited computerised tomographic resources? Br J Cancer 1994;70:1156–60.

[116] Koch MO. Cost-effective strategies for the follow-up of patients with germ cell tumors. Urol Clin North Am 1998;25:495–502.

[117] Mykletun A, Dahl AA, Haaland CF, et al. Side effects and cancer-related stress determine quality of life in long-term survivors of testicular cancer. J Clin Oncol 2005;23:3061–8.

[118] Thorsen L, Nystad W, Dahl O, et al. The level of physical activity in long-term survivors of testicular cancer. Eur J Cancer 2003;39:1216–21.

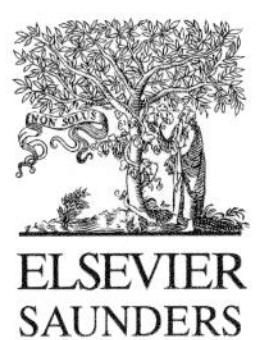

ELSEVIER
SAUNDERS

Urol Clin N Am 34 (2007) 269–277

UROLOGIC
CLINICS
of North America

Infertility and Testis Cancer

Sarah M. Lambert, MD, Harry Fisch, MD*

Male Reproductive Center, Department of Urology, Columbia University, College of Physicians and Surgeons, New York Presbyterian Hospital, 944 Park Avenue, New York, NY 10028, USA

Testicular cancer is one of the few malignancies that affect men in their reproductive years. Testicular cancer represents the most common solid organ tumor in young men between 20 and 35 years of age. The National Cancer Society predicted that 8250 new cases of testicular cancer would be diagnosed in the United States in 2006 [1]. Fortunately, testicular cancer is also one of the most curable malignancies with 370 testicular cancer-specific deaths predicted for 2006. The incidence of testicular cancer therefore correlates with a 1 in 300 lifetime risk for developing testicular cancer and a 1 in 5000 lifetime risk for dying from testicular cancer. The objective of superior testicular cancer treatment includes not only cure but also the preservation of quality of life. The preservation of fertility and sexual function represent important quality-of-life parameters in these young men. To determine how testicular cancer impacts fertility it is important to understand how infertility is assessed and how infertility and testicular cancer are interrelated.

Development of infertility and testicular cancer may arise from congenital abnormalities in testicular maturation, such as gonadal dysgenesis, cryptorchidism, or carcinoma in situ. Additionally, exposure to certain gonadal toxins or trauma impacts testicular integrity, including spermatogenesis and the blood–testis barrier. As a result of these factors, many men presenting with testicular cancer are found to have abnormal semen analysis parameters before initiation of treatment. With the increase in delayed childbearing and the use of assisted reproductive technologies, men presenting with a primary complaint of infertility can be found to have incidental testicular neoplasms [2].

The presence of a testicular neoplasm affects the local testis environment, the pituitary–gonadal hormonal milieu, and the body systemically. Aberrations in any of these factors can adversely affect spermatogenesis. The psychologic impact inherent in the diagnosis of testicular cancer can also affect sexual function and fertility as a result. These tumor-related effects on fertility are compounded by the potentially deleterious effects of treatment modalities, such as pelvic radiation, chemotherapy, and retroperitoneal lymph node dissection (RPLND).

Despite these risk factors for infertility, it is important to stress to patients the preventive methods and treatments for infertility associated with testicular cancer and treatment. In patients who have successfully treated testicular cancer and preserved fertility, the potential effects on genetic integrity must be evaluated. This article reviews the causative factors for infertility in men who have testicular cancer and the treatments available for preserving or restoring fertility.

Diagnosis of infertility

Infertility is defined as the inability to conceive after 1 year of unprotected intercourse, with 75% of patients able to conceive after 6 months and 90% of patients able to conceive after 1 year [3]. This inability to conceive can be caused by male or female factors. Twenty percent of cases result from solely male factors, whereas 40% of cases are caused by male and female factors combined; therefore, male-factor infertility affects 60% of infertile couples [4]. The evaluation of male

* Corresponding author.
E-mail address: hf4@columbia.edu (H. Fisch).

0094-0143/07/$ - see front matter
doi:10.1016/j.ucl.2007.02.002

infertility begins with a thorough history that includes a sexual history, past medical history, and family history. Pertinent information garnered from the sexual history includes frequency and timing of coitus and potency. A patient's past medical history is equally important and provides information regarding congenital abnormalities, cryptorchidism, inguinal or retroperitoneal surgery, radiation, infections, medications, toxic exposures, and past pregnancies. A family history may reveal cystic fibrosis, congenital anomalies, or hormonal abnormalities. Once a satisfactory history has been obtained, the physician can proceed to a physical examination. The physical examination should be directed to evidence of hormonal imbalances, testicular volume, paratesticular pathology, and prostate abnormalities. The physical examination is supplemented with the semen analysis evaluating volume, sperm concentration, motility, and morphology. Hormonal analysis includes serum follicle stimulating hormone, luteinizing hormone, testosterone, and prolactin. Finally, a scrotal ultrasound and transrectal ultrasound are included if indicated. It is only after the completion of this evaluation that a decision can be made regarding treatment options. Patients who have testicular cancer presenting with infertility should be evaluated using these parameters to ensure an accurate diagnosis and appropriate treatment regimen.

Relationship between infertility and testicular cancer

Theoretically, any cause that adversely affects testicular function can result in infertility and testicular tumorigenesis. Many studies evaluating testicular cancer have documented an increased risk for abnormal semen analysis parameters in patients who have testicular tumors. Of 15 patients presenting with germ cell tumors, 10 (66%) had evidence of abnormal spermatogenesis, including poor motility, low sperm concentration, or low semen volume [5]. Conversely, studies have been published documenting an increased risk for testicular cancer in patients presenting with infertility. This connection is clearly documented in a large population-based study in Denmark including 32,442 men who underwent semen analysis from 1963 to 1995. Men who had abnormal semen analyses had a 1.6-fold increased risk for developing testicular cancer compared with the general Danish population. In evaluation of specific semen analysis parameters, a low sperm concentration, decreased motility, and increased abnormal motility were specifically associated with increased development of testicular cancer [6]. An evaluation of 3800 men presenting with infertility and abnormal semen analyses in the United States revealed a 20-fold increased risk for testicular tumors when compared with the population based on the SEER database [7].

These observational studies are confirmed with evaluation of testicular histopathology. Carroll and colleagues [8] examined testicular tissue from eight patients who had mediastinal or retroperitoneal germ cell tumors and found abnormal testicular tissue in all patients, including fibrosis, decreased spermatogenesis, interstitial edema, Sertoli cell only, and Leydig hyperplasia. On retrospective review, these patients had a well-documented history of infertility. These studies provide evidence for a common cause responsible for low semen quality and tumorigenesis. Evaluation of these potential causes is essential to understanding the association between infertility and testis cancer.

Abnormal testicular development

During fetal development, male and female embryos begin to differentiate at the end of the sixth gestational week [9]. Early in the seventh week testicular development begins and depends on many factors, including chromosomal integrity and normal endocrine function. Abnormalities in testicular maturation, such as cryptorchidism, are often associated with infertility and tumorigenesis. Cryptorchid testes have abnormal germ cell morphology, varying degrees of gonadal dysgenesis, and are exposed to elevated intra-abdominal temperatures. As early as 3 years of age abnormal spermatogonia and Sertoli cells can be found in cryptorchid testes. This abnormal development progresses to fibrosis, basement membrane degeneration, and deposition of myelin and lipids [10].

The association between cryptorchidism and tumorigenesis was first described in 1851 by Le Comete [11]. Subsequently many population-based studies have confirmed this relationship. The reported relative risk for testicular cancer in patients who have cryptorchidism is 3 to 14 times higher than the expected incidence [12–14]. Additionally, the detrimental effect of cryptorchidism on fertility is also well documented. A multicenter retrospective review of 162 patients who had cryptorchidism revealed significantly lower sperm concentrations and morphology compared with normal controls. Patients who had retractile testes also had decreased sperm concentration and morphology. Despite these abnormal semen analysis parameters in patients who had retractile testes, the risk for azoospermia was significantly higher in patients who had cryptorchidism [15].

Impaired spermatogenesis, cryptorchidism, and germ cell tumors represent a spectrum of abnormal testicular development and are often interrelated. Andersson and Skakkebaek and colleagues propose that this spectrum of testicular maldevelopment should be classified as testicular dysgenesis syndrome [16]. Their hypothesis advocates a common cause, either genetic or environmental, for cryptorchidism, hypospadias, impaired spermatogenesis, and testis cancer. An evaluation of contralateral testis biopsies in patients who had germ cell tumors including 218 specimens revealed carcinoma in situ in 8.7%, immature seminiferous tubules in 4.6%, and Sertoli cell only pattern in 13.8% of patients. Ultimately 25.2% of patients who had germ cell tumors had evidence of testicular dysgenesis in the contralateral testis [17].

Estrogen exposure in utero represents one such factor proposed as a cause for male genital abnormalities. This hypothesis is supported by animal studies demonstrating the teratogenic effect of estrogen exposure during early embryonic development. Murine embryos exposed to ethinyl oestradiol at embryonic day 13 had a higher risk for cryptorchidism and a trend toward increased testicular teratomas [18]. A case-control study of 108 men who had testicular cancer demonstrated that maternal exposure to exogenous estrogens during the early first trimester was associated with an eightfold increased risk for testicular cancer [19]. The development of testicular cancer or infertility is multifactorial and depends on a series of alterations in the developmental process. At times these alterations may result from a single causal factor during development. Despite this common origin, the association between germ cell tumors and infertility may result from the factors relating to systemic imbalances produced by the tumor itself.

Systemic cancer effects

Malignancy has a wide range of effects on the body, including metabolic derangements, hormonal imbalances, and thermoregulatory changes. These alterations may result from the tumor itself or the body's cytokine response, including increased interleukins and tumor necrosis factors. Investigations of young men who have testicular cancer and Hodgkin's disease suggest that the systemic effects of malignancy alter testicular function and impair spermatogenesis. This evidence results from studies documenting decreased fertility before the initiation of treatment. An evaluation of 158 men at the time of diagnosis of Hodgkin's disease revealed abnormal semen analyses in 70% of men with 8% of patients having azoospermia. The risk for impaired spermatogenesis increased with elevated acute phase reactants and advanced clinical stage [20].

Local tumor effects

Tumors of advanced stage not only produce a heightened systemic reaction but also disrupt the local architecture and functioning of the testis itself. Presumably, more advanced tumors cause a greater disturbance in testicular structure. Invasive germ cell tumors of higher stage are associated with worse semen quality than germ cell tumors of lower stage [21]. This finding may be caused in part by perturbation of the blood–testis barrier. The integrity of this barrier prevents formation of antisperm antibodies that may adversely impact fertility. Although normal fertile men have a 5%–8% incidence of antisperm antibodies, studies have reported men who have testicular cancer to have an 18%, 21%, and 73% incidence suggesting that germ cell tumors disturb the blood–testis barrier [22–24].

This disruption in testicular architecture corresponds to a disruption in testicular function. A review of radical orchiectomy specimens in 28 patients revealed impaired spermatogenesis most apparent within 3 mm of the tumor margin [25]. This local effect of germ cell tumors is supported by a histologic comparison of orchiectomy specimens removed for malignant tumors versus benign tumors; testes with benign tumors revealed significantly fewer abnormalities in spermatogenesis versus testes with malignant tumors. In the presence of malignant tumors, abnormalities in spermatogenesis increased with decreasing distance from the tumor margin [26]. Confirmatory evidence for a direct effect of the cancer process itself exists in the many reports documenting an improvement in fertility after orchiectomy. One such study, evaluating semen analyses in nonrelapsing men on a surveillance protocol for stage I nonseminomatous germ cell tumors (NSGCT) revealed a significant increase in mean sperm concentrations from 26 to 39 $\times$ 10^6/mL in the year postorchiectomy [27].

Endocrine factors

Normal spermatogenesis depends on normal hormonal equilibrium. Hormonally active tumors can disrupt the hormonal balance and adversely affect spermatogenesis. Germ cell tumors are often hormonally active and can produce β–human chorionic gonadotropin (β-HCG) and α-fetoprotein (AFP). A quantitative analysis of biopsy specimens in 53 men who had seminoma demonstrated a correlation between increased β-HCG and decreased spermatogenesis in the contralateral testis [28]. A paracrine–endocrine mechanism is described in which β-HCG stimulation of intratesticular estradiol production impairs spermatogenesis [29]. Hansen and colleagues [30], using multiregression analysis, determined that an elevated AFP was associated with a decreased total sperm count in patients who had nonseminomatous germ cell tumors. In addition, the authors noted that 33% of patients presenting with germ cell tumors had an elevated serum follicle stimulating hormone (FSH).

The subfertility documented in patients who have malignancy can also be attributed to disruption of the hypothalamic-pituitary-gonadal axis. FSH and luteinizing hormone (LH) are often abnormal in men who have malignancy. Men who have untreated Hodgkin's disease were found to have significant hypogonadism with low FSH and serum testosterone when compared with normal controls. Despite abnormally low serum testosterone, these patients had normal levels of LH suggestive of pituitary or hypothalamic dysfunction [31]. Men who had testicular cancer and an elevated FSH before initiation of therapy are noted to have lower posttreatment fertility than men who had normal FSH before initiation of treatment irrespective of treatment modality [32]. Klingmuller and colleagues [33] confirmed this correlation in patients who had seminoma and suggest using pretreatment FSH as a prognostic indicator for predicting posttreatment spermatogenesis.

Cancer treatment and fertility

The association between the development of testicular germ cell cancer and infertility is well known although the causative factors are still being investigated. Also documented is the potential for improved fertility after the primary tumor is removed at radical orchiectomy. Cancer treatment therefore has the potential to reverse impaired spermatogenesis associated with testicular neoplasia. The treatment of testicular neoplasm is a complex paradigm involving histology, stage, and patient selection. After radical orchiectomy, four treatment options are currently available; surveillance, RPLND, radiation, and chemotherapy. These treatments impact reproductive function and have distinct implications for posttreatment fertility.

Surveillance

Postorchiectomy surveillance is a viable treatment option for men who have stage I testis tumors for patients who are willing to adhere to a strict follow-up regimen. Surveillance protocols allow patients to avoid post-RPLND ejaculatory disturbances and gonadotoxic therapies but approximately 20% of men relapse and ultimately require additional treatment. Men who relapse on surveillance protocols and require gonadotoxic treatments may be at greater risk for infertility than men initially treated with nerve-sparing RPLND [34].

In men who are monitored on a surveillance policy without relapse, semen analysis parameters, including sperm concentrations, may remain stable or actually improve after orchiectomy. Carroll and colleagues [35] noted that 50% of patients who have stage I NSGCT and initial oligospermia or azoospermia recovered normal sperm concentrations within 4 to 19 months postorchiectomy. This finding is supported by Jacobsen and colleagues [27] who evaluated repeat semen analyses of 80 men on surveillance for stage I NSGCT and found a significant increase in mean sperm concentrations at 1 year postorchiectomy. At baseline, 40% of these men had sperm counts less than 10 $\times$ 10^6/mL and 5 of the 28 men who attempted to conceive before malignant diagnosis had been evaluated for infertility. Men successfully followed on surveillance can expect a stable or improved semen quality postorchiectomy.

Retroperitoneal lymph node dissection

The removal of retroperitoneal lymph nodes entails a delicate dissection of tissues and structures surrounding the aorta and inferior vena cava, including the retroperitoneal postganglionic sympathetic nerves. These nerves overlie the aorta and join to form the hypogastric plexus in the pelvis. The ampullary vas deferens seminal vesicles, periurethral glands, internal sphincter, bulbourethral, and periurethral musculature receive innervation from these nerves. The surgical disruption of these nerves during RPLND or pelvic node dissection can result in retrograde ejaculation or anejaculation depending on the severity of the nerve injury. The presence or extent of retroperitoneal disease often dictates the type of lymph node dissection performed and affects the preservation of ejaculatory function. Unilateral and nerve-sparing RPLND techniques [36] provide the greatest potential for normal ejaculatory function. In comparing patients who underwent postchemotherapy modified bilateral template RPLND [37] versus postchemotherapy nerve-sparing technique in Norway from 1980 to 1994, antegrade ejaculation was preserved in 11% versus 89% of patients, respectively. Anejaculation was documented in 75% of patients after modified bilateral template RPLND versus 5% of patients after nerve-sparing RPLND. Median ejaculatory volume decreased from 4.4 mL before RPLND to 2.5 mL post-RPLND with the largest decrease observed in patients undergoing modified bilateral template RPLND [38]. Donohue and colleagues [39] documented 76% of men status post nerve-sparing RPLND for stage 1 NSGCT who attempted to conceive were successful. In summary, advances in surgical techniques have allowed for the preservation of ejaculatory function and significantly reduced the risk for infertility associated with RPLND.

Radiotherapy

In rats, testicular irradiation results in transient intratesticular edema and spermatogonial arrest but recovery of spermatogenesis is observed 4 weeks postradiation [40]. Human studies that include testicular biopsies reveal that spermatogonia are the most sensitive germ cells to radiation and can be affected by doses as low as 10 cGy [41]. In men receiving radiotherapy for Hodgkin's lymphoma, the testicular dose ranged from 6 to 70 cGy. Patients who received greater than or equal to 20 cGy were documented to have a transient dose-dependent increase in FSH in the first 2 years following radiotherapy. This finding correlated with transient oligospermia that recovered within 18 months posttreatment [42].

Men diagnosed with stage 1 and 2a seminoma often receive adjuvant infradiaphragmatic radiation therapy. Although gonadal shielding minimizes irradiation of the testis, unintended gonadal exposure doses occur [43]. Centola and colleagues [44] documented a mean testicular radiation dose of 44 cGy with a range from 28 cGy to 90 cGy in men receiving infradiaphragmatic radiation treatment of seminoma with gonadal shielding. In patients receiving pelvic and periaortic radiotherapy, declines in sperm counts are often seen in the first year after radiotherapy but can gradually improve within 2 to 3 years following treatment [45]. Buchholz and colleagues [46] performed a retrospective analysis of 212 patients who had stage 1 or 2a seminoma treated with orchiectomy and adjuvant radiotherapy with gonadal shielding from 1975 to 1997 with a mean follow-up time of 8 years. All patients received ipsilateral pelvic and periaortic radiation with a median total dose of 2611 cGy and 2702 cGy in patients who had stage 1 and stage 2a, respectively. An evaluation of semen analyses revealed no correlation between increased radiation dose and abnormal sperm concentration, with 56% of men having a normal sperm concentration. Seventy-three patients responded to a retrospective questionnaire; of these patients, 15% attempted to conceive children postradiotherapy. Seven of 11 couples (64%) were successful in achieving pregnancy without assisted reproduction and 6 of 7 couples delivered healthy infants with one spontaneous abortion. Men receiving infradiaphragmatic radiotherapy for seminoma may experience a transient decrease in sperm counts but can anticipate a recovery of spermatogenesis.

Chemotherapy

The current chemotherapy regimens for testicular cancer have significantly increased survival. The side effects of chemotherapy therefore have become increasingly important. Because systemic chemotherapy targets rapidly dividing cells, disruption of spermatogenesis represents a common side effect of chemotherapeutics. Chemotherapy-related oligospermia and azoospermia are not unique to patients who have germ cell malignancies and have been documented in patients treated for leukemia, lymphoma, and other solid organ malignancies. An evaluation of 314 patients status post gonadotoxic treatment of these malignancies revealed a significant decrease in sperm concentration and semen volume. Patients who had germ cell tumors had the lowest pretreatment sperm concentration (40.6×10^6/mL) and the highest percentage of posttreatment oligospermia but the lowest incidence of posttreatment azoospermia. The predisposition toward gonadal dysfunction in men who have germ cell tumors continues to impact posttreatment fertility, but less intensive chemotherapy regimens may minimize the risk for posttreatment azoospermia [47].

Bleomycin, etoposide, and cisplatin (BEP) regimens are used as adjuvant therapy for nonseminomatous germ cell tumors and for treatment of metastatic seminomas. Rats treated with BEP had decreased testicular and epididymal weight, decreased sperm count, and decreased motility, but treatment did not affect fertility, pregnancy loss, litter size, or sex ratio [48]. Additionally, rats demonstrated decreased serum testosterone, intratesticular testosterone, and numbers of LH receptors and after exposure to cisplatin [49]. Mice exposed to cisplatin demonstrated a dose-dependent loss of differentiating germ cells resulting from apoptosis [50].

Human studies reveal perturbations in serum LH, FSH, and testosterone. In a study of German men treated with cisplatin-based chemotherapy regimens, 89% of men had elevated FSH levels at 12 months postchemotherapy and this elevation persisted for more than 8 years posttreatment in 64.3% of men [51]. This sustained elevation of serum FSH represents long-term damage to Sertoli cell function. An evaluation of men treated for NSGCT demonstrated elevated serum LH levels in 59% of men who received chemotherapy and decreased sperm counts and semen volume in comparison with men treated with orchiectomy alone [52]. Semen analyses obtained from 30 men 24 to 78 months after BEP chemotherapy revealed 23% oligospermia, 20% azoospermia, abnormal morphology, and decreased motility; unfortunately no pretreatment semen analyses were available to establish baseline spermatogenic function [53]. Petersen and colleagues [54] compared semen analyses and hormonal profiles from 33 men treated with conventional-dose BEP to data obtained from 21 men treated with high-dose BEP and found azoospermia in 19% and 47% of men treated with conventional-dose BEP and high-dose BEP, respectively. In addition, FSH levels were significantly higher in men who received high-dose BEP. No difference in testosterone or LH was noted between the groups.

These abnormalities in semen analyses and hormone levels are not necessarily permanent and the potential for normalization of endocrine and spermatogenic function exists. A review of semen analyses from patients who had germ cell neoplasms treated with cisplatin-based chemotherapy at the Royal Marsden Hospital demonstrated that improved sperm counts were present in 48% and 80% of patients at 2 and 5 years postchemotherapy, respectively. Even more encouraging, the probability of achieving normal sperm counts was 22% and 58% at 2 and 5 years, respectively. High pretreatment sperm counts and the use of carboplatin versus cisplatin were associated with an increased probability of improved fertility postchemotherapy [55]. In summary, systemic chemotherapy for germ cell malignancies affects both Sertoli cell and Leydig cell function and has the potential to permanently impair spermatogenesis. Recovery of spermatogenesis is possible but men who have elevated FSH, high-dose cisplatin therapy, and low pretreatment sperm counts are at increased risk for long-term infertility.

Preservation and restoration of fertility

Currently, men who have testicular cancer have many options available to preserve fertility and potential paternity. The availability of sperm cryopreservation, advances in assisted reproductive techniques (ART), and testicular sperm extraction (TESE) provide the potential for fatherhood for men unable to conceive as a result of testicular cancer treatments. It should be noted that men who have testicular cancer status post chemotherapy have decreased fertilization rates per in vitro fertilization (IVF) or intracytoplasmic sperm injection (ICSI) cycle and a decreased pregnancy rate compared with men who have testicular cancer treated without chemotherapy [56]. Sperm cryopreservation should therefore be recommended to men who have germ cell neoplasms before the initiation of treatment when possible.

Records of 67 couples referred for ART for male factor infertility following treatment of malignancies, including testicular cancer and lymphoma, were reviewed to determine the options used and success of various treatment modalities. Eighty-two percent of men cryopreserved sperm before treatment and 58% of men used cryopreserved sperm for ART. A total of 151 cycles of ART were completed, including 55 intrauterine inseminations (IUI), 82 ICSI, and 14 ICSI-frozen embryo replacements, with a corresponding delivery rate of 11.1%, 30.5%, and 21%, respectively [57]. A separate study evaluating the viability of cryopreserved sperm obtained from men before antineoplastic treatment revealed an overall 18.3% pregnancy rate and 7% IUI, 23% IVF, and 37% ICSI pregnancy rates [58]. In men who have true anejaculation or azoospermia, TESE can provide viable sperm for ICSI. An evaluation of 12 men who had azoospermia status post chemotherapy documented motile spermatozoa in 41.6% of men after TESE [59]. In 17 azoospermic men postchemotherapy, testicular biopsies performed at the time of TESE revealed Sertoli cell only in 76% of patients and hypospermatogenesis in 24% if patients. Of these patients, 45% had successful sperm extraction that resulted in live births in 22% of couples [60]. The ability to preserve fertility through ART is an option for men who have persistent azoospermia or anejaculation after treatment of testicular cancer and cryopreservation should always be recommended to enhance the potential for paternity.

Teratogenic potential

Current cancer treatment regimens and reproductive technologies allow many men to be cancer survivors and new fathers. In the setting of malignant testicular dysgenesis and potentially gonadotoxic therapies, many of these men are concerned regarding the potential risk for increased congenital anomalies. Exposure to etoposide in mice resulted in disomy, centromeric abnormalities, and increased diploid sperm in comparison with controls [61]. Mice treated with BEP did not demonstrate an increased risk for pregnancy loss, but offspring of mice treated with BEP for 9 weeks had a significantly higher rate of neonatal mortality than offspring of mice treated for only 6 weeks [48].

In humans, assessment of sperm integrity before and after treatment of germ cell neoplasms did not reveal a higher DNA fragmentation index after diagnosis of germ cell tumors in comparison with controls but did reveal a higher DNA fragmentation index up to 2 years after radiotherapy. This increased DNA fragmentation index was not noted after chemotherapy [62]. Fluorescence in situ hybridization (FISH) of semen specimens from five men after BEP treatment revealed a significantly increased frequency of diploidy and disomy 16, 18, and XY in comparison with healthy controls at 6 to 17 months after treatment [63]. Conversely, another study using FISH to assess the risk for disomy for chromosomes 1, 12, X, Y, and XY in men treated with BEP found no increased risk for numerical chromosomal abnormalities [64].

Many retrospective studies involving patient-reported pregnancy outcomes have investigated the risk for early pregnancy loss and perinatal morbidity and mortality in children fathered by men who had testicular cancer and found no increased risk for pregnancy loss or congenital anomalies [65]. Spermon and colleagues [66] sent questionnaires to 305 men who had germ cell tumors from 1982 to 1999, 226 of whom responded to evaluate fertility before and after treatment. Using patient questionnaires, Spermon and colleagues [66] documented a 66% and 43% conception rate in patients attempting to conceive within 1 year before the diagnosis of testicular cancer and after treatment, respectively. The rate of congenital anomalies was approximately 4% before and after treatment of germ cell neoplasms. Given this data regarding the potential for chromosomal abnormalities in the posttreatment period, sperm cryopreservation should be performed before the initiation of gonadotoxic treatment. Additionally, men should be counseled to postpone conception for approximately 12 to 18 months after treatment to minimize the risk for potential fetal anomalies [67].

References

[1] American Cancer Society. Cancer facts and figures 2006. Available at: http://www.cancer.org. Accessed July 20, 2005.

[2] Tal R, Holland R, Belenky A, et al. Incidental testicular tumors in infertile men. Fertil Steril 2004;82(2): 469–71.

[3] Spira A. Epidemiology of human reproduction. Hum Reprod 1986;1:111–5.

[4] Mosher WD, Pratt WF. Fecundity and infertility in the United States: incidence and trends. Fertil Steril 1991;56:192–3.

[5] Carroll PR, Whitmore WR Jr, Herr HW, et al. Endocrine and exocrine profiles of men with testicular tumors before orchiectomy. J Urol 1987;137(3): 420–3.

[6] Jacobsen R, Bostofte E, Engholm G, et al. Risk of testicular cancer in men with abnormal semen characteristics: cohort study. BMJ 2000;321:789–92.

[7] Raman JD, Nobert CF, Goldstein M. Increased incidence of testicular cancer in men presenting with infertility and abnormal semen analysis. J Urol 2005;174(5):1819–22.

[8] Carroll PR, Whitmore WF Jr, Richardson M, et al. Testicular failure in patients with extragonadal germ cell tumors. Cancer 1987;60(1):108–13.

[9] Larsen WJ. Development of the urogenital systemHuman embryology. New York: Churchill Livingstone; 1997. p. 261–306.
[10] Mengel W, Wronecki K, Schroeder J, et al. Histopathology of the cryptorchid testis. Urol Clin North Am 1982;9:331–8.
[11] Grove JS. The cryptorchid problem. J Urol 1954;71: 735–41.
[12] Henderson BE, Benton B, Jing J, et al. Risk factors for cancer of the testis in young men. Int J Cancer 1979;23(5):598–602.
[13] Schottenfeld D, Warshauer ME, Sherlock S, et al. The epidemiology of testicular cancer in young adults. Am J Epidemiol 1980;112(2):232–46.
[14] Farrer JH, Walker AH, Rajfer J. Management of the postpubertal cryptorchid testis: a statistical review. J Urol 1985;134:1071–6.
[15] Caroppo E, Niederberger C, Elhanbly S, et al. Effect of cryptorchidism and retractile testes on male factor infertility: a multicenter, retrospective, chart review. Fertil Steril 2005;83:1581–4.
[16] Bay K, Asklund C, Skakkebaek NE, et al. Testicular dysgenesis syndrome: possible role of endocrine disruptors. Best Pract Res Clin Endocrinol Metab 2006;20(1):77–90.
[17] Hoei-Hansen CE, Holm M, Rajpert-De Meyts E, et al. Histological evidence of testicular dysgenesis in contra lateral biopsies from 218 patients with testicular germ cell cancer. J Pathol 2003;200(3): 370–4.
[18] Walker AH, Bernstein L, Warren DW, et al. The effect of in utero ethinyl oestradiol exposure on the risk of cyptorchid testis and testicular teratoma in mice. Br J Cancer 1990;62(4):599–602.
[19] Depue RH, Pike MC, Henderson BE. Estrogen exposure during gestation and risk of testicular cancer. J Natl Cancer Inst 1983;71(6):1151–5.
[20] Rueffer U, Breuer K, Josting A, et al. Male gonadal dysfunction in patients with Hodgkin's disease prior to treatment. Ann Oncol 2001;12(9):1307–11.
[21] Agarwal A, Tolentino MV Jr, Sidhu RS, et al. Effect of cryopreservation on semen quality in patients with testicular cancer. Urology 1995;46(3): 382–9.
[22] Hobarth K, Klingler HC, Maier U, et al. Incidence of antisperm antibodies in patients with carcinoma of the testis and subfertile men with normogonadotropic oligoasthenoteratozoospermia. Urol Int 1994;52(3):162–5.
[23] Guazzieri S, Lembo A, Ferro G, et al. Sperm antibodies an infertility in patients with testicular cancer. Urology 1985;26(2):139–42.
[24] Foster RS, Rubin LR, McNulty A, et al. Detection of antisperm-antibodies in patients with primary testicular cancer. Int J Androl 1991;14(3): 179–85.
[25] Ho GT, Gardner H, Mostofi K, et al. Influence of testicular carcinoma on ipsilateral spermatogenesis. J Urol 1992;148(3):821–5.
[26] Ho GT, Gardner H, Mostofi K, et al. The effect of testicular nongerm cell tumors on local spermatogenesis. Fertil Steril 1994;62(1):162–6.
[27] Jacobsen KD, Theodorsen L, Fossa SD. Spermatogenesis after unilateral orchiectomy for testicular cancer in patients following surveillance policy. J Urol 2001;165(1):93–6.
[28] Hayashi T, Arai G, Hyochi N, et al. Suppression of spermatogenesis in ipsilateral and contra lateral testicular tissues in patients with seminoma by human chorionic gonadotropin beta subunit. Urology 2001;58(2):251–7.
[29] Morrish DW, Venner PM, Siy O, et al. Mechanisms of endocrine dysfunction in patients with testicular cancer. J Natl Cancer Inst 1990;82(5):412–8.
[30] Hansen PV, Trykker J, Andersen J, et al. Germ cell function and hormonal status in patients with testicular cancer. Cancer 1989;64(4):956–61.
[31] Vigersky RA, Chapman RM, Berenberg J, et al. Testicular dysfunction in untreated Hodgkin's disease. Am J Med 1982;73(4):482–6.
[32] Fossa SD, Theodorsen L, Norman N, et al. Recovery of impaired pretreatment spermatogenesis in testicular cancer. Fertil Steril 1990;54(3):493–6.
[33] Brennemann W, Stoffel-Wagner B, Wichers M, et al. Pretreatment follicle-stimulating hormone: a prognostic serum marker of spermatogenesis status in patients treated for germ cell cancer. J Urol 1998; 159(6):1942–6.
[34] Herr HW, Bar-Chama N, O'Sullivan M, et al. Paternity in men with stage I testis tumors on surveillance. J Clin Oncol 1998;16(2):733–4.
[35] Carroll PR, Morse MJ, Whitmore WF Jr, et al. Fertility status of patients with clinical stage I testis tumors on a surveillance protocol. J Urol 1987; 138(1):70–2.
[36] Donohue JP, Foster RS, Rowland RG, et al. Nerve-sparing retroperitoneal lymphadenectomy with preservation of ejaculation. J Urol 1990;144:178–82.
[37] Whitmore WF Jr. Surgical treatment of adult germinal testis tumors. Semin Oncol 1979;6:55–68.
[38] Jacobsen KD, Ous S, Waehre H, et al. Ejaculation in testicular cancer patients after post-chemotherapy retroperitoneal lymph node dissection. Br J Cancer 1999;80(1–2):249–55.
[39] Foster RS, McNulty A, Rubin LR, et al. The fertility of patients with clinical stage 1 testis cancer managed by nerve sparing retroperitoneal lymph node dissection. J Urol 1994;152(4):1150–1.
[40] Porter KL, Shetty G, Meistrich ML. Testicular edema is associated with spermatogonial arrest in irradiated rats. Endocrinology 2006;147(3):1297–305.
[41] Rowley MJ, Leach DR, Earner GA, et al. Effect of graded doses of ionizing radiation on the human testis. Radiat Res 1974;59(3):665–78.
[42] Kinsella TJ, Trivette G, Rowland J, et al. Long-term follow-up of testicular function following radiation therapy for early-stage Hodgkin's disease. J Clin Oncol 1989;7(6):718–24.

[43] Hahn EW, Feingold SM, Simpson L, et al. Recovery from aspermia induced by low-dose radiation in seminoma patients. Cancer 1982;50(2):337–40.
[44] Centola GM, Keller JW, Henzler M, et al. Effect of low-dose testicular irradiation on sperm count and fertility in patients with testicular seminoma. J Androl 1994;15(6):608–13.
[45] Fossa SD, Abyholm T, Normann N, et al. Post-treatment fertility in patients with testicular cancer. III. Influence of radiotherapy in seminoma patients. Br J Urol 1986;58(3):315–9.
[46] Nalesnik JG, Sabanegh ES, Eng TY, et al. Fertility in men after treatment for stage 1 and 2a seminoma. Am J Clin Oncol 2004;27(6):584–8.
[47] Bahadur G, Ozturk O, Muneer A, et al. Semen quality before and after gonadotoxic treatment. Hum Reprod 2005;20(3):774–81.
[48] Bieber AM, Marcon L, Hales BF, et al. Effects of chemotherapeutic agents for testicular cancer on the male rate reproductive system, spermatozoa, and fertility. J Androl 2006;27(2):189–200.
[49] Maines MD, Sluss PM, Iscan M. Cis-platinum-mediated decrease in serum testosterone is associated with depression of luteinizing hormone receptors and cytochrome P-450 in rat testis. Endocrinology 1990;126(5):2398–406.
[50] Sawhney P, Giammona CJ, Meistrich ML, et al. Cisplatin-induced long-term failure of spermatogenesis in adult C57/B!/6J mice. J Androl 2005;26(1):136–45.
[51] Brennemann W, Stoffel-Wagner B, Helmers A, et al. Gonadal function of patients treated with cisplatin based chemotherapy for germ cell cancer. J Urol 1997;158(3):844–50.
[52] Hansen SW, Berthelsen JG, von der Maase H. Long-term fertility and Leydig cell function in patients treated for germ cell cancer with cisplatin, vinblastine, and bleomycin versus surveillance. J Clin Oncol 1990;8(10):1695–8.
[53] Stephenson WT, Poirier SM, Rubin L, et al. Evaluation of reproductive capacity in germ cell tumor patients following treatment with cisplatin, etoposide, and bleomycin. J Clin Oncol 1995;13(9):2278–80.
[54] Petersen PM, Hansen SW, Giwercman A, et al. Dose-dependent impairment of testicular function in patients treated with cisplatin-based chemotherapy for germ cell cancer. Ann Oncol 1994;5(4):355–8.
[55] Lampe H, Horwich A, Norman A, et al. Fertility after chemotherapy for testicular germ cell cancers. J Clin Oncol 1997;15(1):239–45.
[56] Hakim LS, Lobel SM, Oates RD. The achievement of pregnancies using assisted reproductive technologies for male factor infertility after retroperitoneal lymph node dissection for testicular carcinoma. Fertil Steril 1995;64(6):1141–6.
[57] Schmidt KL, Larsen E, Bangsboll S, et al. Assisted reproduction in male cancer survivors: fertility treatment and outcome in 67 couples. Hum Reprod 2004; 19(12):2806–10.
[58] Agarwal A, Ranganathan P, Kattal N, et al. Fertility after cancer: a prospective review of assisted reproductive outcomes with banked semen specimens. Fertil Steril 2004;81(2):342–8.
[59] Mesequer M, Garride N, Remohi J, et al. Testicular sperm extraction (TESE) and ICSI in patients with permanent azoospermia after chemotherapy. Hum Reprod 2003;18(6):1281–5.
[60] Chan PT, Palermo GD, Veeck LL, et al. Testicular sperm extraction combined with intracytoplasmic sperm injection in the treatment of men with persistent azoospermia postchemotherapy. Cancer 2001; 92(6):1632–7.
[61] Marchetti F, Pearson FS, Bishop JB, et al. Etoposide induces chromosomal abnormalities in mouse spermatocytes and stem cell spermatogonia. Nat Genet 1997;16(1):74–8.
[62] Stahl O, Eberhard J, Jepson K, et al. The impact of testicular carcinoma and its treatment on sperm DNA integrity. Cancer 2004;100(6):1137–44.
[63] De Mas P, Daudin M, Vincent MC, et al. Increased aneuploidy in spermatozoa from testicular tumour patients after chemotherapy with cisplatin, etoposide and bleomycin. Hum Reprod 2006;16(6): 1204–8.
[64] Martin RH, Ernst S, Rademaker A, et al. Chromosomal abnormalities in sperm from testicular cancer patients before and after chemotherapy. Hum Genet 1997;99(2):214–8.
[65] Hartmann JT, Albrecht C, Schmoll HJ, et al. Long-term effects on sexual function and fertility after treatment of testicular cancer. Br J Cancer 1999; 80(5–6):801–7.
[66] Spermon JR, Kiemeney L, Meuleman E, et al. Fertility in men with testicular germ cell tumors. Fertil Steril 2003;79(3):1543–9.
[67] Wyrobek AJ, Schmid TE, Marchetti F. Relative susceptibilities of male germ cells to genetic defects induced by cancer chemotherapies. J Natl Cancer Inst Monogr 2005;34:31–5.

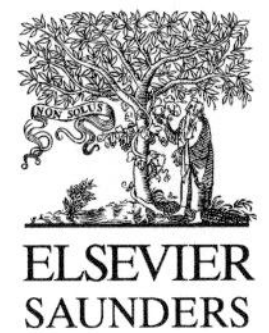

ELSEVIER
SAUNDERS

Urol Clin N Am 34 (2007) 279–285

UROLOGIC
CLINICS
of North America

Index

Note: Page numbers of article titles are in **boldface** type.

doi:10.1016/S0094-0143(07)00028-6

R

S

T

U

V